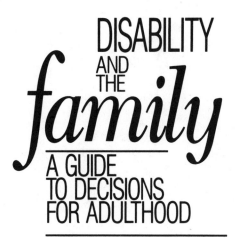

DISABILITY
AND
THE
family

A GUIDE
TO DECISIONS
FOR ADULTHOOD

DISABILITY
AND
THE
family
A GUIDE
TO DECISIONS
FOR ADULTHOOD

by

H. Rutherford Turnbull III, LL.B., LL.M.
Ann P. Turnbull, Ed.D.
G.J. Bronicki, M.A.
Jean Ann Summers, Ph.D.
and
Constance Roeder-Gordon, B.A.

The Beach Center on Families and Disability,
the Bureau of Child Research,
and the Department of Special Education,
The University of Kansas, Lawrence

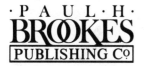

Baltimore · London · Toronto · Sydney

Paul H. Brookes Publishing Co.
Post Office Box 10624
Baltimore, Maryland 21285-0624

Typeset by Brushwood Graphics, Inc., Baltimore, Maryland.
Manufactured in the United States of America by
The Maple Press Company, York, Pennsylvania.

First printing, September, 1988.
Second printing, September, 1990.

Library of Congress Cataloging-in-Publication Data

Disability and the family: a guide to decisions for adulthood / by H. Ruther-
ford Turnbull III . . . [et al.].
    p.   cm.
  Bibliography: p.
  Includes index.
  ISBN 1-557-66004-2
    1. Handicapped—United States—Life skills guides. 2. Handicapped—
Services for—United States. 3. Decision-making. I. Turnbull, H.
Rutherford.
HV1553.D546   1988
362.4'048'0973—dc 19

                                         88-22661
                                             CIP

CONTENTS

PREFACE

If you are a parent with a son or daughter who has a disability, you face a future filled with different questions. What kind of relationships will your son or daughter have? Where will he or she live? What kind of work will occupy the days? When work is finished, what kind of enjoyable leisure activities will be available? If your son or daughter has a mental disability, will he or she be mentally competent to make decisions, or will a guardian be needed?

As you know, answers to these questions affect not just your son or daughter, but every member of your family. What obligations will other family members be willing to assume for your son or daughter with a disability? What is the fairest way to allocate responsibility and resources among the members of your family?

You may also have questions about what your son or daughter wants—after all, it's his or her life that you and others are planning. What are your son's or daughter's preferences? How can you know what they are? Do other members of the family share those preferences?

In this book, we try to help you answer these and related questions. Our efforts are based on six premises:

1. People with disabilities and their families should have freedom of choice concerning every aspect of their lives—friends and assistants, where to live and work, whom to live and work with, and what sorts of recreation to pursue, among other things.

2. The quality of life of people with disabilities and their families is enhanced when choices are available and when the means for carrying out these choices are expanded by careful planning for the future.

3. Future planning can be difficult. It can be stressful and fraught with uncertainty, and can demand a tremendous amount of your time and energy.

4. However, future planning can also help you recognize and act upon the choices that you, your son or daughter with a disability, and other members of your family have. Future planning can thereby improve the quality of your lives.

5. Because so many families affected by disability tend to live a day at a time, they need a future planning guidebook, a companion that they can refer to as they seek to give some shape to the future.

6. This future planning book is for families, but it is also for professionals who will work with families and who need to know as much as families do about future planning, if not more.

We've organized this book into four sections. Section I deals with your son's or daughter's ability to make decisions, the meaning of *mental competence*, the legal issues surrounding mental competence, and the alternative of *guardianship* (what it is, its appropriateness, and alternatives to it).

Section II provides a discussion of the government benefits that can help you put your plans into effect, particularly Social Security programs, and provides a description of how you can use your own resources in combination with government benefits.

Section III introduces the concept of *choice*, shows how you can identify your son's or daughter's preferences, and helps you learn how to build interpersonal relationships and select residences, jobs, and leisure activities on the basis of the preferences of your son or daughter with a disability and other family members.

Section IV provides a discussion of the concept of *advocacy* and includes hints on how to advocate within existing service systems, how to create new programs, and how to incorporate self-advocacy into daily living.

We are optimists about the future. We are especially optimistic about how you, other families, and other professionals can build the future and enhance the quality of life of your son or daughter with a disability and the rest of your family by seeking to create a life based on choice.

ACKNOWLEDGMENTS

This book would not have been possible without the insights of the many families we met throughout the United States while conducting research into future planning at The University of Kansas, Lawrence. Although families from across the United States provided insight and inspiration at various times, two groups were especially helpful. A group of about 20 families from the Topeka, Kansas, area was involved in a demonstration and research activity, the Future Planning Project, which was funded in part by Grant No. G008302983 from the U.S. Department of Education. A second, larger group of families in the Hawaiian Islands helped field-test much of the material in this book. To a lesser extent, we also worked with families in Maine and other states. To each of these families, and to the Kansas Association for Retarded Citizens, the Topeka and Lawrence ARCs, the National Conference of Executives of Associations for Retarded Citizens, the Special Parents Information Network in Hawaii, Susan Rocco and Rick Hoogs in that state, the technical assistance project of The Association for Persons with Severe Handicaps (TASH), Dottie Kelly (who coordinated that project), the Maine Developmental Disabilities Planning Council, and the many families whom we contacted and worked with through these and other associations, we give our deep thanks. This work would not have been as valid without your help.

This book is the first product of efforts by researchers associated with the new Beach Center on Families and Disability at The University of Kansas. The Beach Center, a rehabilitation, research, and training center funded by the National Institute on Disability and Rehabilitation Research, U.S. Department of Education, is extraordinarily fortunate to have Naomi Karp as its project officer. Her high standards of performance, commitment, and integrity, and the support she deservedly has received from Assistant Secretary Madeleine Will and Deputy Assistant Secretary Patricia McGill Smith, are benchmarks for the staff of The Beach Center to emulate.

The development of the Preference Checklist was supported in part by Grant No. HD-01090 from the Mental Retardation Research Center, The University of Kansas, Lawrence. A major contribution was provided by Simha Ruben during all phases of the development of the instrument. Development of materials to help families formulate individual future plans was funded in part by a supplement to the core grant for the Kansas University Affiliated Facility, Project No. 07DD0262.

The opinions expressed in this book do not necessarily reflect the positions or policies of the U.S. Department of Education, the Administration on Developmental

Disabilities, or the Mental Retardation Research Center, The University of Kansas at Lawrence. No official endorsement by these agencies should be inferred.

We acknowledge the substantive contributions in the beginning stages of this book provided by the following colleagues (listed alphabetically): Holly A. Benson, Mary Jane Brotherson, Gary Brunk, Stephen J. Goodfriend, Doug Guess, Joan Houghton, Kathy H. McGinley, Simha Ruben, and Marie P. Shahan.

Special thanks go to Larry Elmquist and Sharon Kekaha for their review of sections of the book and suggestions for improvement, and to Webb Golden of Lawrence for special counsel.

Editorial assistance was generously and competently provided by Opal Folkes and Mary Beth Johnston, with assistance from Carol Brown, Thelma Dillon, Jon Gaines, Lori Llewellyn, and Gwen McKillip. Once again, Dorothy Johanning was particularly helpful to the senior authors.

As always, a young man who graduated in June 1988 from Walt Whitman High School, Bethesda, Maryland, has been our best teacher and has provided the living laboratory in which many of our ideas are born. Jay Turnbull has made many positive contributions to our work, and you too will benefit from his life.

Finally, our parents, brothers, sisters, and other relatives also have been instrumental in shaping this book.

H.R. and Ann P. Turnbull

To Ryan Gray and Kevin Lisbon
and their families,
who know why

1 WHY IS PLANNING FOR THE FUTURE BOTH IMPORTANT AND DIFFICULT?

Jack and Rose Stuart have been married 21 years. They live in Wheatland, Kansas, population 42,000, where Jack works as a finish carpenter for a construction company. Rose works part-time as a continuing education coordinator for the parish of Good Shepherd Church, also in Wheatland.

Jack and Rose have three children—Sally, 16 years old; Steve, 17; and Theresa, 12. Sally is a junior at South High School. Theresa is in the seventh grade and is enrolled in the special program for gifted students. Steve is enrolled in the special education program at the Wheatland Education Center for students with severe and multiple handicaps.

Steve Stuart is nonverbal and cannot communicate or understand very well. He can walk, but with a slow and awkward gait. He also has autism, which has led to some behavior problems.

Despite Steve's disabilities, the Stuarts pretty much lead the normal life of an American family with three teen-agers. One Friday morning started out much like any other day. Breakfast found the family chattering about the day's anticipated activities. Theresa was already talking about the family's summer vacation, which was still months away. Sally mentioned Craig Anderson again, the boy in her third-hour study hall. This was the second week in a row that his name had come up at breakfast. As near as Jack could figure, the reason the Anderson boy was attracting so much of his daughter's attention was simply because he had not yet spoken to her since the new semester had begun.

Because it was Friday, Steve was waiting by the front door. The man who delivered the dry cleaning collected his money every Friday morning. Steve would wait by the front door, clutching the envelope with the money and the list of dry cleaning for delivery. When the route man arrived, Steve would greet him and the weekly transaction would begin.

"Ah, thank you, Mr. Stuart, sir. Yes, I see the money is all here. And, let's see, what'll you need to be done next week?," the delivery man would ask.

Steve, not thoroughly understanding the words but feeling the warmth in the man's voice, would beam and laugh. That was his communication. It was enough. Then they would shake hands as they always did and the delivery man would leave.

Steve enjoyed the routine. Every Friday he would get the sense of taking care of his family's dry cleaning needs for yet another week. In the relative calm of this Friday morning, Steve was waiting to do what had been his task for many months. This morning there was no reason to suspect that things would ever change. It was "just another Friday."

As Jack drove to work, his mind drifted to some financial concerns that had been bothering him. Their situation was not terribly serious, but he and Rose had allowed themselves to become overextended as a result of some recent major purchases. They had dipped into their savings, and Jack was worried about possible unexpected expenses. In his mind he could envision the family car stranded on the roadside, requiring a major engine overhaul. He also thought about Steve's financial security. It was satisfactory now, but what about the retirement years, the other kids' education, and, hardest of all, Jack's and Rose's death? Who would be the breadwinner for Steve? Jack turned up the car radio to shake such thoughts from his mind. Just take things one day at a time, and the future would work itself out. It always had.

Two hours later, Jack and four coworkers were putting up a prefabricated wall on an office expansion. It never became clear exactly what happened, but Jack found himself being crushed beneath the falling side wall. Later, the safety investigators called it a freak event, a one-chance-in-a-thousand accident.

After the accident, Jack found himself dwelling on the future more than ever. A severe concussion, four broken ribs, and a punctured lung had left him laid up, with little to do but think. That falling wall and the suddenness with which his life had been rearranged was an all-too-abrupt reminder of his own mortality and of the uncertainties of life. That was scary enough. But added to all this was Steve. The accident could have been worse, much worse. What would have happened to his family—especially Steve—if Jack died? Even more frightening, what would happen to Steve if both he and Rose were killed in, say, a car wreck? Who would look after the children, and how could the money be found to take care of them?

Jack couldn't stop thinking these ugly thoughts the last few days of his hospital stay. Even after he came home to recuperate, he couldn't shake the feeling of gloom. He spent much of his time in his recliner chair, brooding, not talking much, just staring unseeingly at the television.

Rose was worried. She tried everything to cheer her husband up, from cooking his favorite meals to shooing the kids away so he could have his rest when he needed it. Finally, one evening after the kids were in bed, she couldn't take it anymore. She switched off the TV and faced him.

"What are you doing, Jack? Feeling sorry for yourself over a few broken ribs? That isn't like you."

Jack shook his head like a man clearing cobwebs from his mind, and looked at her, puzzled, anticipating. She stared back at him half-tenderly, half-exasperated, but with total concern. He smiled, but his expression held something back. "I haven't been much good to you lately, have I, honey?" he said. He paused, then, surprising her, blurted out, "Frankly, I've been thinking about Steve." He pushed the recliner arm forward; the footrest snapped into place as Jack sat bolt upright. "Rose, we have to plan what to do with Steve."

Rose's jaw dropped and she sank to the couch next to Jack's chair. She had expected money worries, maybe fear for his job security, maybe just frustration at this forced inactivity. But not this. "Do with him?," she gasped. "But he's only 17 years old! He belongs right here with us!"

"I know that, honey," Jack said reaching over to take her hand. "I'm talking about 4 or 5 years down the line. I'm talking about having something in mind in case . . . " He squeezed her hand. "Well, you know."

"Four or 5 years down the line?" Rose felt foolish, just dumbly repeating what Jack was saying. She shook her head. "I can take care of Steve. I know everything to do for him. I know what he likes and I know the girls do, too. Nothing's going to happen to us! Jack, we've always taken care of our own in this family!" Rose's outburst suddenly subsided, as she realized her voice had been getting a little shrill.

Jack sighed. "Don't you think I feel that, too? Haven't I thought about that myself? Jack Stuart is a lot of things, but he's no quitter, and he provides for his family. Always has, always will." He let go of her hand and sat back in his chair.

Rose just chewed her lip and stared at her lap. Jack went on in a rush before she could think of something else to say. "Honey," he began, "there's all sorts of things we want to do. You want to work full-time. We want to take the camper and get out on the road, just you and me. And what about the girls? Can we really ask them to take care of Steve? They didn't bring him into this world—they have a right to their own lives."

Rose felt the prickle of tears behind her eyes. "But, but . . . oh, Jack, nobody will love Steve as we do!"

Jack paused for a minute. Rose's tears always melted him. But this time he couldn't let that happen. This was too important. He pushed on. "Yes, and what about Steve? Doesn't he have a right to a life of his own, just like the girls? If we really love him, won't we have to let him go?"

The room was silent, except for a furtive sniffle from Rose. Jack's words had brought back a memory from her childhood, of a puppy she had once found. She had kept the little dog securely locked in the garage for days. When her mother asked why she wasn't allowing the little dog to experience life, she said she had to protect him; she was afraid that he would be hurt. Her mother, Emma, explained that growing and living sometimes included pain. The puppy had a right to a life that included her, but that also involved things, other people, and other animals.

Emma had been right. Rose had let the puppy go and the little dog grew, developing its own personality. It sometimes wandered off, but it always came back. She remembered the day her little "friend" died. She had learned from her experience that each living thing has a purpose, and a right to its own life—a right to try, to succeed, and, yes, at times to fail. But from the failure comes knowledge and growth. Her dear Steven certainly had these rights, too, just as Sally, Theresa, and any other child did.

But Rose couldn't give up quite that easily. "Okay. Granted, you're right." She looked at her hands as they kneaded a wad of Kleenex in her lap. "But what's there to plan for, for heaven's sake? He's got all he needs in school now, but what's out there after that?" She looked fiercely at Jack. "You know as well as I do what happened to the Wilsons when their boy turned 22. They had an awful time, turned away from this place and that. It was touch and go whether they'd even be able to get him on a waiting list. And their Sam has mental retardation, but he doesn't have Steve's other problems." She touched her husband's arm. "Jack, there might not even be any services for Steve after he leaves school. Those people don't have to serve him if they don't want to!"

Jack moved over to the couch next to his wife and took her in his arms. "I know, babe, I know," he whispered into her soft auburn hair. "That's why we have to start now, don't you see?"

There was nothing to say to that. Rose did see—there were some long, hard battles ahead. She thought back to other battles already fought, with this teacher, that doctor, this administrator, that program. While there had been some good, caring people over the years, there had also been a few painful confrontations. All that pain came rushing back as she thought of the struggle that might lie ahead, just to make sure Steve could have a life that other people took for granted. She sighed. It didn't matter that it wasn't fair. It didn't matter that it would be difficult or painful or time-consuming. It was just something more they had to do. And just now, sheltered in the crook of Jack's arm, Rose knew they could to it, too. "Okay, you win," she sighed. "Let's get on with it, but not tonight."

*   *   *

The Stuarts are typical of many families that have sons or daughters with disabilities. The exact circumstances may differ, but their feelings about the future and their recognition that they must somehow plan for it have been replicated by families from all over the United States who have talked with us. In this book, we present the steps we have developed to help you plan. First, however, we want to share some of our beliefs about the importance and difficulty of planning for the future of your son and daughter.

It is both important and frightening to plan for the future. For any family, planning for the future of a young person is important. Often, planning begins at a very early age, when children ponder that all-important question, "What do I want to do when I grow up?" They read or hear about different career options. They dream about meeting and marrying someone.

Parents think about their children's future right along with them, giving guidance about how to think and act grown-up, helping them mull over their choices, and —when they can—setting aside money for their education or a start in business. Parents also think about what they want to do when their children leave home. As in the case of the Stuarts, the planning might include taking on a new job, traveling, or perhaps simply spending more time together as a couple. For the whole family, planning for the future is important to helping make those dreams come true.

When one of the young people in a family has a disability, however, planning for the future takes on even greater importance. A person with a disability may need some type of lifelong assistance in order to have an acceptable place to live, to get around and participate in the community, and to hold down a job. Like the Stuarts, many parents assume they will be the ones to provide that assistance. And also like the Stuarts, many parents would like their sons and daughters to be as independent as possible. And like Jack Stuart, they wonder who will take care of their son or daughter when they die, where the money will come from, and how it will be spent. Planning for the future becomes more than planning to make dreams come true. It becomes a matter of planning for survival. Planning, then, it not only important, but frightening.

In our conversations with families, probably the most pervasive theme to emerge is that families with members with disabilities, like most other families, have a tremendous need to live a day at a time. Jack Stuart had pushed aside his worries about everything from bills to his son's future in an effort to cope with those worries. Convincing oneself that things will work out is a way of minimizing the frightening aspects of the future. Living in the present seems to keep fears of the future at bay. But it never really can. For most families, those concerns about the future linger at the back of the mind.

Another impetus to live in the present is that the present is itself so full of things to be done. Most families are as busy as they can possibly be. Think of the Stuarts. In an active household of three teen-aged children, where both parents hold jobs, when is there time to think about the future? The thought of looking ahead and planning months or years in advance means that time today has to be invested in the future. Yet the future must be planned for if it is to be at least as meaningful as the present for your son or daughter. Being torn between living a day at a time and preparing for the future creates a constant dilemma for most families.

Ironically, even as it reduces anxiety, planning can also increase it. Professionals may urge families to engage in future planning because they rightly believe it is absolutely necessary to future well-being. Often these professionals do not realize, however, how much anxiety that planning can produce. Planning for the future may mean confronting all those worries about what might happen after we die. As in the case of Jack Stuart, those confrontations can trigger anxiety or depression. Also, as Rose Stuart experienced, for some parents planning might cause painful memories to resurface. It is sometimes hard to realize that peace of mind can lie at the end of that confrontation and planning process. Planning for the future is an investment in emotions as well as in time.

Adult services are a rights roulette. Many parents of young children or adolescents with special needs have become accustomed to the idea that a free and appropriate public education is guaranteed. They also have learned to use the tools of parental consent and due process to make sure their children's needs are met as parents see them. But there are no such guaranteed rights in adult service programs. Adult programs may restrict their services to those residing in their jurisdiction or having certain types of disabilities. Or they may exclude "troublesome" adults—such as those like Steve Stuart who have behavior problems. And unless the adult has been assigned a guardian by a judge, there is no one beyond the adult herself or himself with the legal authority to say yes or no to a service plan.

Many new and exciting services are being developed to give adults their rightful chance at a meaningful job, a family-like home atmosphere, and a high-quality life in the community. Unfortunately, in too many parts of the United States, those new services have not yet become established. And all too often, the not-so-subtle message from some service providers is that parents should be thankful for what they have and that their sons or daughters risk being released from the program if they or their parents advocate change or express dissatisfaction. It is little wonder that some parents ask, "Future planning for what?"

Another reason that we call adult services a "rights roulette" is that the law regards the status of an adult with a disability ambivalently. It is not always clear who will make decisions about important matters. When someone is a child (under the age of 18 in most states), that person's parents, for many reasons, are legally entitled to make decisions on his or her behalf. One reason is that children generally lack the knowledge, experience, and judgment that would make it possible and safe for them to make decisions on their own. The law therefore presumes that minors are mentally unable ("incompetent") to make decisions. When Steve Stuart turns 18—even though he will still have disabilities—the law will automatically presume that Steve is competent, and his parents will have little, if any, authority to act on his behalf. But in reality, for some people with disabilities, especially those with more severe problems like Steve's, reaching adulthood will not make them competent to make and communicate decisions on their own. Adult service agencies often recognize this, and may informally grant parents the right to continue making decisions for their adult sons and daughters. In the case of a conflict with an agency, however, the agency may choose to disregard the parents' wishes. Unless a court has formally ruled that an adult is incompetent, and has also appointed the parents (or someone else) as guardians, there may be little basis for assuring the legal rights of an adult with a disability. For all these reasons, it becomes imperative to understand fully what the law may and may not allow you to do on behalf of your adult son or daughter.

   You also need to know what you can and cannot do in the case of conflict with an adult service agency, and to plan ahead to gain the greatest amount of negotiating strength the law will allow. You also need to be fully up to date on the best services that are possible for your son or daughter, so that you can knowledgeably advocate change, if necessary. Knowledge of what's possible, plus knowledge of the law, equals the strength and power to assure a quality adult life for your son or daughter. You may never need to use that strength if you are fortunate enough to live in a community where the adult service system is highly progressive. But such communities are currently few and far between. It is precisely because the adult service system is in such a state of change that future planning is so important. Adults with disabilities and their families must be armed with the knowledge of what they want, and the legal power to get it, if they are to effect change. In light of all this, future planning is very much worth all the emotional commitment and time you can give.

2 WHAT ARE THE VALUES AND GOALS OF THE FUTURE PLANNING PROCESS?

Odessa Harris, age 35, is a department supervisor at one of the many textile mills in Georgia's Chattahoochee Valley. Her only child, Jolene, age 17, has Down syndrome and moderate mental retardation, as well as a congenital heart condition. The Harrises, a black family, live in West Point, Georgia, population about 4,500. Odessa's late husband, Staff Sergeant Joseph Harris, was killed in action in Vietnam.

Odessa has chosen to remain in her small hometown not only because of the relative security of employment in the textile mills, but also because of the strong network of family support in the immediate area. She maintains close relationships with her mother and father, Eula Mae and Alvin Weeks, as well as her grandmother, Laurie Grant, and her aunt, Jewell Weeks. Aunt Jewell, who lives nearby, keeps an eye on Jolene after school when Odessa has to work.

Jolene's heart condition has required more frequent visits to a cardiologist in recent years. The nearest one is in Columbus, Georgia, less than an hour's drive away. After appointments with the cardiologist, Odessa and Jolene often visit with Odessa's only sibling, her brother Owen Weeks, who lives in Columbus.

One particular Saturday, however, it was Odessa's brother who drove up to West Point to see her. As he came bounding up the walk to his sister's house, he noticed what a fine spring morning it was—birds singing and the sun dappling the grass through the big old live oak in Odessa's front yard. Owen had a definite purpose in mind. He was a social worker and had frequently observed families who had relatives with disabilities running into all kinds of problems with "the system." Owen had often thought that many of those problems might have been averted by planning. This led him to think about his niece, Jolene. Owen didn't want her and Odessa to go through the same anxieties some of his clients experienced. Owen thought his sister needed a man to help her plan ahead and get things straight. And who else but her own brother? Owen knew all about family and extended family. Now, it was time to put his knowledge to work. From theory to practice—that was his mission that day.

Odessa and Jolene were in the kitchen doing the Saturday baking. Jolene was sitting at the kitchen table sorting out blackberries, meticulously picking out the leaves and stems and unripe berries. It was the sort of task that drives many people crazy, but Jolene loved it. She was humming as she worked.

Odessa was making pie dough at the counter by the sink. Behind her a big pan of bread dough was set to rise on the back of the stove. Owen sat down at the kitchen table with his coffee and a freshly baked cinnamon roll and put his briefcase on the floor beside him.

"Odessa," Owen said, "there's something I want to discuss with you." He shifted in his chair and looked meaningfully in Jolene's direction.

Odessa caught his glance. "There's nothing I want to hear that can't be said in front of my Jolene," she said placidly.

"But this is about Jolene."

"All the more so, then. Isn't that right, Jolene?" Jolene stopped humming and smiled at Uncle Owen. "Go on and say what's on your mind," Odessa continued, "we're listening."

Owen cleared his throat. He could see this wasn't going to go quite the way he'd planned it. "Well," he said, "I just think you need to start thinking about Jolene's future, here and now. It's not always easy to get into these adult programs, you know. They don't have to take just everybody, like the schools do."

"I know all that," said Odessa. "Aunt Jewell and I were talking about it just the other day."

"You do? You were?" Owen looked at her dumbfounded for a moment, then smiled. "Well, then, I want you to know I'm planning a big workshop for parents down in Columbus, and I want you to come, too. I've ordered some training manuals, and . . ."

"Training manuals? Workshop? Humph." Odessa commenced rolling out dough with perhaps more energy than she needed. "I've been to some of those workshops. You sit on those metal folding chairs till your backside goes to sleep. So does my mind. Oh, I know some people like workshops, but I don't. I just feel out of place." Owen held up his hand to protest, but Odessa went on talking without looking at him. "Besides, I know what's in that manual. Some professional telling me what's best for my Jolene without even knowing her."

"Now wait, Odessa," Owen said. "You've got it all wrong. This information I've got doesn't tell you what to do, it tells you *how*. I know about these adult programs, and believe me, it's like threading your way through a rabbit warren. There's a bunch of new professionals, like vocational counselors, and new rules and new initials for everything that are all different from the school's. And you have to think about finances and legal things and so on. You really need to sit down and think it through step by step."

Odessa put her hands on her hips and frowned at her brother. "I thought you knew me better than that, Owen. I'm a doer, not a thinker, and I'm going to do what feels right, not what some expert tells me I ought to do. And anyway," Odessa said, as she picked up her rolling pin and went back to her pie dough, "What's all this 'You've got to plan' stuff? Whose life is it anyway? It's Jolene's life, that's whose. Doesn't she have a say about what she wants to do when she grows up?"

"I know," Jolene piped up. "When I grow up I'm going to get married and have babies. I like babies. And I'm going to sing in the choir with the other ladies. Going to a shopping mall in Columbus, too."

"There you go, Owen." Odessa folded her arms and grinned at her brother. "Your vocational counselors going to help Jolene do all that, are they?"

"Well, er, no." Owen paused to take a sip of coffee and recover himself. "Maybe not the vocational people, but there are others, you know. Sex education people and recreational therapists, and . . ." He could see Odessa gathering up steam and he rushed on quickly. "And the minister, too. And then there's the family. Mom and Dad and Aunt Jewell. And me. You know this family sticks together, Odessa. You've said so yourself. And if everybody's going to pitch in, everybody's got to have their say."

Odessa deftly slipped the pie dough into a pan and, taking the bowl of blackberries from Jolene, poured them into the pie shell. "All right," she said. "We're agreed we have to plan, and we're agreed that we have to do it together. Now, did you get what you came for?"

"Not quite." Owen tipped his chair on its back legs and winked at Jolene. "I have to wait till the pie's out of the oven to get the rest of what I came for."

* * *

The conversation between Odessa Harris and her brother illustrates many of the values and beliefs we bring to the process of planning for the future of a son or daughter with a disability.

Families differ about the procedures they prefer to follow in doing future planning. People also go about making decisions in widely different ways. Some may follow a series of rational, carefully thought-out steps, gathering information and evaluating every option. Others may prefer to take a more intuitive approach, and choosing options that "feel right." Some people enjoy attending workshops and learning with others. Other people, like Odessa Harris, do not find workshops helpful and would prefer to have materials to read and think about in the privacy of their own homes.

The steps to future planning outlined in this book are guided by a rational, problem-solving process. However, we do not intend to suggest there is only one way to go about planning for the future. We hope you will use the materials and exercises in this book in the way that is most comfortable for you.

Planning involves thinking about a whole range of factors related to a quality adult life. Many professionals think of future planning and vocational planning as synonymous. They define the transition to adulthood as leaving the world of school and entering the world of work. We believe, however, that the goal of planning should be a high-quality life that provides the opportunity to live, work, and play in the community, and to have meaningful personal relationships. Many young people like Jolene Harris think of being grown up as being an active participant in the community. In Jolene's case, it specifically means having a family of her own and enjoying the fellowship and amenities of the community. This book is organized with an eye to helping you plan for *all* the needs of your son or daughter with a disability. This broad planning will help you think about how to help your son or daughter make plans that are legally effective. It will help you think about financial plans. It will encourage you to think about social, sexual, and leisure options, residential options, and vocational options. It will help you think about all of this from your son's or daughter's perspective, from your own, and from other family members' perspectives. It will also help you think about next year and about the years down the road. These are the pieces and people that go together to make a truly high-quality life.

To the greatest extent possible, planning should include consideration of the choices and preferences of the person with the disability. As Odessa Harris said, "Whose life is it, anyway?" We had a conversation once with a young man whose special education instructor was teaching him how to do laundry, a task he hated. He said his mother hated doing laundry, too, and always sent it out. That was what he wanted to be able to do someday—earn enough money to pay someone else to do his laundry. To the special education teacher, being an independent adult included being able to do one's own laundry. But to this young man, being an independent adult included having the ability to choose not to do one's own laundry.

We recognize that many adults with disabilities do need some help with decision-making as they go through life. For example, we would not expect Steve Stuart to weigh the pros and cons of a surgical procedure and then decide whether to consent to medical care. But we do believe that people with disabilities are far more capable than most people think they are—capable of doing, and perhaps more important, of having and expressing their own preferences. We also believe that a large part of what we mean by "quality of life" and "independence" is having those preferences respected as much as possible. In Jolene Harris's case, it is not too difficult for her family to understand her preferences—all they have to do is listen and bring their knowledge of her, and their experience with her, into consideration. However, it may be more difficult to understand the preferences of people like Steve Stuart, who are nonverbal or have other communication problems.

Plans for the future should consider the needs of the whole family. Although this planning focuses on your son or daughter with a disability, it is important to remember that other people in the family have needs, too. Consider Jack and Rose Stuart and their dream of traveling during their retirement. Consider also that Steve Stuart's two sisters may someday have families of their own and may not be in a position to care for their brother, even if they want to. It is not inconceivable that Odessa Harris may someday remarry and need to balance her responsibilities to Jolene with her responsibilities toward a new husband.

But just as all family members have their own needs, they can also serve as resources for future planning. It is important to think beyond the professional service system to meet the needs of adults with disabilities. Jolene's minister, for example, might be involved in the planning process, and the church might provide services such as companions from the youth group to go on shopping trips with Jolene. As we noted in Chapter 1, adult service programs may be severely underequipped, and it may require some creative efforts to pull resources from your own family and community. You can do this as long as everyone's needs are considered and respected.

All of this is not to say, of course, that meeting everyone's needs is a simple matter, nor that it is even possible all the time. There are occasions in any family when needs conflict. Suppose, for example, that Odessa Harris may fully understand that Jolene wants to have children. But suppose Odessa is afraid that her potential grandchildren would not have a very good life unless Odessa herself took a major share of the responsibility for raising them, and that she doesn't really want to do that. In such a case the family might try to balance the conflicting needs. In this example we could imagine Jolene in a job that involved working with children in a supervised situation, or Jolene having plenty of opportunities to be with her Uncle Owen's children or grandchildren. A *whole-family approach* means finding a middle ground in some cases.

Family members may also disagree when it comes to their beliefs about what is right for the person with the disability. Imagine, for example, that Jack and Rose Stuart consider placing Steve in a public residential facility and have decided to leave him absolutely no money in their Wills. As his legal guardians, they may have the authority to do this (although they may need a court order in most states to institutionalize him as an adult, even if they are declared Steve's legal guardians). But imagine further that Sally and Theresa, as well as Grandmother Emma, are outraged that Jack and Rose are thinking of institutionalizing Steve and cutting him out of their Wills. In this case there is a conflict among family members about what is the ethical or "right" thing to do.

Such cases cannot be easily resolved without a great deal of careful discussion among the family members to establish a consensus about what "doing the right thing" means. A consensus about what is right is vital to sound, whole-family decisions.

Planning for the future means involving both the school and adult service agencies. A high school student with dreams of going to medical school will probably take many science and math courses. Similarly, a student with a disability should be learning skills that are truly relevant to his or her future. This may include learning how to make decisions and express them appropriately, and learning social skills and specific job skills. To do that, it is vital to know what the individual student's future plans are. But it is also vital for school personnel to know what skills the student must learn to achieve those plans. It is also important for the adult service program (if one is involved) to understand the young person's needs and make appropriate plans to meet them. This means that school staff and adult service staff should begin communicating with one another. As strange as it may seem, however, collaboration between schools and adult service programs is not something parents can take for granted in most communities. It is one more thing you will have to make sure of as you formulate your plans.

We have just introduced you to the principles that guided us as we wrote this book. They have helped us form the structure and steps to be followed in planning, and have helped us determine the specific areas of adult life for which you will need to plan.

We have divided this book into four sections. In Section I ("Decision-Making," Chapters 3–8), we discuss decision-making by your son or daughter with a disability. The ability to make decisions and adapt to changes lays the foundation for security and quality throughout life. Some adults with disabilities will need no help at all in making decisions, some will need some help, and still others will need a great deal. In Section I we also discuss the major factors to consider in choosing the right decision-making options for your son or daughter. We discuss those issues first because your knowledge about them will help you answer a fundamental question: *Just who is going to be making the decisions about my son's or daughter's future?*

Section II ("Financial Planning and Government Benefits," Chapters 9–16) concerns some of the financial issues that you may need to consider as you plan. These include taxes, estate planning, Trusts, and the relationship of your private financial resources to government benefits. In Section II, we discuss government benefits such as Social Security and health care benefits. Our intention is to help you determine whether your son or daughter might be eligible for these benefits and, if so, how you might apply. Section II is designed to help you answer the question: *Who will pay for the future options my family might choose?*

With these two basic questions (about the nature of the future, and how it will be financed) answered, you will then be ready to consider the actual life-styles your son or daughter may want as an adult. In Section III ("Planning for Life in the Community," Chapters 17–35), we begin with a general consideration of the needs and preferences that must be addressed if your young adult is to have a high-quality life in the community—rights as a citizen with a disability to be an autonomous adult with as much control over life as possible, to speak on his or her own behalf, and to be meaningfully involved in decisions about adult services and programs. Next, we consider needs and preferences in the area of interpersonal relationships—social needs, sexuality, and the possibility of a meaningful marriage and family life. With these basics in mind, we then turn to residential options. We discuss what options are available, what each one is like, how to identify preferences, and how to evaluate options. Finally, we consider employment—types of programs available to help your son or daughter find meaningful work, how to determine your son's or daughter's vocational preferences, and how to use vocational rehabilitation programs and other strategies to help you meet vocational goals. By the end of Section III, we hope you will have a fairly clear idea of the future life-style—community participation, interpersonal relationships, where to live and to work—that your son or daughter may want.

Because there still may be a great deal of work to do to ensure that your goals are met, Section IV ("Advocacy," Chapters 36–39) presents some advocacy strategies you may want to use to implement your plan. First, it may be important for you as an advocate to ensure that established programs are addressing your son's or daughter's preferences. Second, it may be important to advocate the establishment of new programs that are more suitable for your son or daughter than existing ones. Third, we discuss how your daughter or son can learn to stand up for herself or himself in resolving problems.

DECISION-MAKING

The chapters in this section (3–8) are concerned with decision-making by people with disabilities. You and your son or daughter may have always handled decisions in a way uniquely suited to your individual styles and needs as the situations arose. Commenting on their decision-making style, the father of an adolescent with moderate mental retardation said, "My son and I share the responsibility, but if there is danger involved, I naturally have the last word. It's worked well, we've never had problems." The man's son is 16 years old, that is, a minor under the law, so at this point, there are no legal questions about the father's rights and responsibilities to act on the boy's behalf.

The situation will change when the boy becomes a legal adult, and the decision-making style that worked in the past may no longer meet everyday needs. Legal definitions of mental competence exist that will determine how and when a person with a disability may act in his or her own behalf. The laws concerning decision-making require families to plan carefully and early to ensure that preferences and needs are protected. This section will help you plan for the decision-making that inevitably will be an important aspect of your son's or daughter's life.

In this section, we discuss and investigate the law regarding mental competence, the implications of your son's or daughter's ability or inability to give consent, and, the issue of guardianship. Both the positive and negative aspects of guardianship are presented, and alternatives to guardianship are reviewed. The procedures for establishing guardianship are discussed in Chapter 8, the last chapter of this section. Important considerations such as choosing a guardian are fully explored in that chapter.

This section is not designed to replace the counsel of qualified legal professionals. It does, however, provide information that will enable you to work more effectively with adult service agencies regarding your son's or daughter's preferences and choices in the future. If seeking guardianship is necessary, the information in this section will help you in your dealings with both attorneys and the courts.

Finally, this section may be useful to legal professionals who deal with family issues relevant to guardianship. It offers insights into the family dynamics that affect decision-making. A better understanding of what the family is experiencing, what the family wants, and what the person with the disability wants will help legal professionals best serve the total family.

WHAT DECISION-MAKING RESPONSIBILITIES WILL YOUR SON OR DAUGHTER HAVE AS AN ADULT?

3

As the Levine family drove across Chicago toward their North Shore home, a silence settled over the car. Today had been a joyous occasion—Arnold, their 25-year-old son, had married Saundra, his beautiful childhood sweetheart, in a fairy tale wedding. Both had just finished school, Arnold with his law degree and Saundra with her MBA. Arnold had already landed a job with a prestigious Chicago law firm. Prospects for the young couple were brilliant. Yet as the evening twilight deepened, so did the gloom in the car. Ruth Levine, 48, Arnold's mother, stared out the window at her right, drumming her fingers on the armrest. Her husband Ben, 55, gripped the steering wheel and gazed steadily at the road. Had they spoken, they would have realized they were thinking about the same thing.

Ruth stared at the megalithic Sears Tower that anchored the sprawling skyline. Just as this building dominated her native Chicago, thoughts of her daughter Anna, who was 19 years old, dominated her mind this evening, as on countless occasions in recent months.

Arnold's wedding had only pointed out to them all the bright prospects that appeared beyond Anna's reach. Anna was in a special education program for students with educable mental handicaps. Her reading and writing skills weren't bad, although her math and money-handling abilities were very poor. So too were what her teacher called her social skills; she was very shy and withdrawn, and could seldom be coaxed to speak above a whisper. Ruth stole a glance at Anna, sitting quietly in the back seat with her hands folded in her lap, lost in her own thoughts. Anna was a striking beauty, a little like herself as a girl, Ruth thought. Her long, glossy black hair reached to the middle of her back, and her startling blue eyes were fringed with long lashes and set in a pale, smooth, oval face. Anna always dressed impeccably, too. No one could tell by looking at her that she had a disability. Yet what was there in Anna's future? Would she ever have a joyous wedding, like her brother? Maybe not. Ruth turned bitterly back to the car window, but all she saw there were images of imagined future sorrow—of Anna, left behind and alone as she often was now, or worse, of Anna being heartlessly used by some man who only wanted . . .

Ben's thoughts about Anna were focusing on Anna's prospects for a job. Arnold was now carrying on the Levine family's passion for achievement. (Ben often joked that his faithfulness to the Chicago Cubs was his one deviation from his normal insistence on excellence.) Ben himself had doubled the size of the family's scrap iron business after taking it over, and had done quite well for himself in a series of investments. Ruth was a buyer of fine crystal, china, and silver for the city's most elegant department store, and had an uncanny sense of what the public would and wouldn't buy. But Anna? What could she do?

It wasn't that Ben wanted her to be a brilliant professional—he had long ago come to accept her as his sweet baby girl, limitations and all. But what was driving him crazy was the thought of Anna sitting at home after she finished school, with nothing to do. She wasn't, after all, without abilities. It would be such a waste! Then a chill passed through him as he thought, "What happens when her mother and I are gone? What can she do with her life? Who will take care of her?"

Ben's business lawyer and friend, Mike McCarthy, had brought up a disquieting issue over lunch earlier that week. Sitting at their usual back table at Miller's Pub on Wabash Street, Mike had just finished explaining the details of the contract that would be signed with a scrap metal dealer from Peoria later that day:

"That's the way he liked things, legal and to the point," crowed Ben, "no room for misunderstandings. Nice job Mike, very nice."

"As a person who likes things crystal clear, you should really do something about your daughter, Ben," Mike said in a voice that was neither threatening nor reassuring.

"I've told you before, I'm taking care of her fine. You just attend to my life and my business, Mike. I don't need any help with Anna," Ben said, his uncertain tone belying his words.

"Ben, she's a woman now, an adult. You're her father and you have to think about both your futures. The law says . . ."

"The law, the law," Ben interrupted, "that's all I hear, if not from you then I get it from my now so smart attorney son . . ."

In the car, Ben again thought of the things Mike McCarthy had often tried to discuss with him. New doubts filled his already-crowded mind. "Who would help Anna make decisions? Could she make her own legal decisions? What should be done?" These thoughts continued to plague him the rest of the drive home.

* * *

One of the distinguishing characteristics of adulthood is that people are generally expected to take more responsibility for making decisions concerning their own lives. This expectation applies to your son or daughter as much as it does to other members of society. Another distinguishing characteristic of adulthood is that adults have the legal right to make decisions on their own. Is that a right your son or daughter will be able to exercise alone, with help, or not at all?

In this chapter we discuss the kinds of decisions your son or daughter will be expected to make, the degree of complexity of different decisions, and the process for making decisions. In the following chapters we focus on whether your son or daughter has the mental competence to make those decisions and, if not, what alternatives are available to facilitate decision-making. As you read this section, we want you to think about this question: *How will my son or daughter get along as a decision-making adult?*

WHAT LIFE-STYLE DECISIONS MUST ADULTS MAKE?

We have identified four major areas in which adults must make decisions about the life-style that appeals to them:

Life in the community
Relationships with other people
The place where one lives
One's job

In each of these areas, adults also need to make decisions about finances—about how to get money and how to spend it, in order to implement decisions associated with these four areas.

In this chapter we provide a brief introduction to each of these decision-making areas. (In Section III, each of these areas is described in greater depth.)

Decisions about Life in the Community

Life in the community includes decisions about legal rights and habilitation programs, about how one is treated as an individual, and about how one uses free time. Getting down to more specifics, we'll first look at legal rights and programs.

Adults with disabilities who are involved with adult service agencies have the right to individualized written programs, usually called individual program plans (IPPs), individualized habilitation programs (IHPs), or individualized work rehabilitation plans (IWRPs). Your son or daughter has the right to, and should be expected to, participate in meetings in which these plans are developed through the identification of instruction and support needs, and options for meeting those needs. Anna Levine, the 19-year-old in the special education program for people with mild mental disabilities, already knows what she wants to do with her life—work in a hotel restaurant, live with her friend Susan in an apartment, date but not have children, take an aerobics class from the city recreation department, and vote. Participating in meetings where plans will be developed to help her do these activities will give Anna a chance to say what she wants to do with her life.

Making decisions about how we are treated as individuals can help us determine how satisfied we are with our lives. This may be particularly true for your son or daughter. Some people may think that individuals with disabilities don't have the same need for respect and self-esteem that people without disabilities have. As a parent, you know this is not true. Consider Jolene Harris. She needs to be prepared to assert herself concerning decisions on matters such as:

The degree of privacy she wants around the house and in her leisure activities
When she needs and does not need permission from others
How to respond to people who ridicule or otherwise treat her rudely

In the area of decisions related to life in the community, how one uses free time is but one very important consideration. What do you do in your free time? Who decides how you use your free time? When do you most enjoy your free time? When does your free time result in more frustration than enjoyment? The answers to these questions all relate to the decisions you make about your free time. The same process of decision-making about free time also applies to your son or daughter. Playing sports or watching movies, riding the bus or walking, being alone or in a group, eating in a restaurant or cooking at home—all of these are examples of decisions about free time that will regularly face your son or daughter.

Decisions about Relationships with Other People

Our lives consist of relationships with other people. These relationships require adults to make decisions continually—about family and friends, sexual needs, and other people and things in one's life. We will briefly examine each of these areas.

Relationships with family and friends are important to everyone, including your son or daughter. In thinking about a group home where Steve might live in the future, Jack and Rose Stuart worry about whether the staff will be able to understand the insecurity Steve sometimes feels when he is separated from his parents and friends. They were distressed to learn that the daughter of a couple they know is only allowed to talk to her parents once a week on the telephone and to visit them only once a month. The staff member at her group home tells her "Don't be such a baby," and discourages her from having more frequent contact with her family. Steve and others will face many decisions about relationships with family and friends, such as:

> Choosing friends who will take their emotions and feelings seriously
> Arranging opportunities to interact with people who do not have a disability
> Choosing people to depend upon for help

An area that is often ignored in the lives of people with disabilities is making decisions about sexual needs. Odessa Harris misses a heartbeat when Jolene says she wants a baby, and Odessa clenches her fist and sets her jaw at the thought of anyone sexually molesting her daughter. The thought is enough to make her want to keep Jolene home forever, and prevent her from ever having a life of her own. Yet Jolene and every other adult with a disability will be faced with a multitude of decisions about sexuality, such as:

> Deciding whether or not to obtain information on birth control
> Deciding whether to have a sexual relationship with a person of the same or opposite sex
> Determining one's own preferences for expressing affection

Decisions must also be made about other people and things. Anna Levine, for example, is struggling with the emotions of living in that gray area between being like other people and being called retarded. She sometimes feels so close to fitting in, and other times hates herself for being such a "klutz." She knows she needs help in handling her feelings, but says she would "die" before telling her parents how she really feels. Anna needs to decide where to get help and how much she can afford to pay for that help. Like Anna, your son or daughter will have to make decisions about:

> His or her own religious views
> A daily schedule that is functional and comfortable
> How he or she will use the telephone and mail

Decisions about Where One Lives

Think for a moment about how much of your activity revolves around your home. Regardless of how involved you might be with a job or community activities, there are still thousands of decisions that you and others make about the things you do at home, where and with whom you live, and the way your home is run. As an adult, your son or daughter will face these same decisions. These decisions are important for your son or daughter whether he or she continues to live in your home, or moves to another home in the community. In Chapters 22–23, we discuss different living options that might suit the needs of your son or daughter, including shared ownership of property, unsupervised and supervised apartments, and group homes operated by a public or private agency.

Regardless of where your son or daughter may live, he or she will need to make decisions about the things that may be done at home. For example, Anna Levine is looking forward to having an apartment of her own and deciding how to arrange the furniture, when to use the telephone, which friends to invite over, and what meals to prepare. In fact, Anna has the misconception that living on her own will mean that she won't have any rules to follow and that no one will be able to tell her what to do. The Levines are struggling with how they can best support Anna so that she can make many of her own decisions, while also recognizing Anna's need for reasonable rules and assistance with decisions that are more difficult, or have potentially threatening consequences. The Levines also know that they need to help Anna decide how she will pay for what she wants to do.

Deciding where and with whom to live is another major area of decision-making. Sometimes families just assume that their son or daughter will always live with them; they may not involve their son or daughter in their planning, or ask them about their preferences or dislikes. Other families assume that their son or daughter will move to a group home after graduating from high school or whenever an opening becomes available. The major problem with this assumption is that numerous related decisions must be made to ensure that this residence is appropriate. These decisions will concern:

The number of housemates, their gender, interests, and level of capability
Whether or not one has a roommate, and, if one does, whether or not one is
    compatible with the roommate
The proximity of the house to one's job, shopping, and recreation

If supervised housing is chosen, the last type of residence-related decision facing your son or daughter involves decisions about the staff and the way the house is run. Earlier, we discussed the Stuarts' concern when they heard about the staff member at the group home who called the young adults who lived there "babies" when they wanted to call or visit their parents. This is just one example of the great influence staff members can have over your son's or daughter's personal decision-making. When you and your young adult are selecting a place to live, the competence, commitment, and interpersonal skills of the staff should be very important considerations.

Decisions about many other home management issues will face your son or daughter. These issues include:

The availability and adequacy of routine and emergency health care
The availability of assistance with personal hygiene, and whether this assistance
    is provided by a male or a female
Whether smoking or alcohol are allowed

Decisions about One's Job

An exciting development in recent years has been the tremendous increase in job opportunities for people with disabilities. Chapters 28–35 describe the progress that has been made and identifies the many services that your son or daughter can use to obtain challenging and rewarding employment. But this surge of job opportunities has increased the number and complexity of decisions that must be made about the kind of job that is desirable, its location, specific duties, pay, and benefits.

A major decision facing your son or daughter is choosing what kind of job to do. Should it be in manufacturing, clerical work, farming, maintenance, human services, or some other area? Jolene Harris has already decided that she would like to have a job helping people, such as children or elderly persons. Her favorite task at school is to assist one of her classmates, Eileen, who uses a wheelchair. Jolene helps Eileen with dining and grooming and has learned from this experience that she would like a job that would allow her to help others.

After decisions are made about the kind of work to do, your son or daughter must then consider the potential workplace and his or her specific job duties. Picking a workplace can involve consideration of many factors, including the proportion of people with and without disabilities who work there, the safety of the work environment, the kind of supervision available, the availability and accessibility of transportation, the noise level, the extent of temperature control, and the opportunity for advancement. The specific duties of the job must also be identified and analyzed so that potential employees can decide if they are capable of completing them, and if they would, in fact, enjoy those specific duties. We all know how important it is to get a feeling of competence and satisfaction from a job. Your son or daughter feels this same need.

Thoughtful job selection is incomplete without consideration of pay and job benefits. A major dilemma facing Jack and Rose Stuart is how to begin planning to ensure Steve's long-term financial security. To help teach Steve the importance of a paycheck to meeting one's needs, Jack and Rose give him money for chores and have him use his own money to pay for recreation and an occasional meal out. Other important decisions in this area concern:

> Obtaining adequate benefits, including worker's compensation, health insurance, and retirement benefits
> Insuring that there is no wage discrimination merely because of the presence of a disability

In summary, we have briefly introduced you to the four kinds of decisions that face all adults, including your son or daughter, about life-style. In Section III, we discuss each of these areas in depth and suggests a process that your son or daughter, working with family and friends, might use in decision-making.

WHAT FINANCIAL PROVISIONS MUST BE MADE FOR ADULTHOOD?

Decisions about your son or daughter's future always must be made with finances in mind. For that reason, Section II of this book focuses exclusively on the process of financial planning and on how you, your son or daughter, and your family can make the most of your resources.

At this point, we want to focus on the two kinds of financial decisions your son or daughter will be expected to make as an adult: decisions about acquiring money and decisions about spending money.

Decisions about Acquiring Money

Decisions must be made about how to acquire enough money to purchase life's necessities—food, shelter, clothing, medical care—as well as how to go beyond these necessities, if possible. Most people acquire money by working. Others have income from Trust funds. Many people with disabilities collect financial benefits from government programs. (These also are discussed in Section II.) There are many means of acquiring money and competent financial decision-making involves considering all of them. We all know the result of not acquiring enough money to meet basic needs. Most parents cringe at the thought of their son or daughter with a disability being without adequate financial resources.

Steve will need to make decisions about a job that will allow him to earn an adequate wage, obtain important financial benefits, and maintain his qualification for government assistance through the Supplemental Security Income (SSI) program. His income may not be sufficient to meet all of his expenses. In Anna's case, she needs to earn enough money to live in an apartment of her own and still meet her other expenses. She also needs to understand the Trust fund that her family is setting up for her and the financial implications of the dividend checks.

Decisions about Spending Money

Many people who make wise decisions about acquiring money nonetheless have poor spending habits. They find that they overspend, extend charge accounts beyond their limits, go into unmanageable debt, get charged exorbitant interest, and even default on rent or mortgages. Others are excellent managers. As an adult, your son or daughter will have to make decisions every day about how to spend money.

Jolene enjoys shopping, but she is unaware of many good habits that help ensure wise decisions, such as knowing a fair price, shopping at sales, knowing how to use credit, and comparison shopping. Going on a shopping trip unassisted would place Jolene in danger of making some injudicious decisions about how to spend her money. Besides routine spending decisions, money management entails many other responsibilities, such as:

Writing and recording checks, and balancing accounts
Completing tax forms
Using charge accounts with discretion
Determining when it is appropriate to sign a contract or lease

Financial decision-making is stressful enough for people who can fully understand the benefits and drawbacks of various financial alternatives. It is no wonder that it poses special challenges and opportunities for your son or daughter and your family as you engage in future planning.

HOW DO DECISIONS VARY IN COMPLEXITY?

As we have just shown, your son or daughter faces a variety of decisions. These include decisions about legal rights, recreation, the location of one's home, and budgeting. These are decisions about what to do, and about life-style. But the complexity of the decisions facing your son or daughter should also be considered. For example, Jolene may make a decision about where to live. She decides about what to do, and about what kind of life-style she wants. But she also has to make a decision about the details of a residence. Not every residence is the same. Her decision, then, takes on a new dimension. We call it *complexity*: Should Jolene live with or without her family? If she wants to live without her family, what kind of residence does she want? As you see, decisions, and decision-making, become complex.

Many factors affect the complexity of decisions. Two of the most important are the potential risk and irreversibility of a decision.

Risk is the potential danger inherent in a situation. Decisions that can have dangerous consequences can be described as having high risk. For example, it would be highly risky to decide to work in an area where toxic substances are present, to work with people who are known to resolve conflict through violence, or to accept a job for which one is not sufficiently qualified. Conversely, deciding to work in a quality-controlled environment, to work with people with a demonstrated record of congeniality and personal support, or to accept a job for which one is well qualified are all examples of low-risk decisions. There is a range of moderately risky decisions between these extremes.

Irreversibility is the other aspect of complexity. A decision is *irreversible* (that is, impossible to reverse) when most of its results cannot be changed or undone, in whole or in part. Thus, the option does not exist to change one's mind or use a different approach. Few decisions in modern life are irreversible, but most of those that are irreversible are in the area of medical care.

When Jolene becomes an adult, she might be forced to decide whether to have surgery to remove a tumor or repair damage to a vital organ. Once surgery is initiated, the decision is irreversible. Often, the results are, too. Other types of medical care, such as bandaging a wound or taking penicillin for an infection, are easily reversible.

Another illustration of reversibility is in the area of contraception. If Anna decides to obtain a sterilization, the results will, at best, be very difficult to reverse. Although medical technology is developing that can reverse some sterilizations, a reversal of sterilization is definitely an exceptional circumstance. On the other hand, Anna might decide to use contraceptives whose results are easily reversible (except in unusual cases), such as birth control pills, a diaphragm, spermicides, or an intrauterine device (IUD). Unlike sterilization, these methods are not permanent.

There is an important middle ground in considering the reversibility of decisions. An example is filing a discrimination grievance against one's boss. Although one can usually withdraw a formal grievance, the fact that a grievance was initially filed probably will influence the nature of relationships with other employees and with employers. Since one cannot totally reverse the results of a decision to file a grievance, it is particularly important to consider carefully the initial decision to file.

There is no exact formula for determining the risk and reversibility of the decisions that face your son or daughter. Indeed, what is highly risky and irreversible for one person may not be so for another. Surgery on an athlete's knee or on a pianist's fingers is different from the same surgery on an accountant with a bad knee or a radio dispatcher with a burned hand. Cosmetic surgery for an actress differs from cosmetic surgery for person with a severe cleft lip. The consequences of any decision—and thus the degree of risk and irreversibility—differ according to a person's present and projected situation, even though the decision to do (or not to do) something may be based on identical needs.

It would be so much easier if gauging risk and reversibility were cut and dried. But we must all determine risk and reversibility individually in making decisions. In the process, it will become increasingly apparent that decisions vary in complexity. In this book, we describe the levels of complexity as:

Simple
Medium
Difficult

Many kinds of decisions must be made about life-style. These are the decisions about:

Life in the community
Relationships with other people
The place where one lives
One's job
Spending money

Second, there are two elements that make any kind of decision more or less complex—risk and irreversibility. Because decisions can have varying degrees of complexity, as determined by the degree of risk and reversibility involved, it is important to ask, "How do I, and how does my son or daughter, make a decision? What process do we use to determine what we want to do and whether we can handle the complexity of our decision (measured by its risk and reversibility)?" Let's look, now, at the process by which all of us, including your son or daughter, usually make decisions. Once we do that, we can put it all together—kind, complexity, and process—and begin to know if your son or daughter can make decisions alone, with help, or not at all.

WHAT IS THE DECISION-MAKING PROCESS?

Regardless of the kind of decisions that face your son or daughter (and their complexity), the process of informed decision-making usually is the same for them and for us. It involves six steps:

Defining the problem or need
Brainstorming
Evaluating and choosing alternatives
Communicating the decision to others
Taking action
Evaluating the outcome of the action

Defining the Problem or Need

Decision-making begins when we recognize that there is a problem or need that warrants our attention. To identify a problem, we might consider the "who, what, when, where, why, and how" of the problem. To do that, however, we need adequate information. Any person making a decision therefore must have the ability to acquire and comprehend information. It is the one thing for Anna Levine to feel "trapped" at her parents' home, and to want to move out. It is another thing, and usually not hard to do, to identify the problem: Anna has matured and, like many other young adults, wants to be on her own. She feels the need to assert herself; she can identify the problem as a conflict between where and with whom she lives, how she lives with them, and her need for independence.

Brainstorming

Brainstorming means thinking of as many different options as possible for resolving a problem or meeting a need. It involves being creative, open-minded, and aware of people and services that may be of help. Brainstorming can be facilitated by asking others for advice and suggestions of options. Anna might discuss her feelings, her need, and her identified problem with her friends and family members, and she might talk to them about how to solve her problem. Arnold and Saundra might suggest one solution—an apartment of Anna's own. Ben and Ruth might suggest another—moving in with Arnold and Saundra. Anna's friends might recommend living in a group home. The purpose of brainstorming is to consider fully all possible solutions in order to be in a position to select the one that is most likely to be successful.

Evaluating and Choosing Alternatives

After all options are identified through brainstorming, the next step in decision-making is to identify the criteria to use in evaluating each option. If Anna is trying to choose which of three apartments to rent, she might decide to base her decision on the criteria of safety, rent, access to public transportation, and size. She must then proceed to evaluate each apartment, based on these criteria, so that she can choose the one that best conforms to her preferences. This same sequence of steps applies to every decision—deciding upon criteria, evaluating each option identified through brainstorming in light of the criteria, and choosing the preferred option for implementation.

Communicating the Decision to Others

Once a decision is made, it is essential to communicate it to others who are affected by it and who have an interest in the decision-maker. Anna realizes that she needs to tell many people about her selection of an apartment—her parents, her brother and his wife, her friends, her teachers, and even her new neighbors. Sharing decisions with others can enable them to offer help with the next step in decision-making—taking action.

Taking Action

Once the preferred option has been identified, the next step is to take action by actually implementing the option. In Anna's case, this would mean going through the necessary steps to rent the apartment of her choice. Anna may stay in one apartment for only a few months or for several years. She may even have to postpone any move—that is, she may have to implement her decision gradually, or she may be able to move out whenever she wants.

Evaluating the Outcomes of an Action

No decision is complete without a careful review of one's satisfaction with it. All of us can learn valuable lessons for improving decision-making in all areas of our lives by carefully reviewing the benefits and drawbacks associated with an action. Anna probably will assess her decision to move, or the apartment she rented, after she takes action. Given her track record of taking all the other steps to make a decision, she (like most of us) probably will reflect on it and decide that it was more or less correct. Identifying the problems or needs that result from the action can then be the basis for beginning again the decision-making process by identifying the problem or need and proceeding through each of the steps.

In summary, the six steps of the decision-making process ideally apply to every decision your son or daughter will need to make. When one considers the three aspects of decision-making—the kinds, complexity, and process of making decisions—it is apparent that adulthood creates great expectations of people with disabilities. Many adults will be able to meet these expectations, and many others will need a wide range of assistance with decision-making.

If you are thinking that this book couldn't possibly be for you because your son or daughter is not at all capable of the kinds of decisions we have outlined, don't despair. Many other parents of people with disabilities (and people without disabilities) are in a similar situation. There are many options available to provide assistance with decision-making, and we get to those in Chapters 6–8. First, however, in Chapters 4–5, we discuss the meaning of mental competence from both a legal and practical perspective, and talk about how you can determine the mental competence of your son or daughter to make decisions.

4 MENTAL COMPETENCE— WHAT ARE ITS LEGAL AND PRACTICAL MEANINGS FOR YOUR SON OR DAUGHTER?

When you engage in future planning, or when your son or daughter makes decisions about life-styles, these questions must be faced: Does he or she have the mental ability (or, to use the term that is most often employed in law and the disability field—*mental competence*) to make a decision? How much mental competence does he or she possess, and for what kinds of decisions? What steps of the decision-making process is he or she competent to handle, and at what level of complexity? Having considered decision-making from a variety of perspectives, we'll apply the information that has been gathered to the idea of mental competence.

Mental competence is the capability to make reasoned decisions. As we said in Chapter 3, the process for making reasoned decisions includes six steps:

Defining the problem or need
Brainstorming
Evaluating and choosing alternatives
Communicating the decision to others
Taking action
Evaluating the outcome of action

Definitions of mental competence, as used in law, vary from state to state. But all definitions address the capability to make reasoned decisions.

Your young adult's degree of mental competence has important legal and practical consequences for you, your son or daughter, and your whole family. You probably have heard people talk about guardianship for adults with mental disabilities, and about the legal determination that a person who has a guardian has been ruled by the courts to be mentally incompetent. A person's mental competence determines if the person will be put "under guardianship" by a court.

Aside from the legal guardianship decision, your son's or daughter's mental competence is the basis for your and other's judgments about how independent your young adult can be when making decisions, and how much assistance he or she needs to make decisions. If your son or daughter cannot make decisions, i.e., is not mentally competent, someone else will have to make them. Perhaps it will be a court-appointed guardian; perhaps it will be family or friends, acting without any power given to them by a court. Perhaps it will be your son or daughter, acting alone or getting help from someone else. In a nutshell, before making actual plans for adulthood, such as where your son or daughter will live or work, you must first determine who will make decisions. The purpose of this chapter is to help you know who should decide about the future of your son or daughter. Is your son or daughter fully mentally competent to make those decisions? If not, what kinds of help, at what level of complexity, will he or she need? By the end of the chapter and after a great deal of thinking, you should be able to answer these questions.

In this chapter, we discuss the law concerning mental competence during childhood and adulthood and the law's approach to levels of mental competence. We also offer a framework you can use to determine your son's or daughter's level of mental competence.

WHAT ARE THE LAW'S PRESUMPTIONS ABOUT MENTAL COMPETENCE?

Legal consequences flow from a determination that your son or daughter has either complete, partial, or no mental competence. Because so much of your decision-making will be affected by the law, it's important to know what the law generally does.

The law makes certain presumptions about people and their mental competence. (A presumption is a previously determined rule that the law applies to all people in similar circumstances. For example, there is a presumption that people are innocent of crime until proven guilty.) The law's presumptions about the mental competence of minors and of adults are very different.

What Are the Presumptions Concerning Minors?

A *minor* is a person who is under age, or not yet an adult in the eyes of the law. The age when a minor becomes an adult varies from state to state. Typically, minors are people under the age of 18, which is usually considered the *age of majority*. The age of majority in the District of Columbia and 43 of the 50 states is 18. The exceptions (with their age of majority listed in parentheses) are Alabama (19), Colorado (21), Mississippi (21), Nebraska (19), Pennsylvania (21), and Wyoming (19). Missouri has not specified a legal age of majority, although people in that state can take on most legal responsibilities at age 18.

Minors are presumed not to have mental competence. When a child is a minor, the law allows parents to make almost all the decisions for the child, just as Jack and Rose Stuart and Odessa Harris have been making decisions for Steve and Jolene, respectively. Because the law presumes minors to be mentally incompetent, it gives parents the legal right to make decisions affecting their minor children. In general, however, the law will not allow parents or other people who have custody of a minor to take action that may or will injure or endanger the child's physical, mental, or emotional health. Indeed, the law is designed to actively prevent such actions. For example, the law will compel blood transfusions for a child despite its parents' religious objections. The law also restricts parents of minors with mental disabilities from placing their minor children in an institution or consenting to have then undergo sterilization.

The law allows parents to make most decisions for their children for many good reasons. One particularly relevant reason is that children generally lack the knowledge, experience, and judgment to use a reasoned process for making decisions. The law therefore presumes that minors are mentally incapable (incompetent) to make decisions. We all know minors who have demonstrated an impressive ability to make sound decisions; even so, they are mentally incompetent in the eyes of the law simply because they are under 18.

What Are the Presumptions Concerning Adults?

While the law presumes that adults have mental competence, it makes exactly the opposite presumption about minors. Thus, when your son or daughter reaches the age of majority, the law presumes that he or she is mentally competent (i.e., has the capacity to make reasoned decisions) regardless of his or her actual competence. This can be an unsettling prospect for the parents of young adults with severe and profound disabilities.

Because an adult is presumed to be mentally competent, parents have very little, if any, authority to act on their adult son's or daughter's behalf. This is so because the law has no special reason to give one adult (a parent) power over another adult (the parent's child). If it did allow parents to continue to have legal power to make decisions for their adult children, it would create a situation in which the son or daughter, even as an adult, might always be treated as a child.

The presumption of the law concerning the mental competence of adults, however, is *rebuttable*. This means that a presumption can be overcome or set aside in individual cases. The rebuttable presumption in favor of the mental competence of adults can be overcome in two ways.

First, the presumption of competence can be overcome *de jure*, which means overcome through law, when a court finds an adult to be incompetent. (In law, the finding that an adult is incompetent is called *adjudication*.) The court's basis for making this decision and rebutting (setting aside) the presumption is that evidence proves that the adult lacks the capacity to make reasoned decisions. We examine *de jure* incompetence in Chapter 6–8, where we discuss guardianship. Suffice it to say that guardianship results from a legal proceeding that rebuts the presumption of mental competence. Guardianship also transfers one person's rights of decision-making to another person because the one person is mentally incompetent and needs the other person to make decisions on his or her behalf.

Second, the presumption of competence can be overcome *de facto*, which means based on particular circumstances. Although a person may not have been formally declared (adjudicated) incompetent by a court, the person may act as if he or she is incompetent. Image that Steve Stuart is now an adult and has not been legally declared incompetent. But he has substantial limitations when it comes to making even simple decisions. Steve is *de facto* incompetent and relies on his family to make all major decisions for him.

It is important to understand the distinction between "having a mental disability" and "being mentally incompetent." A person (such as Anna) may have a mild mental disability. But the same person may be able to make and communicate decisions concerning his or her personal and financial needs. Indeed, like Anna Levine, nearly 85% of people with mental retardation are mildly retarded and probably are able to make and communicate those kinds of decisions. These people frequently are mentally competent.

Another person, however, may have severe mental retardation, like Steve Stuart, or moderate mental retardation, like Jolene Harris. Because of the extent of the person's disability, he or she may not be able to make and communicate any or all decisions about his or her needs. Such a person, perhaps even Jolene, or more likely

Steve, is mentally incompetent. Parents will need to make special plans, within the law's provisions, to safeguard such an individual's personal and financial future.

ARE MENTAL COMPETENCE AND INCOMPETENCE ALL-OR-NOTHING CONDITIONS?

As your own experience shows, mental competence is not an all-or-nothing condition. You may be very competent in languages and not very competent in mathematics, in repairing leaky faucets but not in writing poetry. No one is fully competent in all things, and we doubt that there are more than a few people who are totally incompetent at everything.

For many years, however, the law took the view that a person with a mental disability was completely competent or completely incompetent. It did not make a difference that a disability did not cause a person to be totally incompetent. All that seemed important was for the law to uphold the idea, which we know is wrong, that mental competence is an all-or-nothing condition.

The current trend in the law is toward recognizing that adults with disabilities are often neither wholly competent nor wholly incompetent. An individual may be competent to make some kinds of decisions, but not others. He or she may be competent to make decisions at some levels of complexity, but not at others.

But in law and practice, three "levels" of mental competence are usually recognized:

> Complete competence
> Partial competence
> Complete incompetence

People who are considered completely competent have the capacity to make reasoned decisions across all six kinds of decisions and all three levels of complexity. Being partially competent means having the capacity to make some (but not all) kinds of decisions and/or to make decisions at some (but not all) levels of complexity. Finally, being completely incompetent means having no capacity to make decisions of any kind at even a simple level. There are no clear criteria for classification into these levels. Rather, classification must be approximate rather than precise.

HOW CAN YOU DETERMINE YOUR SON'S OR DAUGHTER'S PRESENT LEVEL OF MENTAL COMPETENCE?

The question arises as to how you can determine the present level of your son's or daughter's competence. This is where the information from the previous chapter on the kinds of decisions, complexity of decisions, and the decision-making process are helpful.

To determine your son's or daughter's level of mental competence, return to the definition of mental competence—the capacity to make reasoned decisions. The decision-making process is a sequence of six steps:

> Defining the problem or need
> Brainstorming
> Evaluating and choosing alternatives
> Communicating the decision to others

Taking action
Evaluating the outcome of the action

Now, let's begin to apply the decision-making process to the kinds of decisions that you or your son or daughter will face. These are decisions about:

Life in the community
Relationships with other people
The place one lives
One's job
The acquisition of money
The spending of money

Figure 4.1 provides a framework you can use to assess your son's or daughter's ability to apply each step in the decision-making process to each kind of decision. The vertical column on the left lists the six steps of decision-making and the horizontal column across the top lists the six kinds of decisions.

Try using the "Mental Competence for Decision-Making" chart to assess Jolene Harris's mental competence to make decisions about spending money (sixth column). You can ask a question about spending money for each step of the decision-making process. Concerning how she will spend money, can Jolene:

Identify her needs?
Brainstorm a range of options?
Evaluate and choose?
Communicate her decision to others?
Take action to implement her decision?
Evaluate the outcome of her decision?

Recognizing that your knowledge of Jolene is limited, try anyway to use the information that you have to answer these questions. Also, ask similar questions for each of the six kinds of decisions. You should ask a question and try to answer it for each box on the chart.

Your answers probably are as vague as ours. We find ourselves saying, "sometimes" more frequently than "yes" or "no." This is because competence varies greatly, depending upon the complexity of the decision.

We can clear up some of the vagueness by adding the third dimension, complexity, to the chart. As we said in the previous chapter, decisions vary in complexity. The two factors that heavily influence the level of complexity are the degree of risk and reversibility of the decision. (As a practical matter, in this illustration the amount of money that Jolene can spend is a fair measure of both the degree of risk and of reversibility. If she has $50 that she can spend, there is less risk and more reversibility than if she is carrying $500 or $5,000 in her pocketbook. *Remember: Risk and reversibility are determined by the person's total context and the kind of decision that needs to be made.* We will come back to this point again and again.

As we noted in Chapter 3, the three levels of complexity are:

Simple
Medium
Difficult

We'll now add complexity to our chart in Figure 4.2. You will see that in each box,

Mental Competence for Decision-Making

	Concerning life in the community	Concerning relationships with other people	Concerning the place one lives	Concerning one's job	Concerning the acquisition of money	Concerning the spending of money
Defining the problem or need						*Can Jolene identify her needs and preferences?*
Brainstorming						*Can Jolene brainstorm a range of options?*
Evaluating and choosing alternatives						*Can Jolene evaluate and choose options?*
Communicating the decision to others						*Can Jolene communicate the decision to others?*
Taking action						*Can Jolene take action to implement her decision?*
Evaluating outcome of the action						*Can Jolene evaluate the outcome of her decision?*

Figure 4.1. Assessing mental competence for decision-making: The six steps of the decision-making process and the six kinds of decisions. Y = "Is able to make reasoned decisions."
S = "Is sometimes able to make reasoned decisions." N = "Is not able to make reasoned decisions."

three lines are drawn. The first level represents simple decisions, the middle represents decisions of medium complexity, and the bottom level in each box represents difficult decisions.

Now we can return to the previous questions about Jolene. But we can ask each of those questions in light of each of the three levels of difficulty. We'll illustrate with the first questions:

> Concerning how she will spend money, can Jolene identify her needs and preferences in simple decisions?
>
> Concerning how she will spend money, can Jolene identify her needs and preferences in decisions involving a medium level of complexity?
>
> Concerning how she will spend money, can Jolene identify her needs and preferences in decisions involving a difficult level of complexity?

Figures 4.3, 4.4, and 4.5 depict the completed charts for Jolene Harris, Steve Stuart, and Anna Levine. Study these charts to learn how mental competence can vary within the same individual and between different individuals. For example, Steve is able to make decisions at a simple level in identifying his needs and preferences for relationships with people. But he is not able to make even simple decisions at most of the steps of the decision-making process concerning how to acquire money. On the other hand, Anna is able to make decisions at difficult levels for all kinds of decisions. Her chart makes it clear that she has a weakness in evaluating the outcomes of her actions.

Before proceeding to the next chapter, we hope you will take time to complete the "Mental Competence for Decision-Making" chart for your son or daughter. Copies for you to fill in appear in Appendix 5. These copies have perforated pages so that you can separate them from the book for use as part of your future planning. Also, we encourage you to involve other family members or friends who are close to your son or daughter in completing the chart on their own or with you. Sometimes several heads are better than one—gaining the perspective of others can help you obtain the most accurate and comprehensive assessment of your son's or daughter's mental competence.

Once you have explored your son's or daughter's mental competence by completing the chart, you will be ready to move on to the next chapter. There, we use information on mental competence to help you determine who is an appropriate person or persons to make decisions (give consent) during your son's or daughter's adult life.

Based on their present capability for decision-making, you should conclude that Steve and Jolene have partial mental competence and that Anna has complete mental competence. Although Steve and Jolene fall into the same category, partial competence, Jolene is substantially more competent than Steve. You learn from the chart that Steve has minimal decision-making capabilities, and you can use the chart to identify his strengths. You therefore can conclude that he is not completely incompetent. Although Anna needs to improve and refine her decision-making, she generally demonstrates that she should not be found even partially incompetent.

Completing the chart is time-consuming. But it is so important to determine your son's or daugher's level of mental competence fully and carefully that this thorough process is well worth your time and effort. It will be worthwhile for you to complete the chart because it will be very unusual for a judge to initiate such a thorough review of the mental competence and decision-making skills of your son or daughter.

Mental Competence for Decision-Making

		Concerning life in the community	Concerning relationships with other people	Concerning the place one lives	Concerning one's job	Concerning the acquisition of money	Concerning the spending of money
Defining the problem or need	Simple						
	Medium						
	Difficult						
Brainstorming	Simple						
	Medium						
	Difficult						
Evaluating and choosing alternatives	Simple						
	Medium						
	Difficult						
Communicating the decision to others	Simple						
	Medium						
	Difficult						
Taking action	Simple						
	Medium						
	Difficult						
Evaluating outcome of the action	Simple						
	Medium						
	Difficult						

Figure 4.2. Assessing mental competence for decision-making: Kinds of decisions, steps in the decision-making process, and the complexity of decisions. Y = "Is able to make reasoned decisions." N = "Is not able to make reasoned decisions."

Mental Competence for Decision-Making

		Concerning life in the community	Concerning relationships with other people	Concerning the place one lives	Concerning one's job	Concerning the acquisition of money	Concerning the spending of money
Defining the problem or need	Simple	Y	Y	Y	Y	Y	Y
	Medium	Y	Y	Y	Y	N	N
	Difficult	N	N	N	N	N	N
Brainstorming	Simple	Y	Y	Y	Y	Y	Y
	Medium	Y	N	N	N	N	N
	Difficult	N	N	N	N	N	N
Evaluating and choosing alternatives	Simple	Y	Y	Y	Y	Y	Y
	Medium	N	N	N	Y	N	N
	Difficult	N	N	N	N	N	N
Communicating the decision to others	Simple	Y	Y	Y	Y	Y	Y
	Medium	Y	Y	Y	Y	Y	Y
	Difficult	N	N	N	N	N	N
Taking action	Simple	Y	Y	Y	Y	Y	Y
	Medium	N	N	N	N	N	N
	Difficult	N	N	N	N	N	N
Evaluating outcome of the action	Simple	Y	N	Y	Y	Y	Y
	Medium	N	N	N	N	N	N
	Difficult	N	N	N	N	N	N

Figure 4.3. Assessment of Jolene Harris's mental competence for decision-making. Y = "Is able to make reasoned decisions." N = "Is not able to make reasoned decisions."

Mental Competence for Decision-Making

		Concerning life in the community	Concerning relationships with other people	Concerning the place one lives	Concerning one's job	Concerning the acquisition of money	Concerning the spending of money
Defining the problem or need	Simple	N	Y	Y	Y	N	Y
	Medium	N	N	N	N	N	N
	Difficult	N	N	N	N	N	N
Brainstorming	Simple	N	Y	N	N	N	N
	Medium	N	N	N	N	N	N
	Difficult	N	N	N	N	N	N
Evaluating and choosing alternatives	Simple	N	N	N	N	N	N
	Medium	N	N	N	N	N	N
	Difficult	N	N	N	N	N	N
Communicating the decision to others	Simple	N	Y	N	N	N	N
	Medium	N	N	N	N	N	N
	Difficult	N	N	N	N	N	N
Taking action	Simple	N	Y	N	N	N	N
	Medium	N	N	N	N	N	N
	Difficult	N	N	N	N	N	N
Evaluating outcome of the action	Simple	N	N	N	N	N	N
	Medium	N	N	N	N	N	N
	Difficult	N	N	N	N	N	N

Figure 4.4. Assessment of Steve Stuart's mental competence for decision-making. Y = "Is able to make reasoned decisions." N = "Is not able to make reasoned decisions."

Mental Competence for Decision-Making

		Concerning life in the community	Concerning relationships with other people	Concerning the place one lives	Concerning one's job	Concerning the acquisition of money	Concerning the spending of money
Defining the problem or need	Simple	Y	Y	Y	Y	Y	Y
	Medium	Y	Y	Y	Y	N	N
	Difficult	Y	Y	Y	Y	Y	Y
Brainstorming	Simple	Y	Y	Y	Y	Y	Y
	Medium	Y	Y	Y	Y	Y	Y
	Difficult	Y	Y	Y	Y	Y	Y
Evaluating and choosing alternatives	Simple	Y	Y	Y	Y	Y	Y
	Medium	Y	Y	Y	Y	Y	Y
	Difficult	Y	Y	Y	N	N	N
Communicating the decision to others	Simple	Y	Y	Y	Y	Y	Y
	Medium	Y	Y	Y	Y	Y	Y
	Difficult	Y	Y	Y	Y	Y	Y
Taking action	Simple	Y	Y	Y	Y	Y	Y
	Medium	Y	Y	Y	Y	Y	Y
	Difficult	Y	Y	Y	Y	N	N
Evaluating outcome of the action	Simple	Y	Y	Y	Y	Y	Y
	Medium	N	N	N	N	N	N
	Difficult	N	N	N	N	N	N

Figure 4.5. Assessment of Anna Levine's mental competence for decision-making. Y = "Is able to make reasoned decisions." N = "Is not able to make reasoned decisions."

Many courts have not seriously considered the demands that will face adults with disabilities. Some courts tend to think that all people with mental disabilities should be legally declared incompetent, and other courts strongly resist ever making such a determination. To get an accurate determination of mental competence, especially in the courts, is very important, as we discuss in Chapter 8. Another reason to use the chart is because it will provide you with documentation to support your choice of the method of decision-making that best suits your son or daughter, and it will enable you to identify your son's or daughter's decision-making strengths and weaknesses. Once you know them, you can use this evaluation for instruction during school years and beyond. The ultimate goal is to help your son or daughter increase his or her decision-making capacity. If your son or daughter is not now performing each of the six steps, we encourage you to ask yourself these questions:

Can he or she be taught to do each step

Fully?
Partially?
Not at all?

If he or she can be taught, is instruction now being provided

In school?
Through adult education?
By family and friends?

Just because your son or daughter doesn't have these skills today doesn't mean the skills can't be learned in the future. We believe that many special education programs have been remiss in the area of decision-making instruction. We encourage you to talk with your young adult's teachers about instruction aimed at building these decision-making skills and ultimately increasing mental competence.

Before proceeding to the next chapter, we hope you will take time to complete the "Mental Competence for Decision-Making" chart for your son or daughter. Copies for you to fill in appear in Appendix 4. These copies have perforated pages so that you can separate them from the book for use as part of your future planning. Also, we encourage you to involve other family members or friends who are close to your son or daughter in completing the chart on their own or with you. Sometimes several heads are better than one—gaining the perspective of others can help you obtain the most accurate and comprehensive assessment of your son's or daughter's mental competence.

Once you have explored your son's or daughter's mental competence by completing the chart, you will be ready to move on to the next chapter. There, we use information on mental competence to help you determine who is an appropriate person or persons to make decisions (give consent) during your son's or daughter's adult life.

CONSENT—WHAT ARE ITS LEGAL AND PRACTICAL MEANINGS FOR YOUR SON OR DAUGHTER?

5

Consent is important to you and your young adult, because once you have put together all the information we have presented, you will still need to determine if your son or daughter can act in a mentally competent way. Can Anna bring her mental competence to bear in her life? Can Jolene and Steve? If any of them cannot use their mental competence by making decisions, who can make decisions for them? Taking action, i.e., making mental competence come alive, is done by consenting or refusing to consent to do or be something in life. If people are mentally competent, they can decide for themselves what they will do or try to become. But if people are mentally incompetent, how can they take action? How can they give or withhold consent to the ordinary or extraordinary events of life? So, consent has very important practical considerations. As we show in Chapter 6, it also has important legal consequences.

Consent refers to a person's action in making a decision. At its most fundamental level, consent involves the approval or disapproval of some action in which an individual is or might become involved. Consent can range from a reasoned process, involving the six steps of decision-making, to a whimsical or snap judgment. The more reasoned and informed the decision-making, the better it is for those affected by the decision—particularly for decisions that are of greater complexity (present greater risks and are less reversible). Let's consider the possibility that Anna Levine wants to buy a condominium with her best friend, because she thinks it makes more sense to own property than to continue to rent. Signing a contract to purchase a condominium has enormous implications for Anna's finances and warrants a highly reasoned, rather than whimsical, approach to consent. It also requires her to have a lot of information.

With this example in mind, let's recall the six steps of the decision-making process:

Defining the problem or need
Brainstorming
Evaluating and choosing alternatives
Communicating the decision to others
Taking action
Evaluating the outcome of action

The act of giving reasoned and well-informed consent involves all of these steps. Two steps that are most closely tied to the act of decision-making are evaluating and choosing alternatives and taking action. As you think about the decision that Anna might make about a condominium, think about whether she can follow the decision-making process. If she can and does, won't her decision be more reasoned, more appropriate, less risky, and more readily reversible? Could Steve make the same decision? Certainly not. Could Jolene? Probably not. If they can't make that decision, who can? Who should?

Now, consider your son or daughter. Is he or she mentally competent enough to follow the six-step decision-making process, and to do so with respect to a particular kind of decision (in one of the four areas of adult life-style decisions and the two areas of financial consideration), given the complexity of the decision (risk and reversibility)? If so, there is mental competence, and your son or daughter can give consent, i.e., buy something (like Anna's condominium). If not, who will make the decision? Who will act for your son or daughter, giving or withholding consent? To answer these questions, you need to know more about consent. As you read on, remember that consent is a legal concept and that the act of giving or withholding consent is the expression of mental competence.

TYPES OF CONSENT

There are three types of consent:

> Direct consent
> Substitute consent
> Concurrent consent

Direct consent is the act of decision-making by the person who is directly affected. Suppose that Anna experiences a sudden loss of appetite and a dramatic weight loss. She goes to her physician and explains her symptoms. The doctor wishes to diagnose her condition through the usual "GI" (gastrointestinal) tract examinations. Anna agrees that he may do so. In agreeing to the diagnostic procedures, Anna is giving her direct consent to treatment—the permission comes directly from Anna.

Substitute consent is a decision made by one person on behalf of another. (Other terms that you may encounter for substitute consent are *indirect consent* and *third-party consent*.) Parents give substitute consent for their minor children, and guardians give substitute consent for adults who have been legally declared completely or partially incompetent.

Steve Stuart's situation helps illustrate substitute consent. Like Anna, Steve has experienced a sudden loss of appetite and weight loss. His mother and father take him to their physician, who wants to do the same diagnostic procedures for Steve that Anna's doctor did for her. Steve's parents agree to those procedures. Steve himself does not give direct consent, because he does not have sufficient mental competence to do so. Instead, his parents substitute their consent for his. Thus, his consent is obtained indirectly.

Concurrent consent is a combination of both direct and substitute consent. Because of this, concurrent consent always involves decision-making by at least two people and the expression of their mental competence by their act in giving joint, or combined, consent. Also, it usually means that a person is helped with decision-making. The person neither makes the decision alone nor has that decision made solely by another. Rather, the decision is made collaboratively. For example, let's say that Jolene is now at the point of graduating from high school and that she has been attending a sex education class. The class provides instruction in physiology, emotional involvement, and social skills. Sexual relations and contraception receive substantial attention, and Jolene decides that she wants to practice birth control by means of the pill. Her physician interviews Jolene concerning her choice and is fairly satisfied that she has used a reasonable process of decision-making to give consent to the pill's prescription and administration. Because the doctor also knows that Odessa is very involved with Jolene, and because the doctor herself is not confident of being able to determine Jolene's mental competence on her own, she also obtains Odessa's consent. Thus, the doctor has obtained, and Jolene and Odessa have given, concurrent consent. The consent is concurrent because it comes from the person with a disability (Jolene) as well as from some other responsible adult (Odessa).

Professionals frequently seek concurrent consent from both the adult with a disability and parents (or other "representatives"), even when the adult is capable of giving direct consent. Often they want to make sure that they are protected from being liable for acting without legally effective consent (from the person with a disability), so they get concurrent consent, especially from family members. We discuss this issue further in Chapter 7 as it relates to criteria you may want to consider in deciding if you need to have your son or daughter declared legally incompetent (partially or completely).

WHAT IS THE RELATIONSHIP BETWEEN LEVELS OF CONSENT AND LEVELS OF MENTAL COMPETENCE?

It is time for a brief review before going any further in deciding who gives consent. You will recall that there are different levels of mental competence. A person such as Anna is completely mentally competent, even though she has a mental disability. Jolene, however, has partial mental competence. Steve, by contrast, is completely incompetent, at least in the law's eyes. Given these facts about these three people, what type of consent in appropriate for each of them? In your young adult's situation, you should be asking: "What is the level of his or her mental competence, and, in light of it, who can give consent?"

One more brief review: The law presumes that minors are mentally incompetent and that adults are mentally competent. Because minors are viewed as mentally incompetent, they are not allowed to give legally sanctioned consent. Rather, parents as guardians have the authority to give consent on behalf of their minor children (substitute consent). Adults, on the other hand, are presumed to be mentally competent, and thus are able to consent directly. When an adult is legally determined to be partially competent or completely incompetent, the court authorizes another adult to consent on his or her behalf. This process is referred to as *guardianship*, and we discuss it more completely in Chapters 6–8. In brief, mental competence refers to the capacity to make decisions, and consent refers to the act of decision-making.

The type of consent usually matches up with the level of competence (see Table 5.1). For example, even though Anna is recognized to have complete mental competence, and thus to be able to give consent for complex decisions about where she will live, a decision to purchase a condominium is one for which she knows to seek the counsel of others. In fact, if she and her family decide that the purchase of the con-

Table 5.1.   The three types of consent generally correspond to the three levels of mental competence

Types of consent	Levels of mental competence
Direct consent	Complete competence
Concurrent consent	Partial competence
Substitute consent	Complete incompetence

dominium is, indeed, the best alternative, it may be preferable for her parents to co-sign the contract with her. This is a situation of concurrent consent for a person who is completely competent. Indeed, it is likely that the person who will sell the con-dominium to her will require her parents to sign the contract. After all, they want to be sure that they have a valid contract, i.e., one made by a legally competent person. So much is at stake—the risk (amount of money) is fairly high, given that Anna has a mental disability, so they may want concurrent consent. If Anna were buying a dress, the risk (amount of money) would be much less, and so the seller probably would not want concurrent consent.

Take Jolene Harris as another example. If she were simply seeing her doctor for treatment of a mild flu, Jolene probably could give direct consent, and the doctor would not need Odessa to give consent too. That is, concurrent consent would not be needed because Jolene's mental competence is partial and the treatment is not risky or irreversible. But if Jolene wanted to be sterilized, the doctor probably would want her direct consent and Odessa's concurrent consent, because sterilization is generally irre-versible and Jolene is only partially competent.

Here is a convenient way of thinking about all this: The greater your son's or daughter's mental incompetence, the greater the need for concurrent or substitute consent. And, the riskier the decision (and the harder it is to reverse it), the greater the need for concurrent or substitute consent.

Once again, it is important to realize that the context of a decision is very impor-tant. A person with partial mental competency might be capable of giving consent for one type of decision by direct consent but not for another without concurrent or sub-stitute consent. You need to consider all three factors together—level of mental com-petence (complete competence, partial competence, or complete incompetence), risk or degree of reversibility, and type of consent (direct, concurrent, or substitute).

At this point, you should review the chart (Figure 4.2) that you completed on your son or daughter in the last chapter. As you review it, you might answer these questions:

> For the types of decisions that you marked with a Y (indicating your son or daughter is able to make them), do you believe your son or daughter can give direct consent?
> For the types of decisions that you marked with an N (indicating your son or daughter is not able to make them), do you believe your son or daughter can provide concurrent consent, or do you believe that substitute con-sent is justified?
> What exceptions to these general guidelines do you want to make in light of the complexity (risk or degree of reversibility) of certain decisions?
> What instruction could be provided that would increase your son's or daugh-ter's competence to give consent?

As you answer these questions, you might make a notation in each box in Figure 4.2 to indicate the kind of consent you believe is appropriate for each type of decision: *D* for direct consent, *C* for concurrent consent, and *S* for substitute consent. Just as we encouraged you in the last chapter to involve other family members or close friends in identifying your son's or daughter's mental competence, you might also ask them to identify the level of consent that they think is appropriate. Completing this analysis will give you a basis for determining the role your son or daughter can assume in decision-making and the extent to which that role will need to be bolstered (concurrent consent) or assumed by others (substitute consent). However, always remember that your son or daughter can continue to develop the mental competence for direct consent. This will ensure that the process of reviewing his or her capabilities is ongoing, so that emerging skills can be identified and used.

If your son or daughter clearly can engage in direct consent, you may want to skip Chapters 6–8. In these chapters we discuss alternatives to direct consent for people who will engage in concurrent or substitute consent. However, if concurrent or substitute consent seem appropriate for your son or daughter, these next 3 chapters will present you with possibilities for devising approaches that meet your unique, individual needs.

6 | WHAT IS GUARDIANSHIP?

In this chapter we provide basic information on guardianship—its definition, its scope, the kinds of decisions it can cover, the individuals or organizations that can serve as guardians, and the duration of guardianship. With this and information provided in later chapters, you can consider whether guardianship is appropriate for your son or daughter. At this point, it is important for you to concentrate on what guardianship is. We urge you not to decide if you want guardianship for your son or daughter until you read Chapter 7.

DEFINITION OF GUARDIANSHIP

Guardianship is a means by which the law deals with the problems of incompetency and consent: how to have someone act (consent) for another who is incompetent. A court first determines if a person has complete competence, partial competence, or complete incompetence. If a court finds that the person has partial competence or complete incompetence (the court's finding is called an adjudication), a competent person (a guardian) is appointed and empowered to consent for the person with partial competence or complete incompetence (the ward).

Guardianship transfers authority to consent from one person to another. It thereby creates a relationship in which the guardian substitutes for the ward and thereby exercises the ward's rights on his or her behalf. Guardianship also allows the transfer of rights only after a court holds a trial and determines if the ward truly has partial competence or complete incompetence.

Guardianship usually should be considered when the person with a disability becomes an adult. Until then, the person's parents are the *natural guardians*. Or, adopting parents, foster parents, or social service agencies are the guardians of a minor. (In this book, we use the terms *guardian* and *ward*. We do so with hesitation, because these terms can seem too technical or even stigmatizing. However, you will encounter them as you do future planning, and it might be helpful in the long run to get accustomed to them. In addition, guardian is less awkward than "substitute decision-maker," and ward is less awkward than "person adjudicated incompetent.")

You will probably note how guardianship is linked to mental competence and consent. If a person is adjudicated incompetent, it is because he or she lacks mental competence, in whole or in part, and therefore cannot give consent. The guardianship adjudication handles the problem by transferring the right to consent from the person who has a mental disability (ward) to another (guardian). (Although the definition of guardianship presented here is the generally accepted one, guardianship can be defined in different ways in the laws of different states. We encourage you to consult an attorney about the definition of guardianship and its application in your state.) In this chapter, we explore the meaning of guardianship and how it might facilitate your future planning. An attorney can help you make specific applications under the laws of your particular state.

You should note the relationship of consent to guardianship. An adult who has not been adjudicated incompetent gives direct consent. Often, as we point out in Chapter 5, the person gives direct consent and another person also gives consent. This is called concurrent consent. However, when a person has been adjudicated to be partially competent or completely incompetent, and a guardian has been appointed, the only legally effective consent is the substitute consent of the guardian. It is good practice for a guardian to try to involve the ward in the decision-making. If a guardian does involve the ward and the ward agrees to the action proposed, this means the ward *gives assent*. The ward cannot give consent because, as a result of the adjudication, he or she has been found legally incapable of giving consent. If the ward gives assent and the guardian gives substitute consent, there is a situation similar to, but not identical to, concurrent consent, in that two people are agreeing to some action. The difference is that assent is legally irrelevant, whereas consent, whether direct or substitute, is legally relevant—it is the only arrangement allowed by law. The law does not recognize assent as legally binding, but guardians may still want to seek their ward's assent so that, as a practical matter, concurrent agreement is expressed.

WHAT IS THE SCOPE OF GUARDIANSHIP?

Guardianship can—and always should—be tailored to the needs of the individual who is incompetent. Because some people (like Steve Stuart) have complete mental incompetence, they need full or complete guardianship. Others, like Jolene Harris, have partial competence and need only limited guardianship. The scope of a person's guardianship, complete or limited, should be tied to the extent of a person's competence. Thus, there are two types of guardianship: *complete* (plenary) and *limited* (partial).

What Is Plenary Guardianship?

Plenary means "full, complete, and unlimited." A plenary guardianship, therefore, is one that gives the guardian full, complete, and unlimited authority to consent on the ward's behalf. Thus, plenary guardianship is an option that is typically considered when a ward has complete incompetence and needs substitute consent. The laws in all states allow a court to establish plenary guardianship.

What Is Limited Guardianship?

A limited guardianship recognizes that the ward has partial competence in at least some areas of decision-making and therefore is able to give direct consent for some kinds of decisions, or for decisions at some levels of complexity. A ward fitting this description is regarded as having neither complete competence nor complete incompetence. Limited guardianship (sometimes also called *partial guardianship*), therefore, gives the guardian some authority to consent on the ward's behalf, and the court specifies the scope of authority. For example, the court may authorize the guardian to make contracts for a certain amount of money (for example, more than $500), but allow the ward to make contracts for any amount less than that. Or, the court may authorize the guardian to consent to surgery, but allow the ward to obtain routine medical care. The laws in many states allow a court to establish limited guardianship. As noted, Jolene is a good candidate for limited guardianship because she has partial mental competence. (Whether Odessa or anyone else should try to have her adjudicated and placed under guardianship is another mattter. Don't rush to judgment about Jolene, and don't decide yet about your own son or daughter.)

WHAT KINDS OF DECISIONS MAY A GUARDIAN MAKE FOR A WARD?

Courts may appoint guardians to give consent for life-style decisions, financial decisions, or both. In Chapter 3, we said the four major areas of life-style decisions concern:

Life in the community
Relationships with other people
The place where one lives
A job

The two areas of financial decisions concerned:

Acquiring money
Spending money

A guardian who has power to give consent for life-style decisions is called a *personal guardian*; the guardianship itself is called a *guardianship of the person*. A guardian who has power to consent for financial decisions is called a *financial guardian* or a *guardian of the estate*; the guardianship itself is called a *financial guardianship* or a *guardianship of the estate* (property). A guardian who has power of personal and financial guardianship is a *general guardian*; the guardianship itself is called a *general guardianship*. Remember, we are concerned here only with the kind of guardianship, as defined by the kind of decisions (personal, financial, or both) that a guardian may make. We are not concerned about the extent of a guardianship—plenary or limited.

What Is Guardianship of the Person?

A guardian of the person may give consent for decisions about the life-style of the ward, as noted previously. A guardian of the person is appointed when the ward has partial competence or complete incompetence in making life-style decisions. For example, the guardian may consent to a transfer from one group home to another (decisions about the place where one lives), or may participate in the development of the ward's individualized program plan (a decision about life in the community).

There are restrictions on the guardian's authority to give consent for life-style decisions. A guardian of the person does not have authority over the ward's financial affairs. Also, some decisions are generally regarded as too personal for a guardian to control. For example, in many states the guardian may not draft the ward's Will, consent to or veto a ward's marriage, decide for whom the ward will vote, donate a ward's organs after death, terminate a ward's life support system, consent to some health procedures, or admit the ward to a residential hospital or institution.

The great advantage of a personal guardianship is the competent, court-supervised oversight of the ward's personal life. This can prevent a ward from being abused, neglected, or simply ignored. The guardian is required to meet certain standards before being appointed by a court. (See Chapter 8 for a discussion of the standards and qualifications for a personal guardian.) The guardian is required to report to a court at least once a year concerning the ward and how the guardian has overseen the ward's life. The guardian also sometimes has to obtain a court's approval before giving consent to certain actions affecting the ward.

Just because a guardian has to meet certain minimum standards, file annual reports, or get special judicial approval does not mean that a guardian or court will always make wise or even defensible decisions. But these requirements at least assure minimum procedures for caretaking, and keep open the possibility that a court will indeed closely monitor the guardian and scrutinize the guardian's decisions. There is also the possibility that people who are interested in the ward will have an opportunity to read the guardian's reports, ask a court to step in if a guardian seems to be derelict in his or her duty to care for the ward, and try to persuade the court to appoint another guardian or to require the guardian to act only in certain, clearly described ways.

Personal guardianship does not guarantee that the guardian will always act in the ward's best interests or that the guardian will try to make decisions that the ward would want to be made if competent to make them directly. Guardianship may even be unwarranted altogether; after all, courts may consider factors other than the person's mental competence. (See Chapter 7 for a discussion of factors that courts, and you, may consider.) Nor is there any guarantee that a court will be diligent in reviewing the guardian's reports or acting if something seems amiss. Finally, as we point out in discussing financial guardianship, there are expenses that must be met if a guardian is appointed.

You yourself will have to weigh the overall advantages and disadvantages of personal guardianship for your son or daughter, remembering that personal guardianship can enhance your young adult's life if it is properly tailored to his or her needs, even though it takes rights away from your son or daughter and gives them to the guardian. What good are rights that cannot be exercised? But remember, too, that too much guardianship can be a dangerous thing, because it does take away rights that your son or daughter just may be able to exercise, either now or later.

What Is Guardianship of the Estate?

A guardian of the estate has authority to consent to decisions that concern finances, but not those concerning the ward's life-style. A financial guardian is responsible for managing, investing, protecting, and preserving the ward's financial assets and can use the financial assets for the ward's benefit only. The guardian may not commingle or combine the ward's property with his or her own.

The guardian must use reasonable care and skill in managing the ward's financial affairs, that is, the care and skill that a person of ordinary prudence would exercise with personal property. Otherwise, the guardian has breached the duty of reasonable care. This means that the guardian may not take undue risks with the ward's assets. The estate guardian is a conservator of assets. For example, a guardian may invest a ward's assets in high-grade corporate bonds or in U.S. Treasury securities in order to earn income safely, but may not make risky investments in a real estate partnership (although the ward could with his or her own money).

In some states, the guardian may not spend or invest any of the ward's funds without first obtaining permission from the court. If a guardian spends the ward's money without prior court approval, the guardian may be required to repay that money from personal funds.

Similarly, many states require the guardian to obtain judicial permission before investing the ward's assets. All guardians have a duty to invest the assets. In some states, if the guardian allows the ward's money to remain uninvested, the court will charge the guardian interest on the uninvested money.

The advantage of a guardianship of an estate, particularly a large one, is the competent, court-supervised management of the ward's assets. This can prevent the ward from wasting his assets or spending them unwisely. The guardian is required to report to the court on the ways in which the guardian has managed the ward's estate. Although the reporting usually is done only on an annual basis, guardians sometimes request special approval to make certain unusual decisions (e.g., to sell a farm or mineral rights that have been income-producing and invest the proceeds in income-yielding bonds).

Annual reporting, and even special reporting that is related to permission to act, does not assure that the court will give highly competent or close attention to the guardian's behavior. But there is at least the possibility that courts will scrutinize the special requests carefully. There is the further possibility that people who are interested in the guardianship (other than the guardian and ward) will have an opportunity to inspect the reports and call for an accounting by the guardian and, if the accounting shows that the guardian has not fulfilled his or her duties in a reasonable and prudent manner, sue the guardian for the money lost because of that fact.

Still, financial guardianship is not as preferable as a carefully constructed Trust as a way of assuring, to the greatest extent possible, that the ward's property is well-managed. (Trusts are discussed in Chapter 10.) This is because court supervision of the guardian's decisions is more routine and perfunctory than careful and eagle-eyed.

There are some disadvantages to having a guardian of the estate. Paperwork and delays in action may be necessary to obtain court permission for investments and expenditures. Restrictions designed to protect the ward's assets may prevent aggressively productive money management. Fees charged by the guardian and the guardian's legal advisor can be expensive. This expense is paid from the assets of the person with a disability unless some other arrangement is made. It may be unwise to pay for financial expertise that cannot be fully used because of conservative investment restrictions.

Another expense is the posting of a "surety" or "performance" bond that provides money which must be forfeited if the guardian makes a mistake or misdeed in the financial management of the ward's estate. (In some states, a judge has discretion to waive the bond requirement. In these states, the bond requirement is usually omitted when either the assets of the ward are minimal or when the guardian of the estate is a bank.)

Finally, most states require a guardian to submit detailed reports (accounts or accountings) to the court about the management and expenditures of the ward's money, stating how much money has been earned, accrued, spent, and invested; explaining how and why these transactions have taken place; and accounting for every transaction made with the ward's money, with the receipts and canceled checks attached.

What Is a General Guardianship?

A general guardianship is a guardianship of both the person and the estate. It becomes appropriate when a person has partial competence or complete incompetence in making personal and financial decisions.

How Does the Scope of Guardianship Apply to the Guardian's Jurisdiction?

The court can establish plenary or limited guardianship for the guardian of the person, guardian of the estate, or general guardian. Figure 6.1 illustrates the various combinations of guardianships that are possible. For example, the guardian of the person can have plenary authority over every kind of life-style decision, or limited authority over only one kind of decision (for example, where one lives). Also, the guardian may have plenary authority over decisions at every level of complexity or limited authority over complex decisions only. A person's own capability and needs for reasoned decisions, as determined by the assessment in Figure 4.6 in Chapter 4, should and usually does determine the scope (plenary or limited) and jurisdiction (personal, financial, or general) of the guardianship.

To get a picture of how limited guardianship might work, think about Jolene Harris. As you can see from Figure 4.3 and our discussion of Jolene in Chapter 4, she has mixed abilities. Clearly, she is not completely competent (like Anna Levine, who nevertheless needs more instruction), nor is she wholly incompetent (like Steve Stuart). What are her areas of competence and incompetence?

| | **Jurisdiction** | | |
Scope	Guardianship of the person	Guardianship of the estate	General guardianship
Plenary	Plenary guardianship of the person	Plenary guardianship of the estate	Plenary general guardianship
Limited	Limited guardianship of the person	Limited guardianship of the estate	Limited general guardianship

Figure 6.1.   Scope of guardianship and guardian's jurisdiction.

To answer this question, and thereby get some guidance about how to tailor her limited guardianship to her special needs, begin by looking at three parts of the chart: first, her decision-making ability, second, her competence in the six areas in which she has to make decisions; and, last, her competence to make decisions that are simple, of medium complexity, and difficult. Overall, Jolene is competent to make simple decisions in all six areas. She is competent to make decisions that are of medium difficulty in only some of the six areas. She cannot make difficult decisons in any of the six areas. You should reach a conclusion that Jolene does not need a guardian for all decision-making. But that is just a general conclusion. How can it be translated into limited guardianship?

To get a better fix on the extent of a limited guardianship, we would have to examine Jolene's competency in *each* of the six areas. For the purposes of illustration, we'll do that for only two.

Relationships with Others   Jolene says she wants to have children. Odessa knows Jolene cannot assume the responsibilities of motherhood, and she fears that someone might take advantage of her daughter. Yet Odessa also wants Jolene to have a life in the community—to have the shopping mall trips, sing with the church choir, etc. Odessa will begin to consider a limited guardianship that allows Jolene to make some choices about her relationships with others, for example, whom to visit, where to go in the community without supervision, with whom to spend weekend "overnights." But Odessa also will begin to consider a limited guardianship that gives her the power to make decisions for Jolene concerning issues such as contraception. As Odessa thinks about Jolene and limited guardianship, she bears in mind the risks or potential irreversibility of Jolene's decisions, because she knows that Jolene's competency to make decisions of medium or difficult complexity is limited, and that risk and reversibility are measured not just by Jolene's competency, but also by the context of any decision that Jolene might make. Thus, Odessa would want the right, acquired through limited guardianship, to veto Jolene's choices about contraception but not about church-related field trips or similar relatively safe activities. Precisely what power Odessa would seek in limited guardianship, and what power a court would give her, then can be tied to the kind and complexity of a decision and to the element of risk and reversibility, all as determined by Jolene's competence, as shown on the chart.

Spending Money   Several facts about Jolene are relevant. She will have Social Security benefits, earn money at her job, want to spend her money on shopping trips, and have most of her needs for food, clothing, housing, and medical care satisfied by family, friends, or government programs. Just how much money will she have? And how much of what she has should she be allowed to spend? Put that last question in a different way: Just how much limited guardianship over Jolene's spending decisions should Odessa have?

There are several factors to consider, namely Jolene's income, needs, and competence, and the risk or reversibility of any of her spending decisions. If we assume that she receives about $250 in government benefits and about $300 in wages each month, has no expenses for food or housing, and gets Medicaid health benefits (we discuss government benefits in Chapters 11–12), we can assume safely that she can spend, without much risk to herself, up to $550 per month, on almost anything she wants. Odessa may be satisfied to let Jolene spend that much, or she may want Jolene to have a small savings account. In either case, it appears (as it did for limited guardianship in relationships with other people) that limited guardianship over the decisions to spend money can be tied to the kind of decision, the complexity of the decision, and the element of risk (does the purchase satisfy a need, or is it for a "nice-to-have" reason?) or reversibility (once the money is spent, is it refundable?), all determined by Jolene's competence, as shown on the chart.

To summarize, the following has been discussed about limited guardianship in this chapter:

It can be used for all or any of six areas of decision-making.

It can be used for all or any levels of complexity in all or any of the six areas of decision-making.

But, it is *not* appropriate if a person can make *no* decisions in any of the six areas, even at a simple level of complexity. Plenary guardianship, however, would be appropriate.

The decision whether to seek either no guardianship (Anna's case), limited guardianship (Jolene's case), or plenary guardianship (Steve's case) is determined *in part* by the combination of a person's decision-making competence in the six areas of adult responsibility, measured by the person's competence to make decisions at the simple, medium or difficult levels, and by the amount of risk or reversibility (or both) resulting from the decision.

WHO MAY SERVE AS A GUARDIAN?

Both individuals and public and private agencies may serve as guardians. In this section we discuss individual, collective, and public guardianship.

What Is an Individual Guardianship?

An individual guardianship exists when a court appoints an individual to be a guardian. Most states now allow one or more individuals to serve at the same time. If only one individual is a guardian (e.g., a mother for a son) there is *sole individual guardianship*. The advantages of individual guardianship are tied to the personal relationship that should and usually does exist between the guardian and the ward. Individual guardianship should be a relationship in which the guardian knows the ward well, is deeply committed to the ward's welfare, responds reasonably to the ward's choices and preferences, works independently of service providers and as an advocate for the ward in service systems, and is sensitive to and comfortable in working with the ward's family, friends, and other guardians. The disadvantages are that a particular guardian may lack the characteristics that are the advantages of an ideal individual guardianship and may be in disagreement with any co-guardians. If there is more than one guardian, there is a *joint guardianship* or *coguardianship* (e.g., two parents for a son). In that case, the division of responsibility for the ward is: 1) Set by the court and determined by the extent of the guardianship (plenary or limited; personal, estate, or general); 2) Is set by the individual guardians; or 3) Is determined both ways. Joint guardianships are helpful for sharing responsibility and maximizing the expertise of the guardians. There can be problems, however, when joint guardians disagree with each other.

What Is a Collective Guardianship?

In some states, laws allow a court to appoint a specially created corporation to be a guardian of the person, guardian of the estate, or a general guardian. This corporation is organized for the principal purpose of serving as a guardian for people with a disability. Usually, the corporation is created by parents who want to pool their assets (often, banks and trust companies decline to be guardians when the assets of a family are small or the person has complicated needs), and usually the corporation operates on a nonprofit basis.

The advantages of collective corporate guardianships are that financial assets are pooled so that even small-estate guardianships can be administered; corporations have strong ties to parent advocacy groups such as local and state Associations for Retarded Citizens, and corporations have professional staffs to help with financial and personal guardianship. Like any other guardianship, collective corporate guardianships are supervised by the court that gives them authority, and continuity is automatically provided for because the corporation has a perpetual or indefinite life.

What Is a Public Guardianship?

In some cases, a child or adult with a disability does not have family or friends. The family may have died in a sudden tragedy, and the parents may not have left a Last Will and Testament designating a guardian for a child or indicating preferences for a guardian for an adult. Or, sometimes parents may have abandoned their children or given up (or been required to surrender and terminate) their rights as parents.

If the person with a disability needs a guardian but there are no options for individual or collective guardianships, courts in all states are authorized to appoint a *public guardian*. This may be an individual (such as a director of social services in the community or superintendent of a state institution where the person resides). It may also be a state or local unit such as a social services, mental retardation, mental health or developmental disabilities agency. Selection of the agency is up to the court.

In a collective or public guardianship, the person who actually performs the duties of a guardian may act as the ideal individual guardian should. But this is not assured because the person will be responsible for many wards. Moreover, in collective guardianships, and particularly in public guardianships, there is a particular risk that the case load of the agency or individuals employed by the guardian will be so large that the ward's needs will not be given enough attention. There also is a risk that the collective or public guardianship will experience conflicts of interest between itself and service providers; the agency may be a service provider or may have to compromise one ward's interests in order to serve other wards who also are involved with the same service provider.

THE NATURE OF THE GUARDIANSHIP RELATIONSHIP

The different options for the guardianship relationship are illustrated in Figure 6.2. If the guardianship is of the person (i.e., the guardian has the authority to give consent for life-style decisions), the guardian should be an individual or group (such as a collective guardianship operated by a parent advocacy group) interested in the ward. Some people may believe that a guardian should be disinterested and objective—someone who will take a somewhat distanced point of view. Others may believe that the guardian should be vitally concerned and interested—someone who will take a highly involved point of view. We believe that the personal guardianship should involve the passionate commitment of the guardian to the ward.

Who	Jurisdiction		
	Guardianship of the person	Guardianship of the estate	General guardianship
Individual			
Collective			
Public			

Figure 6.2. Options for the guardianship relationship.

The personal guardian should be an individual or corporation willing to perform these duties:

Visit the ward

Be available in emergencies

When necessary or appropriate, "step into the ward's shoes" to do something the ward would want to do

Solve problems and deal with service providers, when necessary and appropriate

Have experience with the service provider system

Know the ward's family and family values

Be the ward's friend

Understand the ward's capabilities and limits

Understand the special needs created by the ward's disability

Know how to obtain services that meet the ward's needs, and even how to satisfy those needs directly.

In essence, the guardian must be deeply involved in the life of the ward. Parents may be the personal guardians, but others may also meet these criteria.

Almost by necessity personal guardianship requires an individual to be the personal guardian. It is difficult for corporations (collective guardianship) to serve as personal guardians except in rare cases when there are employees of the corporation who will establish the close relationship that personal guardianship requires.

In some cases, personal guardianship can be shared by two or more individuals, or by an individual and a corporation. If guardianship is shared, it is important for the guardians—either by court order or by informal agreement among themselves—to decide who will have primary and secondary responsibility and authority to consent to certain decisions.

Financial guardianship (guardianship of the estate) does not necessarily require a personal relationship between the guardian and ward. It is possible, for example, for a Trust company to invest, disperse, account for, and file tax returns for a ward's estate, all without any personal knowledge of the ward. This might be the case for a ward who inherits property from a relative. It would make sense for a bank to be the guardian of his or her estate. On the other hand, a financial guardian may be asked from time to time to make extraordinary expenditures on the ward's behalf. For example, the usual monthly or quarterly disbursements from the ward's estate may not be sufficient to cover the costs of necessary hospitalization or a special training program. If that is the case and the guardian does not have some familiarity with the ward, the guardian may refuse to make the necessary expenditure, or at least will not do so without court authority. For this reason, having a guardian of the estate with expertise in financial management and a personal interest in the ward is ideal.

In instances of general guardianship (personal and financial guardianship), the guardian may be one person—usually an individual or, less likely, a corporation. In other instances, the guardianship may be shared by two or more individuals and two or more corporations. In such cases, the guardians must decide, either by court order or informally, how to share responsibility.

When selecting a guardian of the ward's estate, it it helpful to choose one experienced in the administration of estates—investing assets, disbursing funds, filing the necessary accounts with the court, preparing and filing tax returns, and generally managing the estate for the ward's benefit (and not for the benefit of the personal guardian or for anyone who will benefit from the ward's estate after the ward dies).

HOW LONG DOES GUARDIANSHIP LAST?

Guardianship can be permanent or temporary. Normally, an adult with a mental disability who has been judicially declared completely incompetent is subject to guardianship for an indefinite period. This is known as *permanent guardianship*. Actually, that term is somewhat misleading, because the law allows anybody, including the ward, to seek a court order removing the guardianship and restoring the ward to competency. However, the restoration to competency is rarely sought and even more rarely granted. Once adjudicated, a person almost always remains under guardianship permanently.

Other guardianships are temporary. For example, the natural guardianship of parents over children lasts only as long as the children are minors. Temporary guardianship, usually created to deal with a specific life- or health-threatening emergency, lasts only as long as necessary to deal with the emergency.

Typically, guardianship is a permanent arrangement. Therefore, it should be considered with caution, and with the understanding that it is usually easier to establish than to terminate. As children and adults with disabilities get more and better instruction in decision-making, reversals of guardianship may begin to become less rare. For example, it is possible that a 20-year-old might need a guardian of the person, but within 10 years he or she may develop sufficient competence to make decisions so that a personal guardian would no longer be necessary.

Now that we have reviewed the definition of guardianship and some of the important considerations that apply to thinking about various guardianship options, it is time to use this information as you consider whether your son or daughter could benefit from guardianship, and, if so, how you can tailor guardianship to meet his or her needs, as well as the needs of other family members. This is the focus of Chapter 7.

7 WHAT CONSIDERATIONS MUST YOU MAKE WHEN DECIDING ABOUT GUARDIANSHIP?

A variety of factors must be considered when you attempt to determine if guardianship is appropriate for your son or daughter. In this chapter, we highlight many of these considerations and offer guidance on how to proceed toward a decision that is in the best interest of your family.

WHEN IS GUARDIANSHIP NEEDED?

Concerning guardianship, the fundamental issue you face is whether your son or daughter can give direct or concurrent consent for life-style and financial decisions. In Figure 4.2, we provided a guide to determining if your son or daughter has complete mental competence (the capability to make reasoned decisions for each of the six kinds of decisions and at three levels of complexity). If he or she does have complete mental competence, then guardianship is not needed at present. Because the possibility exists that circumstances will change, the question of guardianship may someday need to be asked again, however.

Now, if you have determined that your son or daughter has either partial competence (the capability to make reasoned decisions for some, but not all, kinds of decisions and at some, but not all, levels of complexity) or complete incompetence (no capability to make reasoned decisions of any kind at even a simple level of complexity), you have several guardianship options. If partial competence exists, your son or daughter will likely be able to give some direct consent, or some concurrent consent at the discretion of service providers. But he or she may also need some limited guardianship. If total incompetence exists, your son or daughter will need complete substitute consent (plenary guardianship). Carefully review Figure 4.2 (as it applies to your son or daughter) as you consider these questions:

> For what kinds of decisions does my son or daughter need substitute consent?
> For what steps of the decision-making process does my son or daughter need substitute consent?
> At what level of decision-making complexity does my son or daughter need substitute consent?

The answers to these questions will help you determine the nature and degree of assistance your son or daughter need when making decisions. As you consider these questions, you may find that your answers vary. This is because the level of your son's or daughter's competence depends upon factors such as the instruction given in school or other agencies, periodic behavior problems or depression, and the availability of support services. You need to consider your son's or daughter's general decision-making pattern and acknowledge variations that should be taken into account in your future planning. The nature and degree of assistance needed on both regular and periodic bases will help you determine if guardianship is an appropriate option.

The precise needs of your son or daughter in the area of decision-making should be the major criteria for deciding what options are appropriate for providing the necessary decision-making assistance. Individual needs, however, are not the only consideration in deciding whether to pursue guardianship. Because, unfortunately, the situation is more complicated than that, in the following pages we provide information on options other than guardianship for providing substitute consent. We also suggest factors, in addition to your son's or daughter's needs, to consider in making a guardianship decision. Finally, we review a process you might follow in deciding how to tailor guardianship to your son's or daughter's needs and specific circumstances, if you indeed decide to pursue guardianship.

BESIDES GUARDIANSHIP, WHAT WAYS ARE THERE TO PROVIDE SUBSTITUTE CONSENT?

The four alternatives to guardianship for providing substitute consent are: *protective services, implied consent, a representative payee,* and *Trusts.* Each of these alternatives is a way of substituting the decision-making ability (mental competence) of one person for the decision-making inability (mental incompetence) of another. These alternatives are not as comprehensive and stable as guardianship. But, depending upon your son's or daughter's particular needs for assistance with life-style and financial decisions, these options may offer sufficient means to provide concurrent or substitute consent.

What Are Protective Services?

Most states have laws that allow departments of social services (also known by other names), upon a petition to a court and with court approval, to provide consent for services for a person who, because of disability, is not able to arrange for his or her own food, shelter, clothing, or necessary medical care. In most states, these protective services apply to adults and children alike. They allow anyone to file a report with a department of social services indicating that a person is in need of care or is abused or neglected; authorize an investigation of that report by the department of social services; authorize a petition to a court by the department if it determines that the need for care exists, and allow the court to provide authority to the department to intervene. The department can usually have the judicial proceeding expedited in cases of imminent danger or emergency. Some states also have separate laws allowing for emergency intervention by social services, health services, or mental health services, sometimes without a prior judicial hearing and order. In those states, however, a judicial hearing must be held after the intervention. In some instances, a judicial order allowing the department to intervene may trigger a mandatory guardianship hearing.

If you find that your son or daughter usually has partial or complete competence, but still has a disability that may on occasion result in negligent care or unreasonable decisions, he or she may be able to obtain assistance in consenting to and getting access to necessary services (food, shelter, medical attention) by way of these protective services laws. Protective services can assist with decisions about life-style, but generally do not become involved in financial decisions. However, remember that these laws will not come into play unless someone seeks to bring your son or daughter under the protection of social services agencies. Also, these laws may require the court that allows social services intervention to initiate a guardianship proceeding to determine whether your son or daughter has mental incompetence. Clearly, relying on these laws to provide consent for and access to services when your son or daughter needs help is risky business.

What Is Implied Consent?

Most states have established a *doctrine of implied consent*. That is, the law "implies" the consent of the person with *de facto* incompetence. It assumes that he or she would consent to services, if competent to do so, and it allows services to be provided in some circumstances.

One circumstance is an emergency—a situation in which a person who is unconscious as a result of an accident or stroke is presumed to consent to medical treatment. In such a circumstance, the law "implies" that person's consent. If the person later becomes competent, the implied consent doctrine does not come into play and the person's consent must be obtained directly. For example, assume that while Steve Stuart is watching his community's Fourth of July parade, the grandstand on which he is sitting collapses. (Let's also assume that he is an adult and no decision has been made yet on his guardianship.) He receives serious head injuries, has broken bones, and may have internal injuries. At the hospital, the physicians see that they need to treat Steve immediately, but they cannot obtain his permission because he is unconscious. The doctrine of implied consent to emergency treatment authorizes them to treat him.

Another situation involving implied consent exists when the competent person expresses consent to certain services, but the service provider does more than is expressly authorized. For example, Anna Levine may give direct consent to an operation on a certain part of her body (e.g., a ruptured appendix). During the operation the surgeon may find a diseased condition (say, a cyst on an ovary), and treat it. The surgeon is within his or her right to do so 1) because Anna gave direct consent to one procedure, 2) because the new procedure is closely related to the one for which direct consent was given, and 3) because the new procedure is medically necessary or desirable.

In the past, service providers used the implied consent rule often, and in many circumstances other than medical emergencies. They frequently obtained the consent of the person (direct consent), the family and the person (concurrent consent), or the guardian (substitute consent) for general purposes, and then relied on that general consent to cover almost all specific actions. Or, they obtained consent for one specific action and relied on it for other related actions. In short, they interpreted the scope of the one consent they had obtained very broadly. Nowadays, service providers are much less likely to get "blanket consent" (very broad authority for a large number of actions) or to rely on one consent for related actions. Instead, they tend to seek consent for each specific action, and to avoid the implied consent rule that allowed them so much leeway in the past. This is a positive development because it makes service providers more accountable to the client and other consent-givers, involves the client and other consent-givers more actively in decisions, and creates a stronger basis for any legal action that is taken. In general, we urge you to insist on specific consent. In a medical emergency or when any service provider action is closely and clearly related to a specific consent, implied consent is still viable. Otherwise, it has very little role, and should have an increasingly smaller role, in determining who (among service providers) may do what in the life of a person with a disability.

Protective services and the two types of implied consent have the major disadvantage of being sporadic—neither is a permanent answer to the question of how to supply substitute consent for a person with partial competence or complete incompetence. Also, they address the area of life-style decision-making, but they do not extend to financial decision-making.

What Is a Representative Payee?

A *representative payee* is someone designated by a federal agency to receive the benefit payments from the agency on behalf of a person with a disability. Typically, the agency does not go through the formality of a court hearing to determine that a beneficiary has partial competence or complete incompetence; instead, it relies on the fact that the person has qualified, by reason of a mental disability, for the benefits. In Steve Stuart's case, it is likely that the Social Security Administration would designate his parents as his representative payees to receive his Supplemental Security Income (SSI) payments. (We discuss federal benefits in Chapters 14–15.)

The designation of a representative payee can help families by making it possible for them to avoid the expense and time of adjudication; it also enables them to continue to manage their son's or daughter's financial affairs. One disadvantage, however, is that the designation is not permanent—the agency may revoke it at any time or it may change the payee to the person with a disability or to someone else. This designation also tends to remove a person's rights to control his or her benefits, without a formal court proceeding. Finally, it totally fails to address decision-making related to life-style.

What Is a Trust?

A Trust is a legal agreement in which one person (the donor) gives property to another person (the Trustee) for the benefit of a third person (the beneficiary). Families may create Trusts during their lifetimes or after their deaths (by way of their Wills). The advantage of the Trust is that it can be made permanent; it assures management of the property by the Trustee; and, if the Trust is properly designed, it supplements the government benefits to which the beneficiary may be entitled as a person with a disability. The disadvantage of most Trusts is that the donor loses control of the property and of the way in which the Trustee spends it. We consider Trusts in greater detail in Chapters 14–16.

WHAT FACTORS SHOULD YOU
CONSIDER IN MAKING A GUARDIANSHIP DECISION?

Besides considering the individual needs of your son or daughter relevant to decision-making, you should consider four additional factors: access to services without guardianship, family considerations, and the prevalent ideology in the field of disability. In this section, we discuss each of these factors and point out how they might influence your own decision about guardianship.

What Are Service Considerations?

As we noted in earlier chapters, the law presumes that adults have complete mental competence. This presumption often flies in the face of the reality that the adult with a disability has partial competence or complete incompetence. Moreover, this presumption means that the adult's parents, brothers, sisters, other relatives, or close friends who may have agreed among themselves to continue making decisions for the person usually are not technically authorized, at law, to make those decisions. The only person who lawfully may make decisions is the adult himself or herself, or a court-appointed guardian. Thus, when Steve, Anna, and Jolene become adults, they will be presumed competent to act for themselves, even when it appears that they are more or less unable to do so fully. Likewise, their parents have no clear legal authority to act on their behalfs when they become adults unless courts have appointed the parents to be guardians. This has several important implications for your son's or daughter's access to services.

You may find that your son or daughter can get services without your having to become the legal guardian through a court proceeding. Often, service providers will rely on your son's or daughter's direct consent (e.g., to join a recreation program) or on concurrent consent (e.g., to arrange for contraception), and render services when they know that the ability of your son or daughter to give informed consent is questionable. They usually do this when the services are not unusual or are clearly beneficial (e.g., placement in a group home, employment, or noninvasive and routine medical procedures). Also, service providers usually do this when they are allowed by law to obtain consent from other persons besides a legal (i.e., court-appointed) guardian.

However, your son or daughter may be unable to get services unless he or she has been provided a legal guardian by means of a court proceeding. The reason for this result is that service providers will rely only on substitute consent from a legal guardian, because the services they provide are risky, or irreversible, or governed by laws that require substitute consent from the court-appointed guardian and from no one else. For example, providers typically will want consent from court-appointed guardians when the service includes placement in state institutions, surgery, experimental or research-oriented procedures, or particularly invasive therapies such as electroconvulsive shock treatment. Sometimes, state law requires judicial approval of the decision of a guardian to consent to any of these interventions. Service providers will want not only to comply with these laws, but to get specific consent for these risks.

Professionals and other service providers often rely on direct consent (from Anna directly, for example) or concurrent consent (from Jolene directly and from her mother Odessa, thus from both Jolene and her mother concurrently), before they provide a service to the person with a mental disability.

Sometimes, however, a professional will have a bona fide question as to whether a particular type of consent is legally effective. For example, if Steve needs brain surgery, it is perfectly clear that he lacks the mental competence to consent directly to it. Instead, legally effective consent can be furnished only by his legal guardians. While he is a minor, his parents may give that consent. When he becomes an adult, however, he is presumed competent, even though he is not. When Steve becomes an adult, a surgeon may well refuse to operate, despite his parents' authorization, unless they have been appointed his guardians after a court has adjudicated Steve to be incompetent. The surgeon might feel that Steve's parents (as parents) do not have the legal authority to give substitute consent. Rather, the surgeon may require substitute consent from a person who clearly is legally authorized to give it—such as a court-appointed guardian. Such action will protect not only the surgeon (from a claim that he operated without sufficient legal consent), but also Steve, because the guardian must consider only Steve's interests, not those of others.

The example of psychosurgery is deliberately extreme. Yet it is not the only instance in which intervention is so risky and so hard to reverse, and the person's incompetence so great, that effective substitute consent is required. For example, a service provider might seek legally tight consent in cases of a kidney transfer (e.g., from Steve to Sally, his sister), sterilization (e.g., for Jolene), or placement in a public residential facility for 24-hour, long-term care (e.g., if Jolene needs hospitalization in order to be diagnosed or treated for acting-out behavior related to puberty).

However, there are situations in which a service provider may not be justified in seeking guardianship and legally tight consent for his or her own protection. For example, Jolene may want to leave her mother's home and live in an apartment with some of her friends. This may not be a risky or irreversible decision; also, it is being made by a person who may have an adequate understanding of what it means to live in an apartment, that is, a person who, despite mental retardation, has partial competence to make that particular decision. In such a case, a service provider helping to arrange for the apartment need not seek the additional protection that can be provided by substitute consent through a guardian.

As is the case when parents think about guardianship without the prompting of a service provider, it is probably better to avoid guardianship if it seems that the provider wants it principally to protect himself or herself, not your son or daughter. However, you should not be entirely unreceptive to the service provider's suggestions that guardianship is warranted. Such a suggestion may well be based on a genuine interest in protecting your son or daughter.

You should also be aware of service providers who rely on direct consent from your son or daughter for decisions when he or she lacks competence to make the decision—for example, to withdraw a significant amount of money from his or her checking account. You may encounter service providers who find it easier or more personally beneficial to rely on direct consent (and try to influence or control your son's or daughter's decisions), rather than to obtain the substitute consent of a guardian who may have a greater investment in the well-being of your son or daughter. If your son or daughter is involved with a service provider whose motives for preferring direct consent are questionable, you may want to pursue guardianship as a means of protecting your son's or daughter's rights and preferences.

If emergency medical care is available through your son's or daughter's implied consent or on your approval, his or her immediate health care needs may be satisfied without guardianship. If not, obtaining guardianship may be necessary. You would do well to check with local hospitals about their policy.

What Are Some Important Family Considerations?

Although it is important to assign paramount importance to your son's or daughter's guardianship needs, other family members have needs that you should consider. For example, Steve's sisters may want his guardianship settled so that they will know what their legal duties are to him. This knowledge in turn may relieve them psychologically and allow them more certainty in making their own life plans. Thus, you should carefully consider the guardianship laws in planning the future of your son or daughter with a disability, as well as the future of all other family members. This is true, if for no other reason, because parents also have an obligation to try to minimize the responsibility that the person with a disability will place on other family members, friends, or society. Moreover, when you die or for some other reason can no longer support your son or daughter, he or she may be left without someone designated by you to be legally responsible for his or her care. In such a case, brothers, sisters, and other family members may feel an obligation, possibly accompanied by resentment, to take up your role, and even to go to guardianship although you had refused to do so.

The following family considerations are essential:

The Availability, Willingness, and Ability of Relatives or Friends to Assume the Guardian Role   Are there family members or friends who would be willing to serve as a guardian both now and in the future? In Steve's case, his sisters may be willing to assume this role once they become adults. But what will happen if they want to move far away, or get married and have their own families? What if they grow to resent being responsible for Steve? You and your spouse may be willing to serve as guardians, since this is really a continuation of the responsibilities you have always had for your son or daughter. But what about the future? What are your own retirement plans and how will those plans influence your guardianship decision?

A key consideration is whether family and friends reside in proximity to your son or daughter. Particularly for life-style guardianship, it is important for the guardian to be close by. If you find that you live close to your son or daughter and see him or her on a frequent basis, you may be able to provide support for decision-making informally, without having to pursue a formal (judicially sanctioned) guardianship. The important questions to ask are: "Are there people available to assist my son or daughter on an informal basis?" "Would it be preferable for my son or daughter to have a guardian?" "Why would guardianship be preferable?"

The Life Expectancy and Health of Those Involved   Although life expectancy and health issues are closely related to availability issues, they deserve separate consideration. You need to project how long it is reasonable to assume that family and friends will be available to provide informal support. You can count on growing older and perhaps even becoming disabled yourself, as can your son's or daughter's other relatives. For example, Jolene's mother Odessa and Uncle Owen are about the same age; but her grandparents and great-grandparents are much older and probably will die before Odessa and Owen. Jolene cannot rely on her grandparents and great-grandparents for long-term assistance with decisions in her life. Remember, too, that Jolene doesn't have brothers and sisters. It is helpful for you to consider the general life expectancy and health of the family and friends on whom your son or daughter depends for assistance. Although is may make you uncomfortable, it is also important to anticipate both the unexpected and unthinkable—what would be the needs of your son or daughter if you, other family members, or both died suddenly? Are there certain people in the life of your son or daughter who are indepensible right now? If those people become unavailable now or in the future, how will that influence your guardianship decisions?

The Financial Resources of Your Family and Your Son or Daughter   Anna Levine stands to obtain a substantial sum of money from her parents, Ben and Ruth. In making a plan for the disposition of their property, Ben and Ruth are correct in wanting the plan to have legally tight agreements so that they can be assured that their wishes concerning their estate are carried out and that Anna's financial security can be guaranteed. Ben and Ruth know that Anna is responsible, but they worry that some person she could meet in the future might be able to get control of Anna's money and squander it. They consider financial guardianship for this reason, but they end up deciding to develop a Trust instead. (We discuss trusts in detail in Chapters 14–16).

Another consideration here is the availability of government financial aid (e.g., Social Security or Supplemental Security Income [SSI] benefits). For example, Jolene will benefit from her deceased father's military life insurance policy and will probably also qualify for Social Security benefits. (Social Security and other government benefits are discussed in Chapters 10–12.) The greater the financial resources of your son or daughter both now and in the future and the greater his or her disability, the more you may want to consider financial guardianship to provide for proper management of those resources.

Each family's circumstances are different and the way you respond to these considerations will be different from the way other families respond. Because you know your family better than any "outsider," you are in the best position to identify what is important.

What Are Ideological Considerations?

Ideology can be defined as the prevalent assumptions about groups of people. In the field of disability, different ideologies sometimes exist among various groups of decision-makers. Three of these groups are particularly worthy of your consideration—parent organizations, professional organizations, and the court system.

Parent and Professional Organizations   We are considering parent and professional organizations together because their current ideologies on the issue of substitute consent tend to be similiar. Leading parent organizations (such as the Association of Retarded Citizens of the United States, or ARC-US) and professional organizations (such as the American Association on Mental Retardation and The Association for Persons with Severe Handicaps) generally support the practice of empowering adults with a disability to retain their rights and to be as directly involved as possible in giving direct consent. For example, the ARC-US suggests that parents should ask themselves and others the following questions:

> Why guardianship? Is there some compelling reason for guardianship and will guardianship solve the problem? For example, is there a real danger that a child will a) run away and be totally incompetent to obtain food, clothing and shelter, b) suffer self-inflicted injury or death, c) be physically abused should he or she stay in his or her present living arrangements, d) become involved in serious criminal activity, e) be subject to frequent civil litigation for buying things beyond his or means, f) be forced into prostitution? Is guardianship really necessary now? Is it being suggested only for the convenience of the service provider? Is there an alternative to a court-supervised guardianship? Can parents, or nonretarded children or other relatives or individual trustees after the parents' deaths, continue to assist in making decisions for children with mental retardation who are unable to make those decisions? Under the laws and hospital practices, will the hospital provide emergency surgery and treatment without the informed consent of the person if a parent or other interested person consents? Under the law, can a child who wishes to be sterilized secure this without a guardian being appointed and without court order? Is it really in the best interest of a child with mental retardation for his or her parents to seek guardianship? (1984)

The conventional ideology expressed in the above extract is that guardianship should be pursued as a last resort when other alternatives (protective services, implied consent, a representative payee, and Trusts), informal methods of assisting with decision-making, and concerted efforts to teach decision-making are insufficient. The reason for the "last resort" perspective is that, from an ideological perspective, guardianship can result in a person's loss of rights and disempowerment.

This ideological perspective sometimes overlooks the actuality that a properly tailored guardianship, sought at the appropriate time and for the sole purpose of serving the interests of your son or daughter, may actually be a means for him or her to exercise his or her rights. Particularly if your son or daughter has complete incompetence, you may be able to best ensure reasoned decision-making by seeking to have a person of your choice legally appointed as the only person who can give substitute consent.

However, we also believe that many families pursue guardianship, even a plenary general (life-style and financial) guardianship, when such a drastic measure is not at all necessary.

The Court System   The ideologies of local courts can vary drastically. Many courts have a relaxed attitude toward guardianship and are inclined to grant it. Some courts presume that every person with a label such as "mentally retarded" or "autistic" has complete incompetence. This may be true even though the person has the capacity to make reasoned decisions, and, thus, to give direct consent. Although people both with and without labels may have an impaired capacity to make reasoned decisions, the person with a label is pushed into guardianship, while the person without a label is tolerated as eccentric or highly idiosyncratic, but not considered for guardianship. You should ask a lawyer about judges' attitudes in your area, as well as about applicable state laws concerning the court's prevalent assumptions about people with disabilities and their need for guardianship.

These three considerations—services, family, and ideology—will all influence your decision about the appropriateness of guardianship. You will need to weigh these factors when considering your own unique situation.

WHAT PROCESS CAN YOU FOLLOW WHEN MAKING A GUARDIANSHIP DECISION?

We have discussed in this chapter the factors to consider in determining whether plenary or limited guardianship is an appropriate option for providing substitute consent. We have also identified alternatives to guardianship. The questions and issues we have presented are summarized in Table 7.1. We encourage you to synthesize your thoughts by thinking through these questions and writing answers to them. Writing down your answers may help you make them more focused. As with questions in previous chapters, think about the family members, friends, or professionals who can help you respond to these questions as carefully as possible, and invite them into your planning.

Answering questions about guardianship can be time-consuming and emotionally draining. You may find that you need to mull over these questions for weeks or even months before you are comfortable with making a final decision. One of the major benefits of starting future planning early is that you can take the time to ensure that your decision is right not only in terms of its logic, but in terms of how it feels.

Table 7.1. Should you pursue guardianship for your son or daughter? Take some time to reflect upon and answer the following questions.

A. Individual needs
  1. For what *kinds* of decisions does your son or daughter need substitute consent?
  2. For what *steps of the decision-making process* does your son or daughter need substitute consent?
  3. For decisions at what *level of complexity* does your son or daughter need substitute consent?
  4. Does your son's or daughter's decision-making capability tend to be stable or are there episodes when he or she needs more help than at other times?
  5. What are your son's or daughter's preferences for how substitute consent is obtained?

B. Alternatives to guardianship
  1. Would protective services be sufficient to provide substitute consent in life-style decisions for your son or daughter?
  2. Would implied consent be sufficient to obtain emergency services for your son or daughter?
  3. Would establishing a representative payee be sufficient to provide substitute consent in financial management for your son or daughter?
  4. Would establishing a Trust be sufficient to provide substitute consent in financial management for your son or daughter?

C. Service considerations
  1. Can your son or daughter get access to necessary services without guardianship?
  2. Under what circumstances will guardianship be required for your son or daughter to obtain necessary services?
  3. Under what circumstances might service providers seek unwarranted control over your son or daughter if he or she does not have a guardian?

D. Family considerations
  1. How available, willing, and able are family and friends to provide concurrent or substitute consent in an informal capacity and as a guardian?
  2. What is the life expectancy and health of family and friends who might provide concurrent or substitute consent in an informal capacity and as a guardian?
  3. What are the financial resources of your son or daughter that require concurrent or substitute consent for money management purposes?

E. Ideological considerations
  1. What is the ideology of parent and proiessional organizations concerning guardianship?
  2. What is the ideology of the local courts concerning guardianship?

F. Other considerations
  1. Are there other considerations unique to your family circumstances that are important for you to consider?
  2. Are there other people whom you need to consult?

G. Decision
  1. Should you pursue guardianship for your son or daughter?

If your son or daughter requires substitute consent and you decide not to pursue guardianship, you will need to identify other ways to provide decision-making and consent-giving assistance. We encourage you to think through each of the alternatives to guardianship discussed in this chapter to determine its suitability to your needs.

Given your decision that plenary or limited guardianship is appropriate for your son or daughter as the means for providing substitute consent, this last section of the chapter is designed to help you determine the particular kind of guardianship that will meet the needs of your son or daughter. Essentially, we will guide you in putting together information from previous chapters so that you can apply that information directly to the guardianship decision facing your family.

What Is the Appropriate Jurisdiction
for Guardianship of Your Son or Daughter?

The three categories of the guardian's jurisdiction are *guardianship of the person,*
guardianship of the estate, and *general guardianship.* Selection of a category is based
on the kinds of decisions for which your son or daughter needs concurrent or substitute
consent. Go back to Figure 4.2 and review your son's or daughter's capacity to make
reasoned decisions. First examine his or her needs for life-style decisions. If your son
or daughter needs substitute consent for any of the four kinds of life-style decisions—
decisions about life in the community, decisions about relationships with other people,
decisions about where to live, and decisions about a job—then you should consider
guardianship of the person. If your son or daughter needs substitute consent for either
of the two kinds of financial decisions—decisions about acquiring money and decisions
about spending money—then a guardian of the estate should be appointed. If substitute consent is needed for both life-style and financial decisions, then a general
guardianship may be appropriate. You should keep in mind that making any of the six
kinds of decisions involves following the six steps of the decision-making process—
defining the problem or need, brainstorming, evaluating and choosing alternatives,
communicating the decision to others, taking action, and evaluating the outcome of the
action. You can use Figure 7.1 to indicate the guardianship jurisdiction that you think is
appropriate for your son or daughter.

What Is the Appropriate Scope
of Guardianship for Your Son or Daughter?

Guardianship can either be plenary or limited. A full and complete guardianship is
plenary, while limited guardianship applies to some, but not all, decisions.

Refer again to Figure 4.2. There are two aspects of the chart that must be considered in light of scope. The first is the kinds of life-style and financial decisions. The
second is the complexity of decisions.

If your son or daughter cannot make life-style decisions, he or she will need
plenary guardianship of the person; if he or she is capable of making only some life-
style decisions (for example, decisions about relationships with people but not about
jobs, or simple decisions but not difficult ones), then guardianship of the person can be
limited so that assistance with consent is provided only for the kinds of decisions and
levels of complexity that are problematic. Direct consent could be arranged for the
kinds of life-style decisions and the level of complexity for which your son or daughter
has sufficient capacity.

The same process should be followed for determining plenary or limited guardianship of the estate. Plenary guardianship of the estate is appropriate if your son or
daughter can make neither kind of financial decision, at even a simple level. Limited
guardianship of the estate is appropriate if he or she is capable of one kind of financial
decision but incapable of the other (for example, if he or she has the capability to make
decisions to spend money, but not acquire it) or if he or she can make simple or moderately complex decisions, but not difficult ones.

Finally, plenary general guardianship is appropriate if your son or daughter
needs substitute consent for all six kinds of decisions in the life-style and financial areas
and at all three levels of complexity; whereas limited general guardianship refers to

---

Guardianship Jurisdiction

Take some time to reflect upon and answer the following questions:

A. Guardianship of the person

Does your son or daughter need substitute consent for any of the four kinds of life-style decisions—decisions about life in the community, decisions about relationships with other people, decisions about where to live, and decisions about a job? (Check the box that applies.)

☐ Guardianship of the person   ☐ Guardianship of the estate   ☐ General guardianship

B. Guardianship of the estate

Does your son or daughter need substitute consent for either of the two kinds of financial decisions—acquiring money and spending money? (Check the box that applies.)

☐ Guardianship of the person   ☐ Guardianship of the estate   ☐ General guardianship

C. General guardianship

Does your son or daughter need substitute consent for life-style and financial decisions? (Check the box that applies.)

☐ Guardianship of the person   ☐ Guardianship of the estate   ☐ General guardianship

D. Decision

What guardianship jurisdiction is appropriate for your son or daughter? (Check the box that applies.)

☐ Guardianship of the person   ☐ Guardianship of the estate   ☐ General guardianship

---

Figure 7.1. Which guardianship jurisdiction is appropriate for your son or daughter?

Scope of Guardianship

A. Does your son or daughter need substitute consent for all four kinds of life-style decisions at medium or difficult levels of complexity (limited guardianship of the person)? (Check the box that applies.)

☐ Guardianship of the person   ☐ Guardianship of the estate   ☐ General guardianship

B. Does your son or daughter need substitute consent for the two kinds of financial decisions at medium or difficult levels of complexity (plenary guardianship of the estate), or for only one of the financial decisions at medium or difficult levels of complexity? (Check the box that applies.)

☐ Guardianship of the person   ☐ Guardianship of the estate   ☐ General guardianship

C. Does your son or daughter need substitute consent for the four kinds of personal lifestyle and two kinds of financial decisions at all three levels of complexity (plenary general guardianship), or for only some of the life-style decisions and only one of the financial decisions at medium or difficult levels of complexity (limited general guardianship)? (Check the box that applies.)

☐ Guardianship of the person   ☐ Guardianship of the estate   ☐ General guardianship

---

Figure 7.2. Which scope of guardianship is appropriate for your son or daughter?

assistance with some but not all kinds of decisions and with some but not all levels of complexity.

Figure 7.2 adds the dimension of scope of guardianship, in regard to plenary or limited guardianship of the person, guardianship of the estate, and general guardianship. Use Figure 7.2 to indicate the appropriate scope of guardianship for your son or daughter.

After you check the options in Figure 7.1 and 7.2 to select the appropriate jurisdiction and scope of guardianship, you are ready to proceed to the selection of the guardian. As previously noted, you can consider individual, corporate, and public guardians. In reading this chapter, you have also thought about the availability, willingness, and ability of family and friends to serve as guardian, as well as their life expectancy and health status. Before you select a guardian, however, you will need some more information. In Chapter 8, we focus on what you should do to establish guardianship.

8 WHAT SHOULD YOU DO TO ESTABLISH GUARDIANSHIP?

Once you have decided that guardianship is an appropriate alternative for your son or daughter, you are ready to consider the procedures for establishing guardianship. In this chapter we describe the different ways to have a guardian appointed, and suggest a process for establishing guardianship for your son or daughter.

HOW ARE GUARDIANS APPOINTED?

There are three ways that guardians obtain their powers—through *natural means, testamentary means,* and *judicial means.* The information in this section will help you make the decision on the means to match your circumstances.

What Is Natural Guardianship?

A *natural guardian* is the parent of the child. (Sometimes, in some states, parents are also the natural guardians of an adult son or daughter who has a disability.) Until the child reaches the age of majority, parents do not have to be appointed by a court to be guardians—they are guardians already, by virtue of having given birth to the child. Thus, Jack and Rose Stuart are Steve's natural guardians, and Odessa Harris is Jolene's.

When an individual reaches the age of majority, however, the law generally presumes that he or she is competent, regardless of that individual's actual competence. If your son or daughter with a disability is an adult, your views as a parent will be given great weight by courts and service providers. But in most states you will lack the legal authority of a guardian, such as you would have over your minor child or if you were appointed by a court to be a guardian. Although the general rule of law is that natural guardianship terminates when a child reaches the age of majority, you should still check with an attorney to find if natural guardianship exists in your state for the parents of adults with mental disabilities.

What Is Testamentary Guardianship?

Most parents, especially those whose sons and daughters have a mental disability, wonder how to ensure the well-being of their children after they die. They worry about who will look after their children, and how to control who that person will be. One way to respond to these questions is to recommend a guardian under your Last Will and

Testament. The final appointment is made by the courts, which typically give strong weight to parental recommendations.

Under the laws of most states, parents may use their Last Wills and Testaments to appoint an individual to serve as guardian for their minor children. (In most states, these are children under age 18; see Chapter 4, p. 28, for a list of exceptions.) This right exists whether or not the child has a disability. The person named in a parent's Last Will and Testament is the *testamentary guardian.*

The testamentary guardian assumes the powers and duties of the parent immediately upon the death of the child's last living parent. The testamentary guardianship takes effect only if both parents die before the child reaches age 18. This guardianship usually terminates when the child reaches the age of majority (18 in most states; see Chapter 4, p. 28, for a list of exceptions), since adults are presumed to have complete mental competence. At that time, however, a person who has been acting as guardian for a child with a disability during the child's minority may seek to continue as guardian by asking a court to adjudicate the person as having partial competence or complete incompetence. In this way, the guardianship could be continued.

If your son or daughter is a minor, you should specify a testamentary guardian in your Will so that your intentions may be carried out concerning whom should provide care to your son or daughter (and other children) in the event of your untimely death. This is one of the most difficult situations for parents to contemplate, but it is necessary to consider when making comprehensive future plans. Also, in most states, parents who have already been appointed guardians over their son or daughter during adulthood by a court may, through their Will, name a testamentary guardian to assume the same powers and duties the parents were granted under the original guardianship decision. In this way, parents can strive to ensure the continuity of the guardianship by recommending a person who will continue to serve as guardian in the manner they have established.

A final example of the use of testamentary guardianship is the situation in which parents decline to pursue guardianship of their son or daughter during their lifetime, when parental assistance and support is possible. After the parents die, however, the adult may need a guardian. Parents can make a general statement in their Will designating a person in whom they have confidence to be appointed guardian as soon after their deaths as possible. The person recommended by the parents should then petition the court for guardianship, using the weight of endorsement in the parents' Wills.

Regardless of the circumstances of testamentary guardianship, we do not want to mislead you into thinking that the formal appointment of a guardian can be made through your Will. On the contrary, a testamentary guardian is someone who is recommended in the Will, but the court always holds the power of appointment. Recommending a guardian in your Will offers several advantages: 1) You can select an individual, individuals, or corporation that can serve the best interests and represent the preferences of your son or daughter, 2) You can secure their approval of this role in advance so that the decision can be carefully considered and fully communicated to all family members, 3) You can prevent uncertainty and panic over the well-being of your son or daughter at the time of your death, and 4) You can influence the court's appointment, since parental recommendation carries considerable weight.

What Are the Judicial Procedures for Establishing Guardianship?

The laws of each state detail the ways of obtaining guardianship. Those laws usually are complicated, and always require a judicial proceeding. For these reasons, it is wise— indeed, almost always necessary—to consult a lawyer.

Usually the states' laws have common elements and employ common terms, which a lawyer can explain in fuller detail. These usually include the following:

Petitioner   Anyone may file a petition to adjudicate a person as having partial competence or complete incompetence.

Costs   The costs of the court proceeding, including those of the attorney for the petitioner (person filing the petition), and sometimes those of the attorney for the person with a disability (respondent), usually are billed to the respondent's estate, although they are sometimes billed to the petitioner, or are divided between the petitioner and the respondent.

Contents of Petition   The petition must state who the respondent is, where he or she lives, why he or she is viewed as having partial competence or complete incompetence, what the person's assets are, who might be appointed as guardian, who the person's relatives are, and, sometimes, the interest that the petitioner has in the person (e.g., is a relative or a creditor).

Hearing   The court must always conduct a hearing to determine the person's competence or incompetence, and to determine who should serve as guardian if the person is found to have partial competence or complete incompetence. At the hearing, the person is entitled to be represented by a lawyer and the court usually appoints a lawyer or a guardian *ad litem* (a person who serves as guardian for the purposes of the hearing) to represent the respondent. Sometimes the respondent is entitled to have the hearing before a jury, and sometimes in closed court (in private). The respondent is entitled to be present at the hearing, to be represented by a lawyer, and to present testimony. Usually there will be a mental examination of the respondent and testimony from experts on the issue of competency.

Judgment   The court must find that the respondent has complete competence, partial competence, or complete incompetence. If the judgment is for partial competence or complete incompetence, the court must also appoint a guardian. The court may establish plenary or limited guardianship (in most states), and may appoint a personal or financial guardian, or both.

Appeal   The respondent always has the right to appeal the judgment of the court that hears the petition; so does the petitioner.

Qualifying as Guardian   The guardian must "qualify" by posting a bond (unless the court waives the bond) and taking an oath to perform the duties of a guardian. In another sense, the guardian must be qualified by being a fit and appropriate candidate.

Continued Jurisdiction   The court always has the right to reopen the case on its own initiative and always retains power over the guardianship it has created. Among other things, this means that the guardian is required to file periodic reports with the court.

Restoration to Competence   The respondent or someone representing him or her, or any other person, may petition to have the ward (respondent) restored to competency, that is, to be declared, after another hearing, to be competent and not in need of a guardianship. The usual rights to a hearing and appeal are granted when there is a petition for restoration to competency.

WHAT ARE THE LAWS REGULATING GUARDIANS?

One of the safeguards of guardianship as a means of ensuring reasoned decisions for your son or daughter is that it provides legal oversight. The laws pertain to qualifications, responsibilities, liability, and compensation.

What Qualifications Must Guardians Meet?

Every state has laws that require the guardian to meet certain standards or to do certain acts before becoming eligible to be a guardian. The laws describe these requirements as *qualifications*.

Every state requires a personal guardian to be an adult, mentally capable, free of any convictions of serious crimes or crimes involving "moral turpitude" (i.e., immoral behavior), and willing and able to carry out the duties of a guardian. The same requirements concerning competence and willingness to serve also apply to financial guardians, even if the guardian is a corporation. Every state also requires that a personal and financial guardian post a bond to assure that the ward has funds for protection if the guardian does not perform as required and thereby causes financial or personal injury. In some instances, the court will waive (set aside) the requirement of a bond, as, for example, when parents or close relatives are the guardians or when parents designate a testamentary guardian and request that the bond be waived because the guardian is someone close to the family, for example, a relative.

Besides these fairly standard requirements concerning the moral and financial fitness of the guardian, some states require that a guardian live in the same state as the ward. Other states allow an out-of-state guardian to serve if there also is a person in the state who will be accountable to the court. We already have said that it is advisable to have a guardian who lives close enough to the ward to interact with him or her. This is because the guardian must report to the court and, most important from your son's or daughter's point of view, because the guardian should have a close personal relationship with the ward. Such a relationship can help ensure that your young adult's needs and preferences are addressed. Also, the laws of each state usually prohibit a person from being a guardian if he or she has a conflict of interest with the ward. For example, a conflict of interest might arise when a person's estate, which is quite large and cannot reasonably be expended during his or her lifetime, is administered by the person who will inherit the estate when the ward dies. In that case, there may be a conflict of interest and a court might not appoint as guardian the person who would benefit by accumulating assets in the estate instead of spending them on the ward.

Finally, the courts consider as a legal qualification a guardian's capacity to serve. This means that the courts usually prefer to appoint a guardian who probably will outlive the ward and be capable during the ward's lifetime of performing the guardianship duties. Sometimes that person might be a younger brother or sister; sometimes the guardian might be a corporation (such as a Trust company or collective guardianship with a long-standing and indefinite existence). Of course, courts may appoint parents, even though they may not outlive their children.

What Are the Guardian's Responsibilities?

The general duty of a guardian is to make reasonable and prudent decisions on behalf of the ward, consistent with the amount of authority given in the court order by which he or she was appointed. The guardian's decisions must also be consistent with the responsibilities imposed by state statutes. We'll discuss each of these elements separately.

The requirement that the guardian make reasonable and prudent decisions is part of the law of every state, although it is phrased differently in the different states. The guardian has a special relationship to the ward, because the guardian has been given the power to provide substitute consent on behalf of the ward. With this power comes the duty to serve as a Trustee, steward, and conservator—as a person who acts in a reasonable and prudent (that is, defensible and careful) way on behalf of the ward.

A court order may also assign a guardian some special duties, such as to visit the ward regularly or to ensure that the ward resides in his or her home community if he or she prefers. State laws may also impose special duties on guardians, such as to provide for annual physical and mental examinations of the ward and to conduct an annual review of the ward's habilitation program in cooperation with service providers. Whether the duties are required by court order or by a state's general legislation, the guardian is required to comply with these specific duties in addtion to the general duty of reasonable and prudent care.

Often, a guardian will be exceedingly cautious about exercising any of his or her duties and will seek the approval of the court before undertaking any action about which there is even the slightest doubt. For example, a guardian may have the authority to provide consent for medical treatment. Out of caution, he or she may seek a court's approval for consent to surgery that may have a permanent and perhaps debilitating effect (e.g., heart surgery that, if successful, will extend the lifespan but which, if unsuccessful, may cause death or increased physical disability). It is a wise guardian who seeks judicial approval of any action when there is doubt about the guardian's authority to act or when doubt exists that action would be reasonable and prudent.

The court and state legislation may also impose limitations on the guardian. For example, the court may specify that the guardian has no authority to forbid the ward to spend his or her earnings. In that case, the ward has full discretion over the expenditure of earnings and the guardian may act only in an advisory capacity. As we have noted, state legislation may limit the authority of all guardians to consent to certain types of procedures—for example, electroconvulsive shock therapy, sterilization, abortion, and psychosurgery. In those instances, the guardian may not consent to those procedures. In some states, the law does not absolutely forbid guardians to consent to such procedures, but requires instead that guardians justify them to a court before giving consent.

In all states, a guardian is required to file periodic reports with the court that appointed him or her. Sometimes the reports must be filed annually; sometimes, less often. Sometimes the reports must be highly specific (e.g., it must describe what expenditures were made in the last year, why, and in what amounts; when the guardian last visited the ward; and the results of the most recent annual physical and mental examinations of the ward). The guardian must file these financial and personal reports on time and with the appropriate court. (Some guardians make a practice of filing copies with the ward's interested family members.)

All such reports are regarded as public records that anyone may see simply by inspecting the guardianship file of the court. In rare instances, a guardian will ask the court to seal the report and keep it secret (or to prohibit public access to other papers in the court's file) because of the highly sensitive and personal nature of the material in the report. In those cases, the guardian's report or other papers will not be accessible to the public, or to people particularly interested in the ward, unless they can convince the court to make an exception. For example, a family may not want their daughter's medical evaluations, made in order to obtain short-term hospitalization, available to the public.

What Is the Guardian's Liability?

Generally, a guardian does not have personal responsibility to care for the ward by personal intervention (for example, by actually providing housing) or by the expenditure of personal funds. This is because the guardian is regarded as someone who gives substitute consent for decisions made on behalf of the ward, not someone with direct and personal responsibility for the ward. Thus, a guardian generally is not responsible for taking the ward into his or her own home or to provide clothing for the ward by spending his or her own money on the ward. A guardian also is not liable for the ward's debts. The guardian may do these things, but is not required to.

However, a guardian is personally liable to the ward for *waste*—that is, for spending the ward's money in a manner that exceeds the designated authority provided by the court or by state law. In that case, the guardian may be required to reimburse the ward's estate by the amount of funds, plus interest, that were illegally used. For example, if the local bank that is the guardian of Steve Stuart's estate fails to invest his funds in a reasonable and prudent manner and, for that reason, Steve's funds are dissipated, the bank is responsible for its improper management and would owe him the amount, plus interest, that it should have earned for him by proper investment.

How Is a Guardian Compensated?

Generally, a guardian is compensated from the ward's estate or, if the ward has no assets, by the court itself for the services performed for the ward's benefit. For example, a lawyer who administers a ward's estate, or a Trust company that invests, disperses, and files financial and tax returns, is compensated for this work. Compensation comes from the ward's estate and usually is fixed by state law. In cases where extraordinary amounts of time, service, or expense are involved, a court will authorize the guardian to be compensated in excess of the maximum set by statutes (check with your lawyer to find out the maximum, which varies by state).

A guardian may waive—or decline to receive—the fees to which he or she is entitled. In this case, the fees are simply not paid out of the ward's estate and, in effect, the guardian makes a gift of them (and his or her services) to the ward. The result is that the ward's estate is increased by the amount of the fees that otherwise would be paid to the guardian. Odessa Harris and Owen Weeks, for example, probably would decline to receive a fee for serving as Jolene's guardians.

WHAT SHOULD YOU DO TO ESTABLISH GUARDIANSHIP FOR YOUR SON OR DAUGHTER?

The issues discussed thus far in this chapter provide the background information you need to know the means by which you can establish guardianship (natural, testamentary, and judicial) and the laws that govern guardians in the areas of qualifications, responsibilities, liability, and compensation. What are the decisions that you need to make based on this information? Table 8.1 provides a review of the issues pertinent to your deliberations. As we have done previously, we encourage you to involve appropriate family members and friends in answering these questions and thus determining what to do when you establish guardianship.

After you have had a chance to think about these admittedly very difficult questions, you will have a clearer idea of how to seek guardianship. You also will have a

Table 8.1. What should you do to establish guardianship?

A. Means of establishing guardianship

1. Are you the natural guardian of your son or daughter? (Is your son or daughter a minor? Does your state law allow a parent of an adult who is mentally incompetent to remain a natural guardian, with the same powers as a judicially appointed guardian?)
2. What provisions should you make in your Will for testamentary guardianship?
3. What are the laws in your state concerning judicial proceedings?
4. What means of establishing guardianship are most appropriate for your family?
5. What do you need to do to initiate action to establish guardianship? What is your next step and who can help?

B. Laws regulating guardians

1. Who might be an appropriate guardian for your son or daughter who also meets the legal qualifications?
2. Who might be an appropriate guardian for your son or daughter who is also capable of fulfilling the responsibilities?
3. Who might be an appropriate guardian for your son or daughter who will also accept the liability?
4. Who might be an appropriate guardian for your son or daughter who will also accept the conditions of compensation?
5. Of the people who might meet the legal qualifications for being a guardian, who is the person whom your son or daughter would most prefer to have as his or her guardian?

C. Method of contact

1. What information must you provide to the people who may be appropriate guardians for your son or daughter?
2. What is the best procedure to follow in discussing guardianship with them?

---

clearer understanding of the individuals or corporations you are considering to be guardians. You may determine that you are the appropriate guardian for your son or daughter. Or, you may select another family member, a friend, a professional person, or a corporation. The important point is to select a guardian who will respond to the special considerations of your family, as identified in this chapter and the previous one.

If the person or corporation you choose is someone other than yourself, you will need to consider a plan for talking to the potential guardian about your wishes and the many factors that must be considered before the guardian consents to this role. You might share this book with the potential guardian. It could help that individual understand more fully the whole process of future planning and how the guardian might best assist your son or daughter. You want the potential guardian to make a reasoned decision about guardianship, just as you want that individual to make reasoned decisions in the future as a guardian.

If your first choice for a guardian does not work out, you can always reconsider potential guardians and work to select someone else. Usually the number of potential guardians for any one person is limited. The challenge will be to identify someone willing to assume responsibility, not just narrow down a long list of candidates. If you are unable to identify an individual, consider the corporation option discussed in Chapter 7.

Also, remember that the guardianship needs of your son or daughter will change, and that you will need to review your guardianship decision periodically. Further, guardians' circumstances change, and someone willing to serve this year may be faced with circumstances that would preclude continuation in that role in the future. In future planning, flexibility is the name of the game! No guardianship plan is for the entire future. It must be renegotiated as people and circumstances change.

To summarize, in Section I we have given you information on the process of decision-making in regard to your son or daughter as an adult. We have discussed decision-making from the perspectives of kinds of decisions, steps in the decision-making process, and levels of complexity of decisions. Based on the requirements of decision-making, we have discussed mental competence and the fact that levels of competence are determined on the basis of one's capacity to make reasoned decisions. Consent was then introduced as the act of decision-making, and we generally equated types of consent with levels of mental competence. Next, we analyzed the types of consent and suggested a process you might follow to determine your son's or daughter's capacity to consent. In case your young adult requires substitute consent, we have presented a range of options, including guardianship and alternatives to guardianship. Finally, we have presented information to help you make an informed decision about whether guardianship is appropriate for your son or daughter, and, if so, how you might go about establishing it.

The information in Section I can be tedious and confusing. We hope we have presented it clearly and that at this point you have a good idea of your son's or daughter's decision-making capacity, the type of consent that is appropriate, how to provide opportunities for appropriate consent, and how to work to increase capacity for more direct decision-making in the future.

Determining decision-making methods is the essential first step in future planning. For too long, future planning for adults with disabilities has excluded them from the whole decision-making process. The thesis of the process we present in this book is that adolescents and adults should be actively involved in future planning, consistent with their capacity for decision-making.

Now that you have identified your son's or daughter's capacity for decision-making, you can apply this information to future planning. If your son or daughter is able to provide direct consent for life-style and financial decisions, he or she should do so within the parameters of support that all families should give their members. If concurrent consent is possible, your son or daughter can move with you through the future planning decisions, participating as a partner. Finally, if substitute consent is the appropriate method for decision-making, you can consider selecting the appropriate substitute decision-maker(s) now so that this person or persons can assume responsibility for the future decisions that must be made.

In Chapter 17, we will introduce you to a "Preference Checklist" that you can use to identify your son's and daughter's life-style preferences. When we discuss the checklist, we will encourage the use of the appropriate option for consent that you have determined on the basis of the information you acquired in Section I. Before discussing the checklist, however, we cover financial planning and government benefits in Section II (Chapters 9–16).

section two
FINANCIAL PLANNING AND GOVERNMENT BENEFITS

 S ection II (Chapters 9–16) provides an in-depth exploration of the considerations necessary to your plan for a secure financial future for your son or daughter. Most people with disabilities have access to two general sources of income: 1) salary and wages and 2) government entitlement programs. Still others may have access to the funds of parents or relatives through inheritances or Trusts. Financial planning involves arrangements that will use the various sources of income in ways that enhance the quality of life of the person with a disability.

The chapters in this section will help you understand the financial arrangements you may consider to meet your own needs, the needs of your son or daughter with a disability, and the needs of other family members. Last Wills and Testaments are reviewed and useful information is provided to enable you to formulate a Will to meet your specific needs. Trusts are described, and examples are provided that you may consider for your own purposes.

Government entitlement programs are described and suggestions are offered to help you get access to funds and use them to provide the services your son or daughter needs. Detailed information is offered to help you develop a financial plan that balances government funds and private funds to ensure that your son or daughter remains eligible for some or even all government entitlement programs.

Because this section touches upon complex matters, you may find it useful to read some chapters more than once to understand them fully. Decisions concerning finances can have long-term effects, so they should be made only after you carefully consider all relevant issues. The decision-making approach described earlier applies to financial planning, and you should consider using it. Carefully reviewing the potential benefits and drawbacks of a financial plan is crucial.

This section is not designed to substitute for the services of professionals in financial matters. We strongly recommend getting assistance from a tax lawyer, a certified public accountant, and professionals in the banking industry. The adage, "penny wise, dollar foolish," holds much truth in this situation. The chapters in this section are designed to introduce important issues and help you organize your thinking and energy to pursue a sound financial plan. With the proper professional assistance, your family's financial future can be put on firm footing.

9 WHAT ARE THE MAJOR CONSIDERATIONS INVOLVED IN FINANCIAL PLANNING?

It is a smoggy, humid, spring night in Los Angeles. Luis and Eloisa Rodriguez are sipping lemonade on the back porch of their duplex in one of the city's Hispanic communities. In many ways, it is a typical evening in the neighborhood where they have lived for 20 of the 27 years since they emigrated to the United States from Mexico.

But their conversation is hardly typical—certainly not the usual chit-chat about the Dodgers and their pitching star from Mexico, or about the parties of the wealthy Anglos that Eloisa's employer caters. Instead, they are heatedly discussing their 26-year-old daughter, Maria. For a change, Geraldo, their 24-year-old son, is with them instead of in the newsroom of the *Los Angeles Times*, grinding out stories about the lives, deaths, joys, and sorrows of fellow Angeleños.

What sparked the conversation was Maria's statement, made a few days earlier, that she wanted to quit her job with the local sheltered workshop, move out of her parents' home into an apartment "on my own," and go to work as a technician in the animal labs at California State University-Los Angeles. An attractive, personable, and well-spoken young woman, Maria had graduated from an "educable mental retardation" program several years earlier. As was the custom, she had gone directly into a sheltered workshop. She did so in unenthusiastic obedience to her parents and teachers, who were reluctant to try any other type of job placement.

"I'm tired of being just a scrub woman and working for that workshop. They don't pay me what I'm worth; they take too much of my money for their own purposes; and I can do the lab work without anyone's help. Besides, Geraldo moved out on his own, and so do some of the people at the workshop—they go from their group homes to apartments. So why are you holding me back? Why won't you let me be independent? What good was all that special education—all those EMR classes—if I can't make use of them? Please, mama, please, papa. Let me try."

Luis and Eloisa are adamant—they want Maria to stay with them as long as they live. "For her to leave," says Luis, "would be like a death in the family. It was bad enough when you left, Geraldo. But you had your college degree, and you are more American than Maria. She's still one of us . . . still Mexican. Our tradition is different. We stay together. Always. Why can't Maria understand that?"

Eloisa has other concerns, much more maternal. "Tradition, that's one thing. But my baby . . . *mi niña*. It's tough out there . . . boys, men. You know how they can be."

Geraldo, the first college kid in the family, the sharp reporter, responds, "I tell you, I'm not worried about Maria. She shouldn't have been in special education to begin with. If she were Anglo, not Hispanic, at worst she would've been called a slow learner, not retarded. Look, mama, papa. You know that's true. Sometimes, we don't like to admit that prejudice was a factor 20 years ago. But it was. Now, things are getting better. She can do it by herself. I'm not concerned about that. I'm only worried about Maria being able to keep her government benefits. That Social Security check makes a difference. So does the Medicaid coverage. It's time to look at things more practically. Let's consider the money side of it."

$$*\quad*\quad*$$

On the same day, nearly 1,500 miles away, Ben and Ruth Levine are meeting with Arnold and Saundra in Arnold's law offices on the 40th floor of a downtown glass tower. The surroundings are plush . . . leather chairs, law books, computers, original art, and all the other trappings of money, both old and new. Not surprisingly, it is money that brings that family together this afternoon.

"Arnold," says his father, "your mother and I aren't getting any younger. To be blunt, we probably will live another 10, 15 years at the most. And to be equally candid, we are not exactly poor. We've done well by you . . . college at Northwestern, law school at the University of Chicago. Money won't buy any better. So we have come to talk about us, about money, and about you. And you, too, Saundra."

Ruth, realizing that Ben wasn't being at all clear and was probably offending Saundra, interrupts. "Saundra, Arnold, what your father means is that we're really worried about Anna and how we can help her as we were able to help you. We were coming back from dinner with the Schwartzburgs the other night—you know, the people who always invite Anna to come along when we go there—and it just broke our hearts to look at Anna and think about our future. You know, Mr. Schwartzburg's father recently had a heart attack. Life is so fragile. He made it, though. But it could happen to Ben or me, just like that. And then, what would become of Anna? We need to talk, all of us. We don't want her to be a burden on anyone. And you two young people, why, you've got the world by a string. You don't need any money. Of course, you could use some, but you don't need it. Anna . . . she's a different person. She has different needs. Let's talk. We're a family, all of us, you, too, Saundra. You're part of us now. And such a smart and lovely part, like a fine piece of china or crystal."

"Look, Mom and Dad," says Arnold, ever practical, ever able to cut to the heart of the matter, always unwilling to deal with emotion. "It's simply a matter of business. You tell me you're worried about Anna. Well, we all are. You tell me you've got money. So, what's new? You tell me Saundra and I have great opportunities. We know it. We don't expect any more than you've given already, and that's a lot. So, let me make a proposition, just for discussion. Why don't you disinherit us, put all your money into a Trust for Anna, and kiss the charities goodbye? And let's be sure to ask Anna if that plan suits her. Let's try that for starters."

Saundra sits silently, aghast at the tone and words of her new family.

$$*\quad*\quad*$$

Several hundred miles west, Jack and Rose Stuart are meeting with a lawyer at the offices of the local Association for Retarded Citizens. Like the Rodriguezes and the Levines, they are concerned about the future of their child with a disability and about their other children, too. What they hear from the lawyer was reassuring, informative.

"I know how hard it must be for you to think about the future, about your deaths, about Steve living after you, and about making sure there's enough money for him. But once you know what you want to do, I'm almost sure we can work out a good plan. Many families, like you, have been able to put something away for their children with disabilities. That's what Trusts are all about. And they've also been able to keep that nice package of federal benefits from falling apart. Frankly, if we're very careful, we can do almost anything you want for Steve."

There is audible relief, though no words are spoken. Jack relaxes in his chair; Rose stops wringing her hands. The silence says it all. They know the young lawyer is right. With careful planning, almost anything can be made to happen. One doesn't have to just trust in God, however helpful faith may be.

* * *

Each of these families faces a similar problem: How can they make sure that they "do right" for all their children—those with disabilities and those without—both now and in the future? Like every other parent, especially those who have a son or daughter with a disability, they must face the frightening question sooner or later: "What will happen to my child after I die?" For these families, and probably for you too, the question has many aspects. One has to do with money. How can you put your own assets to use for your son's or daughter's benefit? How can you do that while taking full advantage of all of the government benefits available, assuming you want to use those benefits? And how can you treat all your children fairly, given what you have to leave them and given their different needs and resources?

These are difficult questions. You will be in a better position to answer them if you take into account the five major considerations relevant to financial planning for your family.

WHAT ARE THE FIVE MAJOR CONSIDERATIONS INVOLVED IN FINANCIAL PLANNING?

There are five major considerations you should be concerned with as you do financial planning. We discuss these considerations at various points throughout this and later chapters. This may seem repetitious, but financial planning is so complicated that some repetition may make it easier for you to grasp the points we make. You will note that the five considerations overlap. This is because each major consideration relates to all the others.

When we discuss financial planning, we hope you will think about the two stages that are necessary for any plan. First, what plan do you make and carry out while you are living? Second, what plan do you make for others to execute after you die? Financial planning lets you make both kinds of plans, and we distinguish between them as necessary. Most of what we talk about in this chapter deals with distributing your property after you die. Also, this chapter does not deal with how to plan to meet the daily needs of your son or daughter for living in the community. We address that problem in Section III. After reading the entire section on financial planning (Chapters 9–16), you should have a good idea of how to combine government benefits with your own assets to meet your son's or daughter's needs for a quality life in the community.

How to Provide Money for Your Son or Daughter

In terms of financial planning, it is important to understand that the usual estate planning is not appropriate when you have a son or daughter with a disability. To begin with, you usually cannot make the same assumptions about that child that you can make about your other children. Geraldo Rodriguez went to college, so did Arnold Levine. But Maria Rodriguez did not, nor did Anna Levine. Arnold married; although they may also want to, Maria and Anna may not. Geraldo and Arnold are capable of supporting themselves without help; their sisters are not. People with disabilities usually require special, lifelong assistance.

In addition, your son or daughter with a disability may require special financial considerations. Maria's mother may be worried that Maria will be exploited by men, not just sexually, but financially. Odessa Harris has the same concern about Jolene. Geraldo is worried about whether Maria will be able to remain eligible for government benefits. Owen Weeks is similarly concerned about Jolene. There are, after all, special considerations about how to provide private financial assistance (earning ability or gifts), how to prevent those assets from being exploited or dissipated, and how to keep your son or daughter eligible for government benefits based on financial need. You probably will want to be able to express special wishes for your son or daughter and have them carried out after your death.

How to Distribute Your Estate (Assets) Among All of Your Family

The usual function of your plan, and especially your Last Will and Testament, is to pass accumulated wealth to the next generation or to others (such as the charities the Levines have supported). You probably will face special problems in allocating your estate among your family or among other potential beneficiaries when you must also consider your son or daughter with a disability. How can you balance the interests of all those people? How can you take the "whole family" approach? How can you plan on a "whole life" basis? How long might Maria, Anna, or Steve live? Will there be grandchildren? After all, Steve's grandmother, Emma, and Jolene's grandmother, Eula Mae, have to be taken into account: people do have grandparents. Saundra Levine, who remained silent while her new husband Arnold and her new in-laws, Ben and Ruth, discussed money, must have harbored the thought: "Wouldn't the Levines be surprised if they knew I'm pregnant? Would they want their grandchildren to attend Northwestern and Chicago Law School, too?" And how should the Stuarts allocate their hard-earned property, given that Steve has two sisters?

How to Prevent Government Agencies from Charging for the Cost of Services

Assume that you want to take advantage of the government benefits (these benefits are discussed in Chapters 10–12) that are or might become available to your son or daughter. This may not be a correct assumption in your case, but for other families it is. Many states have laws that require parents of minor children to pay for the services that the state provides, especially if the care is in public residential facilities. Other states have similar laws relating to the cost of services for adults. If a state seeks to recover the cost of services, will the property that you leave to your son or daughter be safe from these charges? Or will your legacy be depleted by the state, with nothing left over for your son or daughter? That is a difficult matter, one on which state laws differ. Yet, it is a special consideration for your family.

How to Prevent the Son or Daughter to Whom You Leave Assets from Being Disqualified from Government Benefits Based on Need

The possibility of Maria's disqualification from government benefits is the matter that Geraldo raised when talking with his parents. Many financial assistance programs require your son or daughter to be financially needy before becoming eligible for the benefits. That is often true even if there is no question about the fact of disability. If your son or daughter has a disability, but also has property such as might have been given by family (the Levines probably will leave a large legacy for Anna), or have been earned (Maria may leave the workshop and earn so much that she will not be needy enough to continue receiving benefits), your son or daughter either will have to "spend down" his or her assets to a very low level, or will have to continue to earn only very little, all to be eligible for government financial benefits.

How to Minimize Federal and State Taxes on Your Estate

Because he is an attorney, Arnold Levine will be able to advise Ben and Ruth about the very complicated matter of taxes. If taxes are an important consideration for you, you should consult a tax lawyer or certified public accountant.

WHAT ARE THE GUIDELINES FOR DEALING WITH FINANCIAL PLANNING ISSUES?

The adage, "The wise family plans," is good advice when you deal with financial planning issues. It is not even important how you plan—informally, as the Rodriguezes are starting to do, or formally, as the Levines are doing. Your family members may disagree about the plan that should be followed, as the Rodriguezes might. There may be different members in charge of the planning, like Ruth and Arnold in the case of the Levines. Regardless of the circumstances, a family like yours is well advised to plan well in advance and plan continually.

You already have taken the first step because you are reading this book and evaluating its advice. You soon will take the second, which is learning the language of estate planning.

The language of estate planning is very specialized. Lawyers, accountants, financial planners, trust officers at banks, tax advisors, and other professionals use it all the time. In order to work with them, you will need to know what their language means. For that reason, you should read the following material carefully, refer often to the glossary at the back of this book, and be willing to use the technical language of estate planning. Not only will the glossary help you, the actual use of the language in this text will, too; familiarity will lead to confidence. Be patient . . . the language is technical, and the subject is difficult, but you can master both.

Take Inventory

First, take an inventory of your family's assets so that will know what type and amount of funds are available to your family members. Because the Levines, Stuarts, Harrises, and Rodriguezes have different types of assets, they will have different *net worths* (the value of all assets minus the amount of all debts equals net worth). Even families with modest incomes will be surprised at how useful it is to take an inventory of their assets and debts. In doing that, you probably will work with various people who can help estimate the value of your property. A good place to start is the local bank, which probably has forms that you can use and perhaps has employees who can help estimate the value of your property. Also, you may want to think about your assets as belonging to one of two major groups of property, *private assets* and *government benefits*.

Private assets include:

1.   Life insurance
2.   Personal residence
3.   Other real property (land and improvements, rights to use of land, water, and minerals)
4.   Personal property
5.   Liquid assets (bank accounts, certificates of deposit)
6.   Stocks and bonds, mutual funds, and tax-sheltered investments
7.   Interests in businesses
8.   Assets in Trusts
9.   Powers of appointment (the rights to designate who will inherit assets left by another person in that person's Will)
10. Retirement programs, pension plans, profit-sharing plans, and individual retirement accounts (IRAs)

Governments benefits are discussed in detail in Chapters 10, 11, 12, 14, and 16.

Involve Many People in Planning

Throughout this book we emphasize, first, that formal, legal decision-making power for your son or daughter must be established (whether or not by guardianship), and, second, that the decision-makers in each family will vary from family to family.

Some families will be very close, such as the Rodriguezes. Others will be extended encompassing a large number of relatives, such as the Stuart and Harris families. Others, such as the Levines, will involve only a few relatives, but a large number of professional advisors.

Some families will have one or two authority figures, people who make the decisions. There is no doubt that Arnold will be consulted, but Ben and Ruth will make the final decision. There is no doubt that Owen and Jolene's grandmother will be consulted, but Odessa will make the final decision. And there is no doubt that Jack and Rose will not only seek the advice of their daughters and of their friends the Wilsons, but will also give serious consideration to what they say.

More than this, each family will involve the person with a disability in the planning in light of the type of consent that has been found appropriate. Each family will want to consider how that person will want to live in the future and how that choice will affect other family members.

"Arnold," says his mother Ruth, "remember Anna. Let's talk about these matters together. But let's be sure to talk *with* her. You know, and you've always told us, that it would be wrong to leave her out of our planning. What was all that talk about when you were in law school, about direct consent? Was it serious? Son, you persuaded me."

Involving a variety of people ensures that your plans, hopes, and intentions for your family are understood and accepted by those who will be affected by and carry out those plans after you die. This suggests that you will want to consider a plan to:

Consult with any guardian(s) appointed for your young adult and with other family members, especially those who will be involved in your son's or daughter's personal or financial future.

Consult with disability professionals who will be service providers or who can give advice about where services can be obtained.

Consult with an attorney, bank trust officer, chartered life underwriter or other insurance broker, accountant, personal financial consultant, and any others (e.g., business partners) who will be involved in the technical planning and administration of your Wills.

Consider the 'Whole Family' Approach to the Future

Throughout this book we state that any future plan for one member of your family almost always affects everyone else in your family. This *whole family* perspective (which we discussed in greater detail in Chapter 2) suggests that you contemplate a plan that:

Considers your son or daughter with a disability

Considers the other members of your family (other brothers and sisters, other family members)

Considers the *whole family* approach

There is no right or wrong process or result. You probably will think about balancing the needs of every family member, realizing that what is fair is a matter of personal judgment having to do with your family's needs, values, beliefs, and traditions.

In consultation with your family and the professionals identified above, consider whether plans should be made into formal legal agreements, through financial guardianship, careful planning of the Will or Trust, or other means. You have already made decisions about direct or substitute consent for your son or daughter. If you have confidence in direct consent, the need for financial guardianship may be reduced or eliminated. But your need for a Will does not depend on your son's or daughter's ability to give direct consent, because a Will has other purposes (see Chapter 13). The same is true of a Trust. If you have decided that your son or daughter needs partial or plenary financial guardianship, you will want a Will or Trust as a way of telling the guardian how to use your property on behalf of your son or daughter.

In the course of your consultations, you should also consider whether plans should be left informal and, unlike formal legal agreements, unenforceable at law. Such plans are called *moral obligations*. If you trust your family to carry out your plans and respect the needs and preferences of your son or daughter, you may not want a Will or Trust. But if you think your family may, for whatever reason, someday disregard your plans and your son's or daughter's preferences, you may want to use a Will or Trust as a way to require your family to carry out your plans and to protect your son or daughter from neglect or abuse by other family members. Your unwritten plans are not enforceable, as a rule. Your written plans, however, usually are.

Consider the personal and financial relationships of the members of your family to each other, particularly as they concern your son or daughter. Are family members unreservedly committed to your son or daughter? If so, you may not need a Will or Trust. Consider the psychological aspects of formal and informal planning for your family. When do moral obligations create guilt or resentment because your family members come to believe that you put too much responsibility on them? When do legal agreements become burdensome to your family? You have no way of knowing the answers for certain, but you may want to think about these issues.

Taxation

Consider the matter of the taxation of your or another family member's estate. State and federal estate and inheritance taxes can be minimized by careful estate planning. You may want to ask yourself whether the most important issue is the personal and financial future of your son or daughter and the relationships within your family after your death, or minimizing estate taxes. The problem essentially is this: You may set up a plan for your family that is based primarily on tax consequences. To do this, you may give less importance to some of the issues involved in the provision of money to your son or daughter. So, you face this question: Is it more important to minimize taxes or to maximize your child's potential income?

For example, in the Levines' case, Ben and Ruth are both professionals, have worked for many years, and have made very profitable investments. With hard work and good luck, Arnold and Saundra are also likely to be financially successful. With the net worth of the parents in excess of $1 million, and with Arnold and Saundra likely to accumulate an estate of comparable value, it is undoubtedly important for the Levines to minimize taxation.

"Dad, Mom," Arnold says, "you've worked hard, been successful, paid your taxes, and haven't used the available tax shelters. You've given lots of money to Associated Jewish Charities, the synagogue, and the universities we attended. Heaven only knows how many times you helped the Boy Scouts, the Fellowship of Christians and Jews, and the Association for Retarded Citizens. You've more than paid your dues. So let's talk about being a bit selfish, about not letting Uncle Sam and the governor take such a big cut from your estate."

"Arnold," Ruth responds, "how can you say such things? Uncle Sam, fried ham! Anna's the most important consideration. Let's try to set up her future; *then* we'll worry about taxes. You young people still haven't figured it out—this is a great country, it's been very good to us, and we have to help it along. That's what taxes are for. So, Anna first, the country next, and you two . . . well, you'll be taken care of. Isn't that so, Ben?"

"Right!," Ben replied, "Your mother's right again."

You may not have the "problem" the Levines face, but you may want to think about the extent to which you plan the future around your son or daughter in light of taxation. Advice on tax planning is beyond the scope of this book. You should consult a tax attorney or certified public accountant for this information.

THE TOOLS OF FINANCIAL PLANNING

When you think about private and public assets, you may also want to think about the basic tools for planning your estate. These include life insurance and the provisions you make to distribute proceeds to beneficiaries (we discuss distribution later); property held in your and others' names (property that belongs to both you and others and that will automatically pass to the co-owners when you die—this property is known as *joint property* or *property held by the entireties*); Wills; Trusts; and financial guardianship. We discuss Wills and Trusts in Chapters 13–16. For now, remember that these are major tools for estate planning and for distributing and controlling your assets during your life or after you die. That is what the Stuarts have in mind.

On their way home from their meeting with the young lawyer who had discussed disabilities and future planning with them, Jack and Rose begin a painful conversation.

"Rose," Jack mutters, "it's hard, harder than I thought it would be. You know, we've never talked about death before. We've always lived each day to the fullest. It's as though we've denied we're mortal. How silly. How natural."

Rose replies, with sadness, "Yes, Jack. That's right. But let's remember, it's all we can do to take life a day at a time. Steven is a wonderful son. He's been so good for us, but not always easy. A day at a time, that's our way."

"True," Jack says. "But now . . . well, it's as though the lawyer put us in our graves and let us see our family, those who live after us, looking down at us and saying, 'Why didn't you plan better?' I don't like that, thinking about death. But he's got a point. What happens if we die today . . . you know, a car wreck. What happens to our family, our property, our Steve?"

What happens when you die? You may want to consider the effect of your death with respect to your estate (your property).

Proceeds from insurance on your life go to the persons designated as the beneficiaries of the insurance policy. Insurance contracts allow flexibility, and you should use that flexibility in designating the beneficiaries. The Levines and Stuarts, for example, own life insurance. They may require the proceeds of the insurance to be paid directly to an individual in a lump sum, to a Trust in a lump sum, or to an individual in installments, for example. The flexibility built into the life insurance contracts allows them to use the proceeds in ways that are tailored to their particular needs. Another advantage of life insurance is that the proceeds are not included in your estate for the *probate* of your Will. We discuss probate in the next chapter, but bear in mind that it can be a slow process in comparison to the payment of life insurance.

Property owned in joint tenancy with rights of survivorship (see the glossary) or as tenants by the entireties (see the glossary) goes to the surviving co-owner. This property usually includes your family home, bank accounts, stocks, bonds, and personal property. This is how the Levines and Stuarts own property. The advantage of jointly owned property is that, like life insurance, it is not included in the probate process. Thus, it can pass from you to the other owners very quickly.

Property put into Trust (see the glossary and Chapter 14) during your life-time (inter vivos Trust) or by Will (testamentary Trust) goes to the Trustee for the benefit of the person named in the Trust. Other property goes to the persons named in the Will. Property in Trust also passes to the Trustee outside of the probate process. It quickly goes to the hands of the Trustee and thus can be used for the beneficiary soon after the Trust is created (while you live or after you die). Trusts have other advantages, which we discuss in Chapter 14. The advantage of having property in a Will is that you can control who gets your property when you die. The disadvantage is that the courts must "probate" your Will. That can be a slow process. We discuss Wills in Chapter 13.

Like the Stuarts, Levines, and other families, you have a great deal to think about. That is why we present the process of financial planning step by step. In the next chapter, we start with the government benefits, and then discuss Wills and Trusts. Remember, you have already thought about financial guardianship. Whatever decision you reached, you have yet to fully consider the other tools of estate planning, so let's begin.

10 HOW DOES THE SOCIAL SECURITY PROGRAM HELP?

Summer had come to New York State. The lush, rolling hills were covered with orchards and gardens. The evenings were cool around Jamestown, cool enough that Henry and Lillian Weber still wore sweaters when they sat on the back porch of their little house to watch the sun set.

One such evening in mid-June, Lillian, a note of caution in her voice, broke the comfortable silence that had enveloped her and her husband. "David had a good day today. The dialysis went well," she said, quietly.

"Good . . . good . . . he's a trouper, a lot tougher than a lot of those truckers coming along today," her husband responded.

Sensing that Henry wanted to avoid talking about David and was trying to shift the subject to the "new breed" of long-distance truckers he dispatched for Jamestown Interstate Movers, Lillian paused a few moments before speaking again.

"Yes, you're right," she nodded in agreement. "He is a courageous young man. And he's got several years more to live, too."

Henry shot a glance at his wife and snapped, "Several? Several years?"

Lillian hesitated before replying. An anxious tone crept into her voice as she continued: "Henry, I know you don't want to talk about it, but we have to. David has a future and it's not all dialysis, transfusions, wheelchairs, medications, and watching that he doesn't start banging his head or biting his hands. Henry, are you going to face the future or not? I can't do it alone. David can get help from us, but he needs you, and I do, too. And he also needs government assistance. Now, I've looked into those programs. For my sake and his, and for your own, put some time aside to learn what I know. It'll give you hope, Henry. It really will. I know your style—turn on the TV, turn off the future. It won't work, not for David and not for me."

She paused, giving Henry time to answer, aware that an uncharacteristic resentment of her lot in life had shown itself. Usually she saw the good parts of David's life, his "positive contributions," as she called them.

When Henry kept his silence, she pleaded, more in dispair than anger, "Help us, please. Help yourself. Just give me some time to explain. Then, after we talk and plan . . . then you can do what you want. Please, Henry!"

Henry remained silent, but his actions spoke for him as he smashed his huge fist into the palm of his other hand. Lillian knew it wasn't David who was on his mind. That gesture, or others like it, meant her husband was raging silently against their other two children.

Gary, now in his early 30s, had moved across the country; no more cold winters for him, only the California sun. And no more resentment of the inordinate amount of time his mother spent on his younger brother, for Gary had made it clear when he left 10 years ago that he wouldn't be back. Henry and Lillian hadn't even met Gary's new wife or their first grandchild, who was already 2½ years old.

Susan, the middle child, also was far away, her beauty, ready smile, and bouncy step having helped her secure a flight attendant's job with a major international airline. From her base in Miami, she would telephone about every other month. But her recent divorce, coupled with the fact that she was "still in the market but not looking for a mate, just for travel and adventure," meant she rarely returned to "Smalltown," as she now called the place where she had grown up. Like Henry, she preferred not to discuss the future; Gary was more like his mother, more open and talkative. Could Susan be counted on to help her brother? Probably not.

Finally, Henry spoke his mind. "Damn it, Lil. Just a couple of birds that we fed and then lost. That's what those two older kids of ours are. And we're now the old birds in our old nest. Problem is, David. Not David, really. Just what we're going to do. Okay, I've put it out of my mind too long. I'll listen. You talk. It's our usual way. No criticism intended, Lillian. Just facts. So, what have you learned? How can we help David? How can the government help?"

So Lillian began to explain.

*   *   *

To plan for the future of a child with disabilities, parents like Lillian and Henry and yourself must be aware of and use the many programs sponsored by the federal government and operated through a federal-state partnership. These are called *entitlement programs*. Some of them are provided for large portions of the population in general, not just for people with disabilities. These are called *generic programs*. Other programs are specifically for people with disabilities. Through a well-planned combination of both generic and specific services, and by supplementing those services with private assets, you can probably establish a relatively secure financial future for your son or daughter.

The key in using government benefits is to create a "package" of benefits. This requires combining several programs authorized by the Social Security laws with programs authorized separately for health, housing, and food stamp assistance. In essence, "packaging" these benefits has the same purpose as "packaging" private assets (we discuss private assets in subsequent chapters) with public benefits. That purpose is to obtain the greatest amount of financial support for the person with a disability. To develop that package and achieve that purpose, you, like the Webers, have to know not only what benefits are available, but also how those various benefits tie in with each other.

*   *   *

"Lil," said Henry, a few minutes into Lillian's explanation, "this business of government benefits seems just too complicated to me. I'm just a trucker. How can anyone except one of those Washington bureaucrats figure out who gets what and how much? I thought the government could really foul things up, what with those new tax forms and all. Now, I'm convinced of it. It's a mess!"

Lillian, in her usual calm way, seemed not nearly as perturbed. "Henry, just relax," she said, soothingly. "I've done some studying on all that. It's complicated, all right. But once you see the links—like a chain-link fence, or, more to my taste, a hand-hooked lap rug—it's not too hard to understand. Just follow the links, Henry, and it'll make sense."

The Social Security Program in General

A clear picture of the eligibility linkages between the federal programs is difficult to draw, as Lillian would be the first to admit. Set out below is a description of these major programs. (We do not discuss vocational rehabilitation, employment training benefits [Job Training Partnership Act], or other job-related programs, because these are discussed in Section III. However, Lillian and Henry will want to take them into account, as you will.

In these chapters on government benefits, we assume that you want to make use of the benefits, as the Webers do. There may be families, however, that do not want to use the programs. They may have enough money that they do not need the programs. Or they may believe that they should use up all of their personal resources before they use government resources. Finally, they may believe that their son or daughter should not be "on welfare" and that the use of the disability benefits programs would violate that belief. These are entirely valid options. If you hold them, you may not want to read the rest of this section on government benefits, or you still may want to read it in order to add support to your opinions.

Original Purposes of Social Security Programs

One of the federal government's most important purposes is to provide for the general welfare of Americans. In the middle 1930s, as the Depression wreaked economic havoc on millions of families, it became clear that the federal government needed to establish a program that would provide basic economic security to financially hard-hit citizens.

The major program was established and financed by the Social Security Act of 1935. Although the Act was first intended to be a vehicle for retirement benefits, it has become the major law for providing benefits to people with disabilities and their families. It now provides a wide range of benefits, including direct payments to persons for "income maintenance," or payments to others who provide medical or nonmedical treatment. In this chapter, we discuss income maintenance programs and, in Chapter 12, medical and nonmedical treatment payments.

Income Maintenance Programs

Social Security programs are directed at all families, whether or not they have members with disabilities. Their purposes, achieved primarily through direct unrestricted money payments to beneficiaries, are:

1. To provide for the material needs of individuals and families
2. To protect those who are elderly or have a disability (or both) against the various illnesses that could exhaust their financial resources
3. To maintain the family structure
4. To increase the opportunity for children to grow up in a safe, healthy environment

To achieve these purposes, Social Security has four major income maintenance components: *retirement insurance, survivor's insurance, disability insurance,* and *Supplemental Security Income (SSI) payments.*

SSDI INCOME MAINTENANCE PROGRAMS

Three of these income maintenance programs provide benefits to people who are disabled at the time when their parents retire, become disabled, or die. These are called *income maintenance programs* because they provide income to the person with a disability to replace the income of a parent who retires, becomes disabled, or dies. The payments are insurance against the loss of income because the person's parents are retired, disabled, or dead. Since the payments go to the person with a disability, they are called Social Security Disability Insurance (SSDI) payments—Social Security payments to a disabled person as a type of insurance. First, we'll discuss what "disability" means. Then we'll discuss the three types of SSDI payments.

What Does 'Disability' Mean?

The term "disabled" means that a person is "unable to engage in substantial gainful activity." This is the *SGA test*—substantial gainful activity (SGA) must be impossible for the person. In addition, the cause of the person's inability to engage in substantial gainful activity must be caused by a mental or physical disability that can be expected to result in death or that has existed or can be expected to exist for 12 months or longer. According to Social Security Administration regulations, the fact that a person has a disability does not necessarily mean that he or she is "disabled" for Social Security purposes. Only if the person cannot engage in "substantial gainful activity" is the person "disabled." Later in this chapter, we discuss how to go about proving that your son or daughter is "disabled."

SSDI for 'Disabled' People

But now, let's consider the SSDI programs—the income maintenance programs that provide Social Security insurance payments to people with disabilities. Remember, there are three types of these programs, all called SSDI programs. Each can provide SSDI payments to your adult or minor son or daughter with a disability when you, a parent, have worked long enough and have paid into the Social Security Trust Fund. This is the *work history* requirement. We discuss the work history rule on p. 95. But first, you should learn how you as a parent can obtain SSDI for your child with a disability. Assuming you have a sufficient work history, your child can obtain SSDI when you retire, die, or become disabled.

    Retirement insurance is meant to replace part of the earnings lost because of retirement. Payments go to the retired worker or eligible dependents, including unmarried children, without regard to their age, who were disabled before becoming 22 years old.

    Survivor's insurance is meant to replace part of earnings lost to dependents because of a worker's death. Payments go to eligible dependents, including minor or disabled children, and all widows, widowers, or surviving divorced spouses under age 60 who have children under their care who are minors or have a disability.

    Disability insurance is meant to replace earnings lost because of a worker's disability. (Disability here does not refer to the disability of your son or daughter, but rather to a disability that you or your spouse might incur.) Payments go to eligible dependents, including some children, especially those of any age who are unmarried and who have a disability.

Social Security Trust Fund

You may wonder where the government (in this case, the Social Security Administration) gets the money to make SSDI payments. Social Security is a social insurance program that provides financial assistance (entitlements) based on the fact that a worker—the parent or the child—has paid premiums into the Social Security Trust Fund. These premiums are usually in the form of mandatory payroll deductions. The source of payment can be either the recipient's parent or child. Either way, the *work history* of the worker must be long enough to qualify for Social Security. Your local Social Security office can tell you how much you or your son or daughter has paid in and whether you or your son or daughter has a sufficient work history.

Usually, you or your spouse will be the worker who pays into the Social Security Trust Fund. Sometimes, however, your son or daughter will be the worker who pays into the fund. In either case, your son or daughter will be eligible to receive payments if he or she is "disabled" and if you retire, die, or are disabled (becomes eligible because you paid into the fund) or when he or she retires (becomes eligible because he or she paid into the fund). We'll first discuss the situation in which you pay into the Social Security Trust Fund, and then the situation in which your son or daughter has worked and paid into the fund.

You (the Parent) as the Person Paying into the Fund   You or your son or daughter are entitled to receive benefits when your employment is interrupted by your retirement, death, or disability. This entitlement exists regardless of your son's or daughter's assets or unearned income from other sources. Henry has paid into the Social Security Trust Fund during each of the 35 years he has worked (the so-called FICA payroll tax is deducted automatically from his bimonthly paycheck). He, Lillian, and David are therefore entitled to benefits when he dies, retires, or becomes disabled. (In the language of the Social Security Administration, Henry is the "primary insured." This indicates that he made the payments and is the main, but not only, insured person; Lillian and David also are insured.)

As already noted, in some circumstances your children are eligible to receive benefits when you die, retire, or become disabled. Fifty percent of your benefit (the *primary insurance amount,* or *PIA*) may be payable in certain situations to your child with a disability, regardless of his or her age, when you retire or become disabled. It is possible for this amount to rise to a maximum of 75% of the PIA when you die. It may not reach this level, however, if there are other family members who receive benefits on your Social Security record. To be eligible, your son or daughter must have been disabled before age 22. Thus, David will be eligible to receive benefits when Henry retires or if Henry becomes disabled. This is because David is "disabled" (unable to engage in "substantial gainful activity") and because his disability occurred before he was 22 years old. Also, his benefits may increase when Henry dies.

If you decide to begin future planning based on your projected Social Security benefits, you can calculate those projected benefits by completing the worksheet titled "Estimating Your Social Security Retirement Check." The worksheet is available from your nearest Social Security district office.

Your Son or Daughter as the Person Paying into the Fund   We said that your son or daughter also may receive Social Security payments if he or she has been employed, and has paid into the trust fund through FICA taxes on earnings. In recent years, adults with developmental disabilities have been able to qualify because of their own earnings being large enough to be covered for FICA taxes, but not large enough to be considered indicative of substantial gainful employment. Thus, David, like Henry, might be eligible to receive Social Security benefits if he is employed and pays into the Social Security Trust Fund from his own wages, through FICA payroll deductions. This also is true for Jolene Harris, Anna Levine, Maria Rodriguez, and Steven Stuart.

Parent and Designated Beneficiary   Your son or daughter may be entitled to SSDI benefits on the basis of either your work record or your spouse's, but not on the basis of both records together. Thus, you should designate your son or daughter as the beneficiary of the parent with the most accrued monies. That is why Henry's work record will be the basis for David's eligibility. Lillian, who has not worked for 17 years, can not pass a Social Security benefit on to David.

You also should consider taking part in other available pension or insurance plans that include benefits for people with a disability, such as those that your employer might offer. Continuing to receive income from several sources will help assure a more financially secure future for your child. For example, Henry's employer has a retirement plan that Henry can use to help David financially.

There probably is not a typical plan offered by employers. But at least three types exist. In one, the employer and the employee both make contributions. In a second, only the employer makes contributions. In a third, only the employee makes contributions. Sometimes an employee may volunteer to participate in these plans. In other cases, the employee *must* participate. You should determine if you are now participating or can participate in a plan, and what benefits will exist for your family, particularly your son or daughter, if you do participate.

Table 10.1.   Evidence of disability and other qualifying information

Social Security card of your son or daughter

Social Security numbers of both parents

Telephone number of the district Social Security office

Birth certificate of your son or daughter

Marriage certificate of the parents, if your son or daughter is one spouse's child by a previous marriage

Guardianship papers (with any provisions for guardianship)

Any Will that names your son or daughter as a beneficiary

Papers concerning your son's or daughter's admission to any residential facility (past or present)

History of your son's or daughter's school placement

Information on any facility where your son or daughter is now or has been a resident, and its status as a skilled nursing facility, intermediate care facility, community residence, or group home, including number of occupants, and public or private and profit or nonprofit status

Phone numbers of social workers you have dealt with through agencies such as a department of social and rehabilitation services and residential or community programs

Record of your son's or daughter's employment and wages currently earned

Last federal income tax return of your son or daughter and parents

Earnings record of your son or daughter

Information on your son's or daughter's present and future income and assets, including income from Trusts and assets of the surviving parent if you are seeking SSDI for a minor

Information on: 1) Social Security or SSDI benefits presently received by your son or daughter or parents, 2) the basis for SSDI payments, and 3) type of living arrangements (where your son or daughter lives)

Any papers which refer to other private or state pension funds that will provide additional income to your son or daughter. You should have certified copies of Trusts and usually an affidavit from the Trustee stating that the intention of the grantor of the Trust was to use the Trust income or principal in addition to basic support provided by the SSDI program

GATHERING EVIDENCE OF
DISABILITY AND OTHER QUALIFYING INFORMATION

Because you are concerned with future planning for your son or daughter, you should gather the materials and information listed in Table 10.1.

Applying for SSDI

After reading this chapter, we recommend that you consider taking the following actions: 1) Read the next five chapters before taking any other step, 2) Consult a lawyer about writing a Will, creating a Trust, and applying for SSDI benefits (try to get an attorney who has experience with Wills, Trusts, and disability law—perhaps your state's protection and advocacy system, developmental disabilities planning council, or association for retarded or other disabled citizens can help you find one), 3) Go to the local office of the Social Security Administration, ask for copies of the pamphlets about SSDI, ask for copies of the SSDI application forms, and read the pamphlets and forms carefully in light of what you have learned in this and subsequent chapters, and 4) Finally apply for SSDI. When you apply, remember to take all necessary documents with you. Be sure to ask the Social Security employee you deal with how long it will be before your son or daughter begins receiving SSDI, and what amout will be paid.

11 WHAT IS SUPPLEMENTAL SECURITY INCOME?

Supplemental Security Income (SSI) is a separate income maintenance program under the Social Security Act. But, unlike Social Security Disability Insurance (SSDI), it is available only to needy individuals who are elderly, blind, or have a disability. The rules on eligibility for SSI change frequently. So do the benefits. This is because Congress amends the SSI laws from time to time, and because the Social Security Administration changes the regulations from time to time. The statements made in this chapter and in Chapters 14 and 16 about SSI and other government benefits were accurate as of January 1990. However, you should check with your local Social Security office to find out if any new laws or regulations have gone into effect since that time.

DISABILITY AND NEED

A person is considered disabled if he or she is unable to engage in substantial gainful activity (SGA) because of a mental or physical impairment that has lasted or can be expected to last at least 12 consecutive months or longer, and that occurred before the person became 22 years old. SSI provides a monthly payment to individuals who are disabled, beginning when they are 18, who have little or no income or resources. The maximum federal SSI payment is $386 per month. David Weber (like Jolene Harris, Anna Levine, Maria Rodriguez, and Steve Stuart) is "disabled," and thus will be eligible if he is also "needy."

SSI therefore is like SSDI in one respect: the recipient must be "disabled." But SSI is different in a major respect: the recipient must also be financially needy. We'll compare and contrast other aspects of the two programs before discussing the factors that affect the amount of benefits paid to a disabled person in financial need.

Although the Social Security Administration manages the SSI program, SSI is not the same as SSDI. As we noted earlier, the money for SSDI retirement, death, and disability benefits comes from individual contributions in the form of FICA taxes to the Social Security Trust Fund. By contrast, SSI benefits come from the general funds of the U.S. Treasury.

Also, unlike SSDI, your son's or daughter's SSI payments can be reduced by other income. This is because SSI payments are based on need, and need is defined by the lack of other income. Because of this, your son or daughter must apply for the SSDI benefits due him or her, and SSDI payments reduce the amount of SSI payments. Lillian and Henry understand this requirement as the "packaging" issue.

Individuals who receive SSI benefits can also be eligible for benefits from the SSDI income maintenance programs. Thus, if your son or daughter receives an SSDI income maintenance check for less than $387 per month, he or she may also be eligible for SSI. This package takes into account the $386 maximum income maintenance SSI payment for your son or daughter and $20 of unearned income which is not counted as income. If Henry dies, retires, or is disabled, David will continue to be eligible for SSI because he himself is "disabled" and "financially needy." He also will be newly eligible for one of the other SSDI income maintenance programs because his father is dead, retired, or disabled.

FACTORS AFFECTING THE SIZE OF SSI PAYMENTS

Several factors affect the size of SSI payments. Unlike SSDI payments, which are based only on the fact that the person is disabled, SSI payments are based on both disability and financial need. The current rule is that a person is needy who has no more than $2,000 in resources and no more than $386 in monthly income. If a person earns a monthly wage of $500 or more (before taxes and after deductions allowed by the Social Security Act), the person is considered able to engage in Substantial Gainful Activity and therefore does not qualify for SSI. To determine a person's financial need, the Social Security Administration considers: 1) the person's place of residence, 2) the parents' employment status, 3) the link to Medicaid (discussed in Chapter 12), and 4) the person's status as a beneficiary of a Trust. We consider each of these in order, with separate chapters devoted to Trusts (Chapters 15, 16).

SSI and Your Son's or Daughter's Place of Residence

Living arrangements may affect the amount of your son's or daughter's SSI benefit. In the first place, SSI payments are reduced by up to one-third if your son or daughter lives in your or another person's household. Since David, Jolene, Anna, and Steve all live with their parents, their SSI benefit payments will be reduced so long as they live with their parents. If, however, they move to an apartment, group home, or other setting, their payments will be for the full amount.

Second, if your son or daughter who is eligible for SSI resides in a hospital, nursing home, or intermediate care facility (ICF; these are discussed in Section V), whether public or private, where bills are paid from Medicaid funds, monthly SSI benefits will be reduced to $25. But the SSI benefit is payable only if your son or daughter has no more than $20 in other income. For example, if David Weber or Steve Stuart become residents of such a facility, their SSI benefits will be reduced to $25 per month if their cost of care in those facilities is reimbursed by Medicaid. Recent law allows a person to continue to receive SSI if his or her stay in an institution is for 1 or 2 full months. If the person stays longer, he or she loses the SSI.

Third, if your son or daughter resides in a public institution not funded by Medicaid, SSI will not be available unless the institution is designated as an educational or vocational school or a community residence for 16 or fewer individuals. This means that if you choose to place your son or daughter in such a program, you may want to choose a small, community-based program that is both private and designated by the

Social Security Administration as a school or community residence. Otherwise, your son or daughter will lose SSI eligibility.

Fourth, if your son or daughter lives in the household of another who provides both board and lodging "in kind," there will be a one-third reduction in SSI. This standard deduction takes the place of setting the exact dollar value of the board and lodging. This deduction will not apply if your son or daughter pays a pro rata (proportionate) share of the costs, nor will it apply in private group homes or foster placements arranged as part of a program administered by a public agency. For example, if David Weber lives in a "board and care" home and pays his pro rata share of the costs of living there, his SSI benefits will not be reduced. But if he does not pay his share, his benefits will be reduced, because he does not need the funds to pay his own way.

If your son or daughter is already getting SSI and needs to be institutionalized, and if the institutional placement is expected to last less than 3 months and the SSI payments are needed to continue your son's or daughter's usual living arrangements, then the SSI payments may continue during the period of institutionalization. This allows a short-term institutionalization without interruption of SSI payments.

Finally, the period your son or daughter may be eligible for SSI while living in a public shelter is now 6 months over any 9-month period.

Parents as Workers

Let us say that you or your spouse is employed. Does that affect the size of your child's SSI payments? The answer depends on how old your son or daughter is.

Usually, SSI can be started for your minor child while you are still employed. This is because you are not yet receiving Social Security retirement or disability payments, and thus your minor child is not receiving SSDI payments. Here is another consideration: your income and resources are *deemed* (counted as belonging) to your child only until age 18. Later, if your child begins to receive SSDI benefits, the SSI benefits may be reduced or terminated. In many cases, if you are still working, and have a son or daughter over the age of 18, SSI will be paid if your son or daughter meets the "needs" test.

Your Son's or Daughter's Earned Income

The Social Security Administration has rules that determine the extent of your son's or daughter's financial need. First and foremost, these rules define income and determine need on the basis of income.

"Income" refers to anything received (earned and unearned) that may be used to meet the needs for food, clothing, or shelter. Thus it includes cash, checks, some items received in kind, such as food and shelter, and many items which would not be considered income for federal or other tax purposes. Wages, net earnings from self-employment, earned income tax credit payments, and income received from sheltered workshops are examples of earned income. Social Security benefits, worker's or veterans compensation, pensions, support and maintenance in kind, in-kind assistance from nonprofit organizations, and income from Trusts, annuities, rent, and interest are examples of unearned income.

Note, however, that income from Trusts is unearned income only if the Trust is not prepared under the rules we discuss in Chapter 14. If the Trust is prepared under those rules and if the Trustees take care to make distributions only in accordance with the rules we discuss later in this chapter, the Trust distributions are not unearned income and will not be counted against the SSI payments.

The items listed in Table 11.1 are *not* defined as income by the Social Security Administration.

Many of the items in Table 11.1 are available under federal or state aid programs, such as food stamps, housing assistance, and vocational rehabilitation assistance. For this reason, it is all the more important to your son's or daughter's future that you put together a package of benefits in which SSI payments are supplemented by other governmental aid and, if you set up a Trust, by payments from the Trust.

In addition, the value of household goods, personal effects, an automobile, property needed for self-support, and burial plots are (subject to certain limits) not included in the determination of resources. The value of a home where your son or daughter lives is also excluded, as is a total of $1,500 for burial, $2,000 in an irrevocable Trust for burial, and life insurance. In Anna Levine's case, for example, much of her personal property (e.g., furniture, clothing, jewelry, stereo, VCR) will not be treated as assets. Moreover, if Ben and Ruth want to give Anna a house to live in, placing the title in her name and perhaps in Arnold's as well (to make sure that Arnold has some control over the use and disposition of the house), that house usually will not be counted as an asset. If you can afford to do so, you will find that giving a house to your son or daughter is a good way of assuring that your child has a suitable place to live and still

Table 11.1. Items *not* defined as income by the Social Security Administration when Supplemental Security Income (SSI) levels are being computed

---

Medical care and services, including reimbursements and payment of health insurance premiums by others

Social services, including reimbursements from programs

Receipts from the sale, exchange, or replacement of resources

Income tax refunds

Payments by credit life or disability insurance

Proceeds from a loan

Bills paid by another individual for things other than food, clothing, or shelter

Replacement of lost or stolen income

Weatherization assistance

Twenty dollars per month of earned or unearned income except for unearned income such as a veteran's pension based on need

Sixty-five dollars per month of earned income plus half of earned income, $85 a month of earned income plus half of the remainder

Irregular or infrequent earned income if it totals no more than $10 per month

Irregular or infrequent unearned income if it totals no more than $20 per month

If the SSI-eligible person is a child, one-third of any payment for the child's support received from an absent parent

Earnings up to $400 per month but not more than $1,620 per year of a child who is blind or has a disability *and* who is a student under age 22

If the SSI-eligible person is visually impaired or has some other disability, the amount of income necessary for the fulfillment of an approved plan to achieve self-support

If the SSI-eligible person has a disability, an amount equal to impairment-related work expenses (Consult the Social Security Administration to determine if this provision applies to your son or daughter.)

Food stamp assistance

Housing assistance from federal housing programs administered by state and local agencies

Incentive allowances and specific types of reimbursements for individuals in certain training programs (Consult the Social Security Administration to determine if this provision applies to your son or daughter.)

---

receives SSI benefits. Indeed, some parents are beginning to take this route as part of their planning for their child's financial future. There are some circumstances in which real property (other than the house) is not counted as an asset. Otherwise, all of your son's or daughter's assets must be "spent down" to the level of $2,000 to meet the "needs" test.

A more extensive listing of income stipulations is available at your local Social Security office, in two pamphlets, "A Guide to Supplemental Security Income," and "SSI for the Aged, Blind and Disabled."

SSI and Your Son or Daughter as a Worker

It is possible for individuals who work to be eligible for SSI benefits. The first $65 of your son's or daughter's earned monthly income does not affect eligibility for, or the amount of, SSI benefits. After that $65, however, SSI benefits will be reduced by $1 for every $2 your son or daughter earns. Apart from earned income, any other unearned income above the first $20 a month will reduce SSI payment amounts. This type of unearned income includes SSDI payments (e.g., to David Weber if Henry dies, retires, or is disabled), veteran's compensation, worker's compensation, pensions, annuities, gifts, payments from Trusts, and other forms of income.

We mentioned earlier that packaging federal benefits is the key for your son or daughter to receive the full benefit of government programs. This is particularly true in the case of SSI (or even SSDI) payments to your son or daughter and his or her eligibility for the federal health insurance program called Medicaid. Although we discuss Medicaid in Chapter 12, you need to know now that the Medicaid program pays for the health care of financially needy people with disabilities. Usually, a person who receives SSI is also eligible for Medicaid. In the past, a person whose earnings were so great that he or she became disqualified for SSI (no longer financially needy) also automatically was disqualified from receiving Medicaid. The result was that the person's income maintenance (SSI) and health insurance (Medicaid) benefits were cut off just at the point where a person became marginally self-sufficient. Being cut off from both SSI and Medicaid became a major disincentive to work; people with disabilities preferred to avoid work to protect their SSI and Medicaid benefits. Congress acted in 1986 to eliminate this disincentive. The 1986 amendments to the Social Security Act (PL 99-643, Employment Opportunities for Disabled Americans Act) make it possible for people who receive SSI to continue to be covered by the Medicaid federal health care program even when their monthly earnings exceed the amount at which they become totally disqualified for SSI. There is a minor exception to this general rule, which we will not discuss here.

The general rule is fairly straightforward. If your son or daughter is eligible for full SSI benefits, he or she may receive $386 per month in SSI benefits, and have $20 unearned income and $65 in earned income; that is, the $20 and $65 will supplement the $386.

As we noted earlier, however, once your son or daughter begins to make more than $65 per month earned income, SSI benefits are reduced on the basis of 2:1. That is, every $2 earned results in a reduction of $1 of SSI. Stated in a different way, SSI benefits are reduced by $1 for every $2 earned. The break-even point where earnings result in a total loss of SSI benefits is roughly $867 of earned income per month.

Under previous law, if your son or daughter earned income in excess of the break-even point, he or she would automatically stop being eligible for Medicaid benefits. As we said, this law effectively discouraged your son or daughter from earning more than the break-even point. It was a disincentive to seeking employment and higher wages.

Recognizing that this disincentive was not consistent with the intent of vocational rehabilitation laws to help people with disabilities obtain work and be self-supporting to the fullest extent possible, the 1986 amendment provides that a person who exceeds the break-even point in earnings and thus loses all SSI benefits will still retain Medicaid coverage. It also provides that a person who receives any SSI benefit (even $1) will still receive Medicaid benefits.

Under that provision, your son or daughter will continue to be eligible for Medicaid if he or she needs the Medicaid coverage in order to continue to work and cannot afford other medical insurance. Thus, the continuation of Medicaid coverage when your son or daughter does not receive SSI (because his or her earnings exceed the $867 per month break-even point) depends on his or her need to have medical insurance in order to continue to work. Coverage depends on employment-related need and financial need.

In order to define when your son's or daughter's need exists, the Social Security Administration apparently will not take a position that the need for insurance depends solely on physical or mental medical needs, such as a need for medical insurance as a means for physical or mental habilitation. Instead, the Social Security Administration is adopting, as a general rule, the position that your son or daughter must have sufficient earnings in order to purchase private insurance that is the equivalent of Medicaid. That is, he or she must be able to use earnings to replace the government's medical insurance. In order to have that amount of earnings, the Social Security Administration estimates that your son or daughter must earn approximately $1,000 per month, or $12,000 per year.

As noted earlier in this chapter, SSDI is similar to SSI only in that your son or daughter must be disabled. Let's reconsider SSDI briefly. So far, we have considered only the SSI program as changed by the 1986 amendments. But, as we have noted, many people with disabilities are covered by SSDI. David Weber might be covered by SSDI if his father Henry dies, retires, or is disabled, since Henry paid into the Social Security Trust Fund with his FICA payroll taxes.

Under the 1986 amendments, the rules for people with SSDI (like David) are different from those for people with SSI. The basic difference is at the break-even point. Under SSDI, the break-even point is $300 per month of earned income. Under SSI, it is greater, about $867 per month of earned income. Although David and perhaps your son or daughter will lose SSDI and Medicaid if their earnings exceed the break-even point, there is a 3-month transition period when Medicaid coverage continues. After that 3-month transition period, David or perhaps your son or daughter may continue in Medicaid only after paying premiums for Medicaid coverage. If a person is working on a "trial work period" (essentially, a 9-month period when the person tests whether he or she can work), the person is eligible to receive Medicare coverage (discussed in the next chapter). If the person who is receiving some Social Security benefits other than SSI (e.g., SSDI) loses those benefits because he or she has engaged in enough work to pass the "break-even" point, normally the person will also lose the Medicare coverage. Recently enacted law permits the Medicare coverage to continue for 39 months after the person ends the trial work period. This provision is an incentive for people to work. Social Security did not always provide such incentives; in fact, it used to include many work disincentives. In the paragraphs below, you will read about one of the disincentives and how it has been reduced.

Plans for Achieving Self-Support

Before recent amendments to the SSI program, an individual with a disability faced two disincentives to working. Both disincentives have been reduced by recent amendments.

One disincentive concerned the person's "assets." Before the amendments, a person with assets over $1,700 was required to spend those assets down to $1,700 before qualifying for SSI payments. Under the recent amendments, a person may set aside money—over the new ceiling of $2,000—for a vocational goal if the Social Security Administration approves. A person can obtain approval by working with the Administration to develop a Plan for Achieving Self-Support (PASS). Under the plan, the Administration and the person agree that he or she may accumulate assets up to a certain level so long as they are used for work purposes, including the purpose of making it possible for the person to get and hold a job.

A second disincentive concerned the person's income and his or her expenses involved in holding a job. As we have noted, if a person has a job, it can affect the size of his or her SSI check. But as we all know, it takes money to make money. So, the law now provides that the Social Security Administration must deduct certain work-related expenses from the disabled person's earnings when it calculates how much a person should receive from the government through SSI.

To be deductible as an Impairment-Related Work Expense (IRWE), a service or material that the person pays for must be necessary because of his or her disability and may not include the expenses that a nondisabled person would incur in order to work. The service or material must be necessary to control a disabling condition, to meet the physical or mental demands of a job, to prepare for the trip to work, to travel to and from work, or to provide assistance immediately upon the return home from work.

Disability-related services or materials that a person needs to work can be deducted from income even if these services or materials are needed for nonwork activities. Examples of such deductible expenses are special transportation, medical devices, work-related equipment and personal assistants, modifications to the person's home, routine drugs or medical services, diagnostic procedures, certain types of attendant care, and job coaches.

Finally, the law now also allows a person to continue receiving monthly payments after he or she earns more than $500 per month, and allows a person to keep Medicaid benefits after he or she stops receiving monthly SSI checks. There are limitations to these general rules that you should review with the Social Security Administration.

* * *

Henry Weber turned to Lillian, shaking his head slowly from side to side, turning his palms up toward the porch ceiling, indicating his confusion.

"Lil," he said apologetically, "I'm having a hard time following you. Let me see if I have the general idea, okay?"

"Sure, darling," replied Lillian. "That'll be fine."

"Well," said Henry, "first, we have to put together two 'packages.' One is the government benefits. The other is our private resources. To get the public benefits package, we can use SSDI or even a combination of them. But then we also have to add medical care, housing, food stamps, and job training programs. Right?"

Lillian replied, "Exactly right. It's not hard to get the big picture."

Henry broke in, "Yes, but then it gets confusing. For David to get SSI, he has to be financially needy. Now, that's where things become confused, because you told me early on that we can use our Wills and Trusts to give him money. If we do that, though, he won't be needy, will he?"

"Well, it all depends on how we give him property. Look, Henry, before we talk about the Wills and Trusts and private property, let's finish talking about the other government benefits. Then, we'll talk about Wills, Trusts, and Trusts plus SSI, in that order. Is that okay?"

"Sure," Henry replied, resigned to the inevitable. "But how about a break? Say . . . about a day?"

"Yes," answered Lillian with determination, "but in 24 hours, we'll resume our talk!"

12 | WHAT OTHER GOVERNMENT PROGRAMS ARE AVAILABLE?

A day later, Henry and Lillian were still talking about the linkages between federal and state assistance programs for David.

"Lillian," Henry said, "I know you're smarter than I about these matters, and you've certainly boned up on them. But I still don't understand how these income maintenance programs and the medical benefits program tie together. Talk about chain-link fences and hand-hooked lap rugs! Them, I understand. Governments . . . no way do I understand them!"

"Henry, just relax," Lillian said, reassuringly. "It's simple enough. If David gets SSI, he also gets Medicaid. It's automatic. Just like a fence, one link is connected to another. Let me explain."

About the same time, halfway across the continent, Arnold Levine turned to his parents and said, "Dad, Mom, I hope you're reassured by our conversations. You have a solid plan, and the Trusts will be written to take into account all the issues we talked about concerning SSI. Anna will have her cake and still be able to eat it, too. Now, let's talk about her medical needs. Not that she has any now, but she might later. There are two major federal programs, Medicare and Medicaid. They're different, but both can help Anna."

*   *   *

MEDICARE

A federal health insurance program, Medicare was created in 1965 in response to growing concerns about the high cost of medical care for older Americans. The program has since grown to protect more than 26 million aged individuals and 2 million adults with disabilities. Like the SSDI and SSI programs, it is part of the Social Security Act.

Medicare should not be confused with another program under the Social Security Act, Medicaid. Medicare is not the same as Medicaid. *The right to benefits under Medicare is established primarily by payroll tax contributions.* In this respect, Medicare is like the SSDI program. The tax is the FICA payroll deduction. *Under Medicaid, however, the right to a benefit is established by financial need.* In this respect, Medicaid is like the SSI program. Also, Medicare is intended to help persons who are elderly and disabled, while Medicaid seeks to help nonelderly people who are financially needy or who have a disability. Thus, Medicare will be useful for your son or daughter and for Jolene, Anna, Maria, Steve, and David because they have disabilities. They will also be eligible for Medicaid if they receive SSI. Let us first consider Medicare.

Medicare Components 'A' and 'B'

Medicare is available to people over 65 and to people with disabilities. This is because any person who receives Social Security benefits based on his or her own disability (i.e., disabled workers, disabled widows and widowers, and adult disabled children) is eligible for Medicare coverage beginning 24 months after he or she begins to receive Social Security benefits. Moreover, all families that have one or two parents who have been engaged in sustained covered employment (i.e., they have been employed and have paid into the Social Security Trust Fund) will become eligible for Social Security, and hence for Medicare, on the retirement, death, or disability of the (currently) working parent.

Medicare has two components. *Part A—Hospital Insurance (HI)* helps pay for inpatient care, inpatient care in a skilled nursing facility, home health care, and hospice care. *Part B—Supplemental Medical Insurance (SMI)* helps pay for physicians' and hospital services no matter where they are received. Part B—Supplemental Medical Insurance also covers outpatient hospital services in connection with diagnosis and treatment, such as emergency room care or care in an outpatient clinic. Under certain conditions, medical insurance can cover an unlimited number of home health visits as well as services and supplies. Moreover, Medicare now also provides unlimited hospital coverage and a "stop loss" on outpatient and physicians' services under Part B. People with incomes below the poverty level will receive these services essentially free because Medicaid will pick up the deductibles and co-insurance (which are part of the "stop loss").

Almost everyone over age 65, as well as many individuals with disabilities, is eligible for Part A—Hospital Insurance and Part B—Supplemental Medical Insurance. Individuals age 18 or over who become disabled before age 22 can be entitled to Part A—Hospital Insurance benefits 24 months after first becoming entitled to SSDI benefits. For example, a person who is 20 years old and who is disabled ("unable to engage in substantial gainful employment" because of a disability that is expected to result in death or to last for 12 months or longer) is eligible for Medicare if he or she is also eligible for SSDI benefits. Thus, your son or daughter can become eligible for Medicare if he or she is also eligible for SSDI. Individuals entitled to Part A—Hospital Insurance benefits are eligible to enroll for Part B—Supplemental Medical Insurance.

Medicare is a voluntary program which requires a monthly payment. In most cases, the monthly premium is deducted from monthly SSDI benefit checks.

SSDI and Medicare are entitlements that do not depend on your son's or daughter's place of residence. Residents of all types of facilities, except prisons, can receive Social Security benefits and medical services covered by Medicare.

Limitations on Medicare

Unfortunately, Medicare does not fully protect your son or daughter against the high cost of health care. Medicare provides extremely limited protection against the cost of long-term care. This is a major concern if you have a son or daughter with a disabling condition. Also, Medicare does not cover catastrophic health care. (The terms "long-term" and "catastrophic" are defined by the U.S. Health Care Financing Agency. You should consult your local Social Security Administration office to determine precisely what Medicare does and does not cover.) By itself, Medicare covers less than half of the total health care bill by individuals with disabilities. Other public programs such as Medicaid can provide some necessary protection for them, and a person may qualify for both Medicare (as an SSDI recipient) and Medicaid (as an SSI recipient). However, it is often necessary for extra medical costs to be paid by the individual. States may provide additional medical services programs and you should inquire into them at your local social services or Social Security Administration office. Local Social Security offices will take your application for Medicare, provide information, and help you file claims.

MEDICAID

As we pointed out earlier, if your son or daughter is eligible for SSI, in most (but not all) states he or she is also eligible for Medicaid. When covered by Medicaid, your son or daughter will receive at least these services:

Inpatient hospital services
Outpatient hospital services
Laboratory and x-ray services
Skilled nursing facilities (SNF) for persons over 21
Home health services for individuals
Medical diagnosis and treatment for persons under 21
Family planning services and supplies
Physician services

These services are all medically oriented. They are typically provided in nursing homes or institutions. Each state decides what services are paid for by Medicaid. Most states reimburse for these services, but there are variations among the states. You can find out which services are eligible for reimbursement in your state by contacting your local social services agency.

Under a program started in 1981, states may establish a waiver of traditional, medically oriented services in favor of services provided in homes and communities. These *home-based and community-based services* include case management, homemaker services, home health aid, personal care, adult day care, habilitation, respite care, and other necessary services. These services are defined by Medicaid regulations. Check with your local social services office to learn precisely what is covered.

The home-based and community-based services program is designed to be an alternative to nursing home or institutional placement and to provide your son or daughter with the opportunity to remain in family settings. Individuals who meet state guidelines are eligible for this program. You can find out your state's guidelines by inquiring at your local social services agency.

Upon acceptance in the home-based and community-based services program, your son or daughter will receive a written plan of care, indicating the required medical and nonmedical services to be provided. The Medicaid program, especially this component, provides many benefits. But because it may not fully cover all of your son's or daughter's medical or habilitative needs, we encourage you to check very carefully into two matters. First, you will want to know if your son or daughter is covered by Medicaid. If not, find out when and under what circumstances he or she might become covered. Second, you will want to know precisely what services Medicaid pays for, and the amount of payment for each service. Again, you should inquire about and apply for Medicaid coverage at your local social services agency.

Once you learn more about Medicaid coverage, you may want to decide whether this coverage is sufficient or, if it is not, what other health insurance you might obtain for your son or daughter, or what he or she might obtain as an employee of a company that provides health insurance benefits. You may find that Medicaid, as good as it is, is not entirely sufficient. Therefore, you may want to find out if you can supplement it with other insurance. That is part of "packaging." It also is just the point that Lillian was making to Henry as they resumed their planning for David's future.

OTHER GOVERNMENT PROGRAMS

"Henry, let's admit that we're in pretty good shape as far as David's future is concerned. He'll get SSI or SSDI—although I hope it's SSI, because, well Henry, neither of us expects you to die or become disabled anytime soon, and I know you don't plan to retire yet. So, that means David'll get Medicaid too. Now the last matters to consider are food and housing programs. Just have a little more patience so I can explain those programs. Then we'll have all the facts on government benefits. Okay?"

"Sure, Lil," said Henry with resignation. "Go right ahead. It's still over my head, but I'm starting to get the drift of it." He paused, then added, "Your're incredible, Lillian—making chain fences and lap rugs out of federal programs. My, oh, my!, what the people in Washington would think if they heard you. You've got more sense then all those bureaucrats combined. Lillian, how about running for Congress?"

"Don't flatter me, silly," his wife said, smiling. "I'm perfectly happy here with you and all our friends in our pretty little town, and you know it! Now, about food stamps and housing," Lillian said, her voice taking on a serious, teacherly tone.

Food Stamps

The Food Stamp Program provides financial assistance by enabling recipients to exchange the stamps for food. It is a major supplement to income if your son or daughter meets income tests. This program is federally funded through the Department of Agriculture's Food and Nutrition Service (FNS). It is administered by state and local social services agencies.

One purpose of the Food Stamp Program is to increase the quality and quantity of food available to low-income households. A household is a group of individuals who live together and share income and expenses. While most households are families, other groups of unrelated individuals may also be considered households, including the residents of group homes.

For your son or daughter to be eligible for food stamps, his or her income and resources must be taken into consideration. If your son or daughter lives with you, your income is counted toward your child's income. Your son or daughter may qualify for food stamps if he or she:

> Works for low wages
> Is unemployed, or works only part-time
> Receives welfare or other assistance payments
> Is elderly or has a disability and is financially needy

In most cases, if your son or daughter is eligible for SSI, food stamps will be available too.

Other special provisions of the Food Stamp Program include the following:

Households with members who are elderly or have a disability may be certified for food stamps for an entire year.

People who are elderly or have a disability may apply for food stamps at the local Social Security office when applying for SSI.

People who are elderly or have a disabilty and who are not mobile may request a home visit or telephone interview, and the stamps can be issued by mail.

People who are elderly or have a disability can name an authorized representative to receive food stamps on their behalf.

More information may be obtained from the booklet, "Food Stamps: Do You Qualify?", available from the Food and Nutrition Service of the U.S. Department of Agriculture, or from your local department of social services.

Housing

"Now, Henry," Lillian said, as Henry's mind obviously began to wander from food stamps to Sunday's slate of baseball games, "there is just one more program I want you to know about. Pay attention. It affects David in a very real way, because we won't be around his whole life."

"I know, Lil," Henry answered. "I'm sorry . . . I'll listen harder. But let's not think about dying before David. It's too . . . . well, let me put it this way. Let's take life one day at a time. Let's talk about what we might do for David tomorrow, while we're alive and kicking."

"That's a deal," concluded Lillian, knowing full well that any other approach would meet with rejection.

For years, after all, she had been trying to get her husband to think about David's life after they died. Maybe it was the nurse in her, accustomed to life, diseases, and death. And maybe it was the mother in her, having taken care of David at home for all of his life. She had developed perspectives on life and mortality that were different from Henry's. Her style of dealing with the future was different, but she knew there was no sense in trying to bring him around to her point of view. She would accommodate him, but only in style. In substance, she would prevail. It had always been that way, but she never let Henry know it.

*   *   *

A variety of publicly supported housing programs are available to your son or daughter if he or she meets the tests of need and disability. You may get the information relating to these programs from the U.S. Department of Housing and Urban Development (HUD), or from local housing authorities.

Section 8   Your son or daughter may get payments to help cover the cost of rent. These payments are made directly to your son or daughter but are restricted in use—they are for rent only. The purpose of this program is to help obtain decent, safe, and sanitary housing in private accommodations. There are income limitations for eligibility for Section 8 housing. These are determined locally.

This rental assistance program is designed to be applied to existing housing, new construction, and to moderately or substantially rehabilitated units. However, new funding is currently unavailable for new construction or substantially rehabilitated projects.

Seven specific steps for applying for rental assistance are outlined below:

1. An application must be completed and filed with the local housing authority.
2. Eligibility is then determined, based on the intended type of occupancy (elderly or disabled) and income.
3. It is then up to your young adult and, perhaps, you, to find suitable housing on the private market.
4. This housing must then be inspected by the local housing authority and meet the mandated quality standards.
5. Once the housing has passed inspection, it must be determined if the landlord is interested in participating in Section 8.
6. The local housing authority fair market rent standards and utility allowance standards must be considered.
7. If it is determined that rent and utilities do not exceed the fair market rent, and the landlord is in agreement, the housing may be leased. If the fair market rent is exceeded, you must seek alternative accommodations.

Section 202   This program provides direct loans for the construction of housing for your son or daughter. Long-term loans are made to eligible, private, nonprofit sponsors who are financially viable and can meet the special needs of the designated tenant groups (in your case, tenants with a disability). Applications are made to the local housing authority.

The Section 202 program is designed to serve three specific populations: individuals with developmental disabilities, chronic mental illness, or physical disabilities. Thus, your son or daughter could qualify as an occupant of housing constructed with Section 202 aid. Projects are designed to meet the specific needs of the particular tenant population. Individuals from one group may not be accepted for occupancy in a project designed for a different tenant group because of the special needs of each population.

Projects intended primarily for individuals with developmental disabilities usually are approved only for the development of small group homes. Although homes for up to 15 persons per site are now permitted, facilities for 6–8 are preferable to assure a more normal, homelike environment.

The Differences and Links between Section 8 and Section 202   Special Section 8 (rental assistance) funds are available to help pay rent for Section 202 (construction assistance) units. These Section 8 funds differ from those discussed previously in that they are not administered through the local housing authority. The income standards and percentages of payment required of tenants are the same but, in this case, the project bills the government directly for the difference.

Participation in this "in-kind" program, provided by Section 8 rent subsidies, as well as access to group homes developed with Section 202 funding, can help give your son or daughter the opportunity for safe, healthy, community-based living environments. This is especially true when these benefits are combined with the income maintenance benefits provided by participation in SSDI and SSI and with the medical care benefits available through Medicare or Medicaid.

SUMMARY

"Now then, Henry, that wasn't too difficult, was it?," Lillian asked, trying to bring him into the planning process and make him feel more competent.

"No, it wasn't, Lillian, and I've got to hand it to you. Like I said before, you made it all seem quite doable. Not that it's easy, but it is possible."

Lillian smiled softly. She had succeeded in mastering the general outline of federal programs and leading Henry into the future. Her smile broadened and reflected her obvious delight as she heard her husband speak.

"Lillian, light of my life, I know you think faster than I do, and you may even get the idea that I don't pay you enough attention. But I've listened carefully. For an old trucker like me, it's sort of like learning a new city and using a new road map. Those programs are the city, and you drew the map. Now let me see if I have it," he added, with a sly grin, knowing full well that his summary would indeed "have it."

*   *   *

If your son or daughter has a low income and a disability, various federal programs must be packaged to assure that income, health care, food, and housing needs are met. In most states, people with a disability who also have a low income usually combine programs. The best package is shown in Table 12.1.

This table shows the "package" that can result. If your son or daughter receives SSDI benefits, then Medicare (Part A and Part B) is available. If your son or daughter receives SSI, then Medicaid, housing aid, and food stamps are available. Finally, your son or daughter may receive both SSDI (based on a parent's retirement, disability, or death) and SSI (based on your son or daughter being financially needy); in that case, all the benefits are available.

Your son or daughter must have both a disability (as defined by these programs) and a financial need to qualify for the SSI and associated programs. You may use every legal means of planning to assure both that your son or daughter meets the financial need requirement and that he or she has access to extra income from your family. The best way to do this is for you to leave money to your son or daughter in a pure discretionary Trust, which you may create by your Will or while you are alive.

All across the United States, families are doing just that. Some families, like the

Table 12.1.   Getting the best benefits package for your son or daughter

If your son or daughter receives:	Then these benefits are available:
	Package 1
Social Security Disability Insurance (SSDI)	Medicare
	Part A—Hospital Insurance
	Part B—Supplemental Medical Insurance
	Package 2
Supplemental Security Income (SSI)	Medicaid
	Housing aid
	Food stamps
	Package 3
Both SSI and SSDI	All the benefits listed in Packages 1 and 2

Remember: Your son or daughter may receive SSDI if you (the parent) are retired, disabled, or deceased. Your son or daughter may receive SSI if he or she is financially needy.

Levines, have substantial personal wealth that they can put into a Trust for their children. Others, like the Harrises, Rodriguezes, Stuarts, and Webers, have limited personal wealth, but even they are finding that there are ways to set up small Trusts so they can face the future with confidence.

*   *   *

Maria Rodriguez had confronted her parents about her work; she wanted to leave the sheltered workshop and get a real job. She wanted to leave her parents' home and get an apartment for herself. The Rodriguezes' cultural traditions and their natural concerns as parents came into conflict with Maria's desires and Geraldo's experiences. But before they resolved that matter, they followed Geraldo's advice to "consider the money side of it."

Ben and Ruth Levine did the same, but with far less reluctance. It was their style to plan deliberately, logically, and even somewhat coolly about the future. That was what made them good at business. And that was what suited Arnold and Saundra. As Arnold had said, "It's simply a matter of business."

Jack and Rose Stuart had listened to the lawyer's advice: "But once you know what you want to do, I am almost sure we can work out a good plan." They set their goals, assessed their personal and financial resources, thought about what Steve would want, and planned accordingly.

Owen Weeks had taken Odessa by surprise; his sister had not been willing to look into the future and think about Jolene's life. Yet he had shown her that, although she had very few worldly assets, she had a great deal of other assets. There were her family, friends and neighbors, her church, the local Association for Retarded Citizens, and many more professionals who could help than Odessa had ever imagined. "Yes," she thought, "it is one thing to have faith; indeed, it is indispensable." But even God planned. "He worked for six days and rested on the seventh," Odessa thought. "That was good planning on His part."

And David Weber now had a recognizable future, thanks to Lillian's persistence in learning about federal programs, explaining them to Henry, and planning to make sure David became eligible for those beneifts. Henry was like so many other New York "upstaters"—self-reliant, hesitant to go "on welfare," even proud that he had "never had my face in the trough." But he was practical, too, and thrifty. He had paid his taxes; his FICA deductions had increased annually. Now it was time for him to "get back what we put in," as he put it. The only thing he needed was information on how to do it. Lillian had found out how, and Henry, knowing that David would be helped, stood up to take a stroll.

"Before you tell me about Wills and Trusts, I want to soak up this beautiful day, Lillian," he said as he started out the door. "The apple trees are beginning to seed up. Soon they'll be ripe and drop their apples, and then their leaves. They're sort of like me—ripening up, about to go into the last stages. It's not so bad for them. And it's not so bad for us, either. David . . . well, he's sort of like a young tree that won't quite grow up, so nature has to give special attention to that little tree's needs. I've seen how you've given David that special attention, Lil; now I want to see how nature does it. Care to come along?"

13 WHAT IS A LAST WILL AND TESTAMENT?

Henry Weber had his stroll through the apple orchards, thinking about the government benefits that Lillian had just explained. He thought about the trees and the benefits—like a young tree, David needed the fertilizer that the benefits provided. But trees also need water . . . maybe Henry's own frugal ways of saving money could be the water in David's case. Of course, water needed a hose to direct it to the trees. Perhaps, Henry thought, a Will and a Trust could be like a hose that puts water on the trees at just the right times and in just the right places. Water, Wills and Trusts; fertilizer and government benefits . . . David as a special tree, needing both. That was how Henry made sense out of Lillian's talk.

* * *

A Last Will and Testament (or Will, as we'll refer to it) is a legal document that comes into effect upon your death. (The person making the Will is called a *testator* if a man or *testatrix* if a woman.) Your Will permits you to designate the person(s), institutions, or both, whom you want to receive your property when you die.

For the Will to be valid, you yourself must:

Be over the age of majority (usually 18)

Have mental competence—this means you must know the nature and extent of your property and the people who are to inherit that property and their relationship to you, and be capable of determining how to dispose of your property

Be acting voluntarily

Also, your Will must have been *executed* (signed) according to certain legal formalities. Usually, there are two such requirements. First, your Will must be written. There is an exception, but it is rarely used. The exception applies to a *nuncupative* Will (see the glossary). Normally, and according to best practice, your written Will is typed or printed. A Will can be handwritten (*holographic*) and signed at the bottom. We strongly encourage you to use a professionally prepared, written Will.

Second, your Will must be witnessed and, in some states, "acknowledged" (i.e., signed in the presence of a notary public). State law usually requires more than one witness, requires the witnesses to sign in the presence of each other, and requires that they have complete mental competence and be "disinterested," that is, not be beneficiaries of your Will.

If you do not have a Will and want one, or if you want a different one from the one you already have, act now. It is clear that Ben and Ruth Levine will properly execute their respective Wills; after all, Arnold is a lawyer and both the Levines and their son take good care of their business affairs. Since Jack and Rose Stuart, Odessa Harris, and Luis and Eloisa Rodriguez all have begun doing careful future planning, it is obvious that they, like the Levines, plan to execute Wills. But planning and actually doing are two different things.

"Dad and Mom," Arnold says, "let's talk about what you want to do, today. Then, let me work on the matter with the person in this law firm who handles these complicated estate-planning issues. Together, we can check out the tax consequences, and the matters related to Anna, if you want to give her money. And then, in, say, a month, all of us will meet again and get the whole package signed, sealed, and delivered, as they say. After all, you don't know what will happen to you in the next month. You're still driving that Chicago Loop, and it's a known killer. I don't want to sound like the voice of doom, but planning and acting must be kept close together in point of time."

IS IT NECESSARY TO HAVE A WILL?

There are two basic answers to the question, "Is it necessary to have a Will?:" yes (the best answer), and no (acceptable in some circumstances).

The answer will be yes if you wish to carry out a carefully planned program of financial care for your son or daughter with a disability, distribution of your estate (assets), and allocation of financial and personal benefits and responsibilities among members of your family (spouse, other children, grandchildren, or other relatives). The Webers, Levines, Stuarts, Rodriguezes, and Harrises all will want to have Wills because they all want to accomplish these goals.

Yes, if you wish to use testamentary guardianship (guardianship under your Last Will and Testament for your minor son or daughter, which we explained in Chapters 6–7).

Yes, if you wish to establish a Trust under your Will.

Yes, if you wish to avoid intestacy laws.

Yes, if you wish to minimize taxes.

The answer will be no if you have little or no concern about the personal or financial decisions affecting your son or daughter, little or no concern with tax minimization, no need for testamentary guardianship, or no desire to establish a Trust, and if you are satisfied to have the intestacy laws distribute your property.

The Webers, Stuarts, Levines, Harrises, and Rodriguezes all decide to make a Will. Each family wants to have a plan, and to carry it out. And each understands that money is simply a means for carrying out a plan. Each understands, too, that the lack of money must be taken into account.

"Owen," protested Odessa Harris to her brother, "you are just plain blockheaded, talking about 'my estate' as if I were a mill owner instead of a mill worker. I don't have anything except this little house and my Social Security, if I live long enough. And a tiny—and I mean tiny—retirement account with the mill."

Does that mean Odessa should not plan? Of course not. She still might want to say who should take care of Jolene after she dies. That is what a testamentary guardianship can do. And, in the case of the Levines, using Trusts to help Anna, and at the same time thinking about minimizing taxes, is another reason for them to plan.

WHAT DOES YOUR WILL DO?

A Will has four essential functions. As Arnold has pointed out to his parents, their Will disposes their property. But it also names somebody to carry out the directions of the Will. This person is called an *administrator* or *executor* of the Will. Next, it gives directions concerning the payment of debts, taxes, burial costs, etc. Finally, it can be used to name a testamentary guardian.

Your Will disposes of your property. Under a Will, you may direct your administrator to make sure that certain gifts of property are carried out. In the Levines' case, here is how Ben might make gifts under his Will:

> I give all of my golf, fishing, and hunting equipment, my sailboat, and the gold-and-diamond ring that my father gave me to my son, Arnold, who shared my hobbies with me and who is named after my father.

This type of gift is called a *specific legacy* because it is a gift of specified property to one (or more) named individual(s) whose identity can be determined at the time that the Will is administered.

Ben then might make another gift, for example:

> I give the sum of $10,000 to my friend and partner, Joseph Behr, and an amount equal to ten percent (10%) of the net value of my estate, after payment of debts and taxes and the execution of my specific legacies, to the Greater Chicago Area Association for Retarded Citizens.

This type of gift—actually, there are two gifts, each of the same type—is called a *general legacy* because it is a gift of money to identifiable persons or organizations. It is unlike a specific legacy in that the specific legacy is specified property other than money.

Finally, Ben might make still another gift, for example:

> I give all the rest and residue of my estate to my wife Ruth, for her life, and then to the First National Bank of Chicago, in trust, for the benefit of my daughter, Anna.

This type of gift is called a *residuary legacy* because it is a gift of whatever is left in Ben's estate after specific and general legacies have been made.

Not only does your Will dispose of property, but it can do so in certain ways. For example, your specific and general legacies are *outright* gifts, because they go straight and directly to the person to whom they are given (the *legatee* or *donee*). Indeed, even the gift to Ruth is an outright gift, even though it is only of a limited period (for her life, i.e., it is a gift of a lifetime interest or estate).

By contrast, Ben's gift under his Will to the First National Bank of Chicago is a gift that creates a trust for Anna's benefit. A gift in trust can include specific, general, or residuary legacies, or all of them. But they all are given to one person (Trustee) for the benefit of another (beneficiary). That is the key element of a Trust. We discuss this more fully in Chapter 14.

Your Will names persons to manage your assets and supervise your dependents. Such persons are *fiduciaries*. This means they have special duties in your estate—to carry out your Will as you requested. Fiduciaries include the following: personal representatives, administrators, or executors, whose duties are to collect the maker's assets, pay the debts and taxes due on your estate, and distribute the remaining assets according to your Will. This process is called *administration* of your Will. The person who administers your Will is a fiduciary.

We use the term, *executor,* to refer to all of the following people:

Trustees, whose duty is to serve for the benefit of others ("beneficiaries")
Testamentary guardians (discussed in Chapter 7)

Thus, Ben's Will names Arnold as his executor and the First National Bank of Chicago as his Trustee for Anna; but it cannot name a testamentary guardian because, as we already have learned, Anna is over the age of majority and has been determined to have complete mental competence.

Your Will generally addresses other matters as well:

Payment of debts
Payment of taxes
Funeral, burial, or cremation arrangements
Gifts of the body or organs
Common disaster and survivorship (*simultaneous death* of yourself and your spouse and distribution of property held in joint tenancy or tenancy by entireties)
Powers of fiduciaries (personal representatives, executors, trustees)
Bonding (insurance performance) of fiduciaries (Bonds can be waived.)
Disinheritance. In some states, a spouse cannot be disinherited unless the spouse agrees to be left out of the Will; if the maker tries to disinherit the spouse, the spouse still has a right to the intestate share as part of a *widow's allowance*, also called the spouse's *election against the Will.*
Your Will appoints a testamentary guardian of your minor children.

HOW MAY YOU LEAVE PROPERTY TO YOUR SONS, DAUGHTERS, OR SPOUSE?

When leaving money, you have three basic options concerning your sons or daughters:

You may provide for specific, general, or residuary legacies to any or all of them
You may provide for a Trust for any or all of them
You may disinherit or make a nominal gift (e.g., $5) to any or all of them. (In most states, a *pretermitted* son or daughter, that is, one born after you execute your Will, inherits the share of your estate that he or she would have inherited if your property had been apportioned by intestate distribution. So, you must re-execute your Will if you want to disinherit or make a nominal gift to a pretermitted child.)

For example, Odessa Harris makes a gift to Jolene of her jewelry, household furniture, and clothing. The Stuarts make a general gift of money ($1,000) to the local Association for Retarded Citizens. And Ben and Ruth Levine give property to each other for the rest of their lives (a *life estate*) and then say the property goes to Anna after they die (a remainderman gift to Anna), in trust.

But none of these family members makes these gifts without first considering very carefully whether they should disinherit their son or daughter with a disability. On first consideration, disinheritance may not seem an acceptable alternative, particularly for someone with a disability. There can be valid reasons for disinheritance, however.

WHAT ARE THE SPECIAL
CONSIDERATIONS RELEVANT TO DISINHERITANCE?

To illustrate why disinheritance may or may not be suitable, we'll examine the example of a parent who has a spouse and several sons or daughters, not just the one with a disability. If you have a spouse or other sons or daughters, you may leave property to any or all of them, disinherit your son or daughter with a disability, and ask your spouse or other sons or daughters to support the one with a disability. There are four advantages to disinheritance.

The first advantage is that your son or daughter with a disability owns no property and therefore has no assets against which governmental agencies may levy for cost of care, and no assets that will disqualify him or her from being eligible for government benefits.

A second advantage is that disinheritance prevents a situation in which a gift to your son or daughter with a disability may require the appointment of a financial guardian to manage the funds. Up to that point, it may have been possible for you to avoid an adjudication and the appointment of a financial guardian.

A third advantage is that disinheritance protects your son or daughter with a disability from unscrupulous people who might seek to use his or her funds solely for their benefit.

A final advantage of disinheritance is that it averts a situation in which your son or daughter with a disability may have to make a Will, but be unable to do so, in order to dispose of the funds after his or her death. Disinheritance also prevents a situation in which a Will might have to be defended in court, which would cause further expense to the estate and a further depletion of your original gift.

However, total disinheritance has disadvantages. One is that it may cause a nonlegal problem for your son or daughter with a disability, which is that he or she may feel unloved. In that case, a small gift (e.g., $1,000) may show your love, particularly if your son or daughter can be made to understand the purpose of your Will (to prevent cost-of-care levies and to prevent disqualification from eligibility for government benefits). Also, a useful function of the *Letters of Intent* (explained in pp. 122–123, this chapter) is to explain why you choose certain options, particularly disinheritance.

Another disadvantage of total disinheritance relates to something the law calls a *morally obligated gift*. Here is what that term means: Assume that you disinherit your son or daughter with a disability, give all of your estate to your spouse or other children, and ask your other children to support your son or daughter with a disability, using the money that you gave them. This request is called a morally obligated gift, but it cannot be enforced at law on behalf of your son or daughter with a disability. Therefore, this is a gift that will leave your other children free to use your assets any way they want, including ways that will not benefit your son or daughter with a disability. For example, if Jack Stuart were to leave half his property to his wife and half to his daughters Sally and Theresa, ask his daughters to use the money to support Steven, and then disinherit Steven entirely, there generally would be no way at law that Steven or a guardian acting on his behalf could require Rose, Sally, or Theresa to use any of that property for Steven. Even Jack's Letter of Intent would not help Steven acquire a legal right to that property. Remember, this is the general rule of law. There may be exceptions, depending on how the request is stated, whether it is contained in a Will, and the law of your state. But generally, your expectation and even your request (depending on how and in what written document it is expressed) create only a legally unenforceable moral obligation.

The morally obligated gift assumes that your spouse and family members will carry out your wishes with respect to your son or daughter. Jack knows that Sally and Theresa care deeply for Steven and that any morally obligated gift from him to them for Steven would cause them great concern and may even make them feel that they must use that property and other property as well for Steven. That is a burden that Jack wants to avoid imposing on them.

As a rule, the smaller your estate, the more sensible it is to disinherit your child. There are several reasons for this. First, your estate is so small that it will not cover the costs of services for your son or daughter, who will rely solely on government benefits instead. Second, the costs of administration will deplete the small amount already available to your son or daughter. Third, your spouse or others may use the funds more effectively, including for the benefit of your son or daughter.

Disinheritance also might be used when your son or daughter is the owner of substantial assets in his or her own name (e.g., owns property and later becomes disabled), or is the beneficiary of a substantial Trust, while, at the same time, other members of a family (e.g., brothers and sisters) do not have equivalent property, or even any property, themselves. Disinheritance in these two cases can result in the even distribution of your property.

WHAT ABOUT PROVISIONS FOR YOUR SPOUSE?

Generally, most states allow your spouse to take a certain portion of your estate (the so-called *widow's allowance*) even if you have tried to disinherit him or her. The law thus provides for support of spouse by allowing for an *election against the Will*. Or, you may make specific, general, or residuary legacies to your spouse. And, of course, you may provide for a Trust for your spouse.

MAY YOUR SON OR DAUGHTER HAVE A WILL?

In some states, if your son or daughter with a disability has sufficient mental competence and acts voluntarily, he or she may make a Will. In some states, however, if your son or daughter has been adjudicated incompetent and there is not a limited guardianship that allows him or her to dispose of property by Will, he or she may not make a Will.

HOW DO YOU ENSURE THE SAFEKEEPING OF YOUR WILL?

It is only wise to keep your Will in a safe place. But this should be a place to which others have immediate access after your death, such as a safe deposit box that is your joint property with your spouse or children, or the safe deposit box of your lawyer or the executor of your Will. Likewise, it is a good idea to provide copies to interested or affected persons (e.g., your spouse, children, lawyer, or executor), telling them where the original copy is. Thus, Ben and Ruth, having executed new Wills, place their original Wills, the ones that they signed, in their safe deposit box. And they give a duplicate copy, without their original signatures, to their son and to the First National Bank of Chicago, which they named as a trustee under their Wills.

IS YOUR WILL PERMANENT?

Your Will is not permanent until you die. It can be amended (and should be reviewed annually for desirable amendments) by a *Codicil* that, like the Will itself, can be made only if you have complete mental competence and are acting voluntarily. Your Codicil must be executed according to the same legal formalities that apply to the execution of your Will. Your Will also can be revoked, usually by your intentional physical destruction or mutilation, combined with your execution of a new Will indicating your intent to revoke your prior Will.

Periodic (annual) review is helpful. Here are some questions you might ask during periodic reviews:

Have my financial objectives changed?
Has the size of my estate changed drastically?
Have the laws changed, especially concerning Wills, taxes, and services for
people with disabilities?
Have any new family members been born or otherwise added?
Have any family members become disabled or died?

Ben already had prepared a Will before meeting with Arnold. In it, he provided for specific, general, and residuary legacies, and he made some of those legacies outright and some in trust. But that Will is several years old, having been executed (written, signed, and witnessed) while Anna was still under the age of majority. Moreover, it was executed when Arnold was still in law school and not yet launched upon his career. Ben and Arnold therefore review Ben's old Will, its provisions, and the circumstances of Ben's life when it was drawn up, and now they decide to change it.

"Dad," Arnold says, "if I were you, I wouldn't amend your Will. Having a Codicil around—you know, the document that amends your Will—can be confusing. Let's just take a clear cut at the whole matter and, on the day you execute your new Will, let's destroy the old one and say in the new one that the old one is revoked."

Arnold is correct to make this recommendation to Ben. After all, Ben's plan is quite different from before, and it calls for a new Will altogether, not an amendment by Codicil.

In Odessa's case, however, a Codicil should suffice. Under her first Will, she left everything to Jolene. Now, to show her gratitude to her brother, Owen, she amends her Will by executing a Codicil that provides for a specific legacy to Owen, namely the Bible that has been passed down in Odessa's family for generations:

"Owen, you know, this is quite a Bible. It not only has the Lord's story in it, it's got ours, too. It shows who our ancestors were. It's quite a story. It's our story, and it's your Bible. Thank you."

WHEN DOES YOUR WILL TAKE EFFECT?

Assuming your Will was valid when you executed it and that you have not revoked it, your Will and any valid Codicils become effective upon your death. Upon your death, your executor presents your Will for *probate*. Probate is the legal process by which a court determines whether your Will is valid, rules on any claims against your estate, and makes sure that your property is distributed according to your Will or by intestacy. Property exempt from the judicial process of probate usually includes life insurance with a designated beneficiary other than your estate, joint property with rights or survivorship or property held as tenants by entireties, and property put into lifetime (inter vivos) Trust.

Probate is a judicial process, requiring the assistance of lawyers and the payment of court and legal fees. Time must be allowed for creditors to file claims, prove claims, and be paid before assets are distributed. Creditors include claimants for taxes, administrative fees and costs (commissions to executors and personal representatives, attorneys, trust administration, guardianship), outstanding debts, and in some states, charges for services provided to your son or daughter.

Probate can take 2 years or even longer if there are disputes among your heirs, problems in locating or placing values on your assets, or tax audits.

WHAT OTHER DOCUMENTS ARE USEFUL?

Sometimes, you will not want to put certain information or instructions in your Will that relate to what you want done after your death. The principal reason for this is that a Will is a document that members of the public—including members of your family and your friends—may see whenever they want, by going to the probate court records. There are, however, two documents that are not open for public inspection but that can supply your instructions and preferences. These are the *Letter of Intent* and *Letter of Instruction.*

Your Letter of Intent can include information or hopes that are not appropriate for your Will itself. For example, it might express in great detail your hopes and concerns about how to take care of your son or daughter financially and personally. Unlike the provisions of your Will, however, these hopes and concerns, even when stated as instructions, are not legally enforceable. That is, nobody may sue the executor of your Will to require that person or anyone else to carry out your hopes, concerns, and instructions as expressed in a Letter of Intent. On the other hand, the administrator of a Will and others can have a much better idea of what you wanted—the "spirit" of the Will—if you also prepared a Letter of Intent.

Jack and Rose Stuart have consulted the lawyer who is familiar with disability matters and received her advice about the usefulness of a Letter of Intent. With her help, Jack has drawn up the Letter of Intent presented in Figure 13.1.

A second document that is just as useful as a Letter of Intent, just as private, and just as legally unenforceable, is a Letter of Instruction. Typically, a Letter of Instruction sets out details concerning your funeral, burial, and other matters of immediate importance, except the donation of your body organs. (A separate written document, available at any hospital or most lawyers' offices, is required for the donation of organs.) In addition, your Letter of Instruction can give directions about how to care

To: Executor of My Last Will and Testament and Trustee Under Trust for Steven Stuart

From: Jack Stuart
222 Spruce Street
Wheatland, Kansas

Date: September 22, 1987

Dear Executor and Trustee:

Today I executed my Last Will and Testament and Trust for the benefit of my son Steven. I put the original of each in the safe deposit box in my name (#222) at the First National Bank of Wheatland, Kansas, put a photocopy of them with my lawyer, Ellen Lisle, and instructed my brother Tom (335 Maple Street, Wheatland, Kansas) concerning where I put my Will and Trust and the contents of each.

I am writing this letter to supplement the provisions of my Will and Trust. In my Will, I disposed of a portion of my estate by giving it to the Trustee under the Trust. In my Trust, I created, to the maximum extent I could, a Trust that would give full and absolute discretion to the Trustee to manage the Trust for the benefit of my son Steven, who has severe mental retardation.

Because the Trust gives no instructions to the Trustee, I want the Trustee to know that my son has been living at home with me and my wife, Rose, for all of his life. He is now 17. His skills are limited for working and living on his own, and in my opinion, he will always need special help to live and work. Because he most likely will be supported financially by the Trust and whatever government benefits may be available to him, it is important that the Trustee and his guardian or other persons responsible for him know what his mother and I have done and what we want for him.

We have always given Steven all the love and strength that God has given us. We have chosen not to send Steven to live in a public residential facility. We have always believed that a family and home like ours would be the best kind of care anyone could provide. We believe we have been right in this decision. That decision was not the one some of our friends made. But what worked for us would not suit them, and vice versa.

Steven likes people and has many good friends in our community. He has received much help and support from local organizations such as the Association for Retarded Citizens and Special Olympics. This town also has good teachers and doctors who work with him and us.

We are planning for him to remain in Wheatland—it's the best place for Steven. Therefore, it is our plan for him to be as familiar with the activities and the people of Wheatland as possible. We want him to be a part of this town. After we die, we want Steven to remain in Wheatland. We do not want him to be placed in some school or institution.

In addition, we want Steven to work at a job where he is a part of Wheatland. That is the goal of his vocational training.

Therefore, the Executor(s) of my Will and the Trustee of my Trust should dispose of the assets I have made available for Steven in ways that assure, to the maximum extent possible, Steven lives and works in Wheatland and has a chance to have the friends he's grown up with as well as new ones who come along.

Very truly yours,

Jack Stuart, the father
of Steven Stuart

Figure 13.1. A sample Letter of Intent.

for your son or daughter immediately after your death and could even instruct family members how to explain that you have died.

Again, Jack and Rose have been advised about the Letter of Instruction and Jack has written one (see Figure 13.2).

WHAT IF YOU DIE WITHOUT A WILL?

If you die without a Will, your property that is not distributed by insurance beneficiary designation, survivorship (joint property or joint tenancy), or a Trust made during your

---

To: Executor of My Last Will and Testament

From: Jack Stuart
       222 Spruce Street
       Wheatland, Kansas

Date: September 22, 1987

Dear Executor:

Today I executed my Last Will and Testament. I placed the executed original copy in the safe deposit box registered in my name (#222) at the First National Bank of Wheatland, Kansas, and placed a photocopy of it with my lawyer, Ellen Lisle. I told my brother Tom (335 Maple Street, Wheatland, Kansas) about the contents of my Will and the accompanying Letter of Intent (addressed to my Executor and the Trustee under the Trust for Steven Stuart, dated today).

Because I do not wish my Will to contain instructions concerning the disposition of my body, I am setting out in this Letter of Instruction those instructions.

1. I wish to be cremated.
2. I wish my ashes to be placed in an urn and the urn buried beside the graves of my parents, John Grason Stuart and Sally Ridgley Stuart, at the Good Shepherd Church, Wheatland, Kansas.
3. I wish the funeral service to be according to the Book of Common Prayer of the Episcopal Church.
4. I wish the hymns to be "The Strife is Over," "Abide with Me," "The Doxology," and "Glory, Glory, Alleluia," in that order.
5. I wish a festival party to be held at my house after my burial, with food, drinks, and merriment. I am not dead—I have simply passed on.
6. I wish my family to tell Steven that I am in Heaven, with Baby Jesus and with Grandfather and Grandmother Stuart. Tell him that I will always be there, and that I will pray for him as I always have done. Tell Steven not to be sad. Give him a photograph of me and him together to hold while we have the funeral and party and to take with him wherever he goes; and tell him that his father loves him more than anybody in the world (Rose and Sally and Theresa know this is partially true—I love Steven in a different way than I love them, not any more).

I appreciate the concern with which you will comply with these requests.

                                    Very sincerely yours,

                                    Jack Stuart

Figure 13.2. A sample Letter of Instruction.

lifetime will be distributed by the state of your residence according to state intestacy laws. In most states, the intestacy laws distribute property as follows:

1. Half goes to your spouse and half to your children (whether minors or adults).
2. If you have no spouse, equal shares go to each son or daughter—if any one of your children has died, his or her share is divided equally among your other children or among any children that they might have (*per stirpes* distribution).
3. If you have no children or grandchildren, etc. ("no other issue"), all goes to your spouse.
4. If you have no sons or daughters and no spouse, all goes to your parents.
5. If you have no sons or daughters, spouse, or parents, all goes to your brothers and sisters in equal portions.
6. If you have no relatives, your estate becomes the property of the state (the *escheat* laws require that your property be deeded to the state).

If you are married, estate planning is even more important. This is because if both spouses died at the same time (*simultaneous death*), the laws concerning joint tenancy and tenancy by the entireties (see Glossary) would not apply if each spouse were a joint tenant of the other. Instead, the laws of intestacy would apply. Both you and your spouse, therefore, should make Wills. Do not rely on intestacy.

Both spouses in the Weber, Stuart, Levine, and Rodriguez families have drawn up Wills. Odessa Harris has also made one. In addition, the Weber, Stuart, Levine, Rodriguez, and Harris families have created or are considering creating Trusts. As Henry Weber might have noted, a Trust is like another hose; it supplements one hose, the Will, and it puts water on a tree (David Weber) that is already fertilized by government benefits.

In the next chapter, we show how this can be done. We use the Levine family as the example, because they are in a position to create a very large Trust. However, we also show that, if they are not careful, they might inadvertently disqualify Anna from government benefits.

14 WHAT IS A TRUST, AND HOW DOES IT HELP IN FINANCIAL PLANNING?

As we pointed out in Chapter 9, the parents of individual with disabilities must make special considerations when they do financial planning These considerations include the following:

1. How to provide money for your son or daughter after your death
2. How your estate (assets) should be distributed after you die
3. How to prevent government agencies from charging you, your son or daughter, or someone else (such as a Trustee) who has control over money available to your son or daughter for the costs of services
4. How to prevent a son or daughter to whom you plan to leave assets from being disqualified from need-based government benefits
5. How to minimize federal and state taxes on your estate

Dealing with these special considerations is not difficult, but it requires special skill. You should consider developing a Trust even if you have even a modest estate and want to ensure that your son or daughter will benefit from it while maintaining eligibility for government benefits. The special skill lies in knowing just what a Trust is and how to create the right kind of Trust.

* * *

The meeting between Ben, Ruth, Arnold, and Saundra in Arnold's law office had moved from the point at which Arnold suggested—"only for the sake of argument," as he put it—that his parents disinherit him, to a point where the subject of discussion is Anna.

"Ben," Ruth said, "don't you have something to tell Arnold and Saundra, now that the pleasantries are over?"

Ben knew that he had no choice but to comply—Ruth almost always stated her requests to Ben in forms of questions, particularly when they were with other people, even family. Her father, a rabbi, had been particularly fond of giving answers by asking questions. His influence was obvious. And it was a good one, for it allowed Ben to be the "businessman" and Ruth, true to her disposition, to be the diplomat if Ben were too blunt.

"Look, Arnold and Saundra, we have been thinking about our Wills and about our deaths. It's no fun to think about dying. And it's not much use for us to wait until we're dead for you and Anna to enjoy what we've earned. So, we want to make a gift now—to the two of you, and to Anna. In your case, it's easy. Arnold, you taught me how: just comply with 'Rule One' of the Lawyer's Rule Book. Remember?"

Arnold, not prone to embarrassment, nonetheless shifted in his chair and cast his eyes downward. "Yes, dad, I remember. Rule One says that the lawyer should get his cash in advance."

"Right," said Ben, as he handed to Saundra—not to Arnold, for Ruth had said he should include Saundra in a very demonstrative way—a check for $100,000. Saundra had the good taste not to look too hard at the check; her alarmed smile, however, told more than any words that she was impressed, to say the least.

"Now," said Ruth, aware of the impact the gift had made, "let's talk about Anna. Can't we give her the same amount—or perhaps more—through a Trust that we can set up now? And then, after we die, she can get the remainder of the life estates we are establishing for each other. Arnold, you need to draft a Trust for Anna; we want to put money into it today. You understand, don't you?"

"Dad and mom," Arnold said, "you certainly have made clear what your intentions are, and far be it from me to do anything except support you fully. Right, Saundra?"

Nodding, Saundra said, "Of course, we wouldn't want it any other way. In fact, I think I would do just what you want to do myself . . . an important charity to take care of, like our synagogue, or a friend to remember by a gift, and a Trust for Anna. It's a sound plan and it helps everyone out, including Arnold and me. It'll be so reassuring to know that Anna has some assets in the hands of a trustee who knows her and her needs, and also understands your intentions."

"Yes," added Arnold, "it will help us to know Anna is set financially. You're very wise, mom and dad. And very generous, too! Saundra's not exactly poker-faced, is she? Let's forget all this business for the moment and look at a draft in a few weeks. Now let's go to dinner, and celebrate life."

The weeks passed as Arnold and his partners prepared a Trust for Ben and Ruth to consider. At another meeting, Arnold explained what a Trust is, what its functions and purposes are, and the factors that his parents should consider as they select trustees. What follows is the substance of his discussion with them, with examples.

WHAT IS A TRUST?

A Trust is created when one person (called a *grantor* or *settlor*) gives property to another person (called a *Trustee*) for the benefit of a third person (called the *beneficiary*). Ben and Ruth, each called a grantor, plan to give $250,000 (the property or *corpus*, meaning *body* or *principal* of the Trust) to the First National Bank of Chicago and Douglas C. Turnbaugh, Jr. (the Trustees) for the benefit of Anna (the beneficiary).

Although an unwritten Trust can be created, it is unusual and can cause problems. This is because an unwritten Trust can easily be challenged by other people seeking the property that was put into Trust. Thus, most lawyers, like Arnold, will advise their clients to create a written Trust.

As the Levines just demonstrated, a Trust can be created during the grantor's lifetime. This is called an *inter vivos* Trust because it is created "between living people" (which is roughly how inter vivos translates). Also, a Trust can be created under a person's Will. This is called a *testamentary Trust* because it is created under the Last Will and Testament and does not come into effect until the maker of the Will dies.

Consider using either or both types of Trusts. Your decision will be based on your capacity to part with money today (inter vivos) and on your perspective concerning all other matters that we discuss in this book.

How large does an estate have to be to justify a Trust? There is no fixed rule. Generally, a Trust can be funded (created) with any reasonable sum (e.g., $10,000 will generate $800–$1,200 annually, depending on the rate of return). Also, the greater the amount available for a Trust, the wiser it is to create a Trust, particularly if the beneficiary has partial competence or complete incompetence. Finally, to keep federal taxes to a minimum, a Trust should be used when the assets of the grantor or grantors exceed $600,000. This is because federal estate taxes apply to a husband-wife estate that exceeds $600,000.

So, the Stuarts, who are not as affluent as the Levines, should consider a Trust for Steven. Odessa Harris, who has a life insurance policy for $25,000, may want to create a Trust for Jolene, using the life insurance. The Stuarts and Webers—who own real estate as well as personal property—may want to consider putting land into the Trust, along with cash.

WHAT ARE THE PURPOSES OF A TRUST?

A properly drafted Trust fulfills many equally important purposes:

To Leave Funds to Benefit a Person Who Cannot, or Who Needs Assistance to, Manage the Funds

For example, you may create a Trust for the benefit of your son or daughter who is a minor or who is an adult with partial competence or complete incompetence. If your son or daughter lacks complete competence in decisions related to acquiring and spending money, it means that he or she needs to have some, if not all, financial decisions made entirely by someone else (i.e., he or she needs substitute decision-making). In these cases, your Trust makes it possible for your son or daughter, the beneficiary, to have the benefit of your money and avoid losing those funds because of partial or full incompetence in managing them.

You may find it helpful to refer back to Figure 4.2 (see Chapter 4), which you used to determine the extent of your son's or daughter's mental competence and the appropriate kind of consent he or she is able to give. If your son or daughter requires substitute consent for decisions related to acquiring or spending money, a Trust is a way of saying who will be the trustee, that is, the person with the power to give substitute consent. A Trust may also be appropriate for people who are capable of giving direct consent when the Trust involves management of a large sum of money, but who are partially competent (i.e., may need special assistance in managing money).

Besides considering the kind of consent appropriate for your son or daughter, you might also reflect on whether your son or daughter already is under financial or general guardianship, whether unscrupulous strangers might try to get his or her assets, and even whether other members of your family might try to get his or her assets.

* * *

"Arnold, you and Saundra are learning what Ruth and I have, unfortunately, known for a long time. There are some very nasty people out there," Ben said, pointing to the streets far below Arnold's law office. "Your mother and I recognize that Anna is mentally competent. In fact, she has a lot of good sense. Common sense, you know, is the least common of the senses. It would be excessive for her to have any kind of court-appointed guardianship. Still, $250,000 isn't chicken feed, and, frankly, her being an attractive woman and wealthy—well, we'd feel better if we could make it possible for Anna to have her own money and keep it out of the hands of someone who might want to marry her or do business with her just to get her money. She's so trusting. And so few people out there are worth that trust."

To Leave Funds to Your Child That Will Supplement Government Support or Other Agency Assistance

The Trust makes it possible for you to provide for the life-style expenses of your son or daughter, over and above any provisions made by government agencies or other organizations. Government benefits may provide only minimum subsistence (e.g., SSI pays $354 per month). You may want your son or daughter to have access to more of life's necessities, and even some privileges.

*   *   *

"Saundra and Arnold," Ruth said, always careful to include her son's new wife in the family circle, "Anna has been a privileged young woman. Like the two of you—camps, nice clothes, music lessons, all the extras that make life so different, so . . . well, special. She doesn't know what it means to go without something she wants. Remember, Arnold, when she was a little girl? When one of her toys broke, she always said, 'Broken, busted, and throwed away. Go to the store and get another.' That's how we want it to be for her as an adult—the extras should be hers. We can't rely on the government programs to provide the extras, and we shouldn't."

To Avoid 'Spend-Down' Requirements

As we just noted, the Trust makes it possible for the Trust funds (income and principal) to cover life-style provisions that other benefits might not. Equally important, the Trust prevents the government or other agencies from using the Trust funds to pay for services they furnish. Federal, state, and local government agencies will sometimes seek to recover the cost of services they furnish to the beneficiary, especially for room and board, clothing, and medical and other habilitation services. They will be especially aggressive if the beneficiary is a resident of a state institution. They will try to make the Trustee spend down the Trust assets in order to get reimbursed for services rendered, and to assure that the person with a disability is also poor enough to qualify for government assistance based on financial need.

*   *   *

"Dad and mom," Arnold said, "I'm glad you decided to use a Trust in order to preserve Anna's property. Illinois is not much different from other states. It wants to avoid having to pay for the services it provides to Anna. It especially wants to be able to charge her for any services it provides in the state institutions. Don't get the idea that Anna belongs in one of them. In my judgment, nobody belongs there, especially Anna. But, for example, she might wind up in a facility as a very old lady, and the state might want to charge her for taking care of her there. If we are careful in writing the Trust for her, she'll be able to avoid those cost-of-care charges and any spend-down claims. After all, you've more than paid into the state's treasury, and even Anna, now that she's working, is paying taxes, too. You're wise to set it up so that the state can't get to the property you're putting into Trust for her."

To Leave Your Child Funds without Disqualifying Him or Her from Benefits

We have just noted that two purposes of a Trust are 1) to provide money over and above what is provided by government benefits, and 2) to prevent the government from requiring your son or daughter to spend down his or her assets to the point of being financially needy. There is another aspect of Trusts that we must discuss now—the rule that government benefits are only for those who are financially needy, and the relationship of that rule to Trusts.

A properly drafted Trust will provide funds to your son or daughter without disqualifying him or her for government benefits that are based on financial need and are set aside for people with a disability. Many government benefits are based on financial need. If the beneficiary of a Trust has enough assets, he or she is not financially needy. The Social Security Administration, which administers the major federal entitlement programs (Social Security Disability Insurance [SSDI], and Supplemental Security Income [SSI]), uses complicated rules to determine if an individual is financially needy, and therefore eligible for SSI. The Social Security Administration will try to require the trustee to spend down the principal of a Trust to a set level ($1,900 for SSI) before it regards the beneficiary as financially needy, and therefore eligible. A successful spend-down claim by Social Security can result in Trust assets being used to pay for services and in the Trust being depleted except for the minimum amount ($1,900). But if the Trust is properly drafted, a spend-down cannot be required. The properly drafted Trust will not be required to pay for services that the government would otherwise provide. Thus, enough money will stay in the Trust to supplement minimum government benefits and provide for unforseeable circumstances.

As we have explained, most people with a disability seek to participate in federal or state aid programs based on financial need. If your son or daughter has assets that he or she can control, the law requires the beneficiary to spend down those assets for self-support. The government's policy in these cases is to conserve its assets and help only those people who are financially needy. If a person has assets, there is no financial need, and therefore no government benefits. The properly drafted Trust can separate the Trust assets from the beneficiary, making a person with a disability financially needy and thereby still eligible for government benefits.

* * *

"Odessa," Owen Weeks said to his sister, "the policy of our governments is to keep people with disabilities off the so-called welfare rolls by helping them get jobs. But sometimes—usually, in fact—a person with a disability needs government help. The Social Security programs, like Supplemental Security Income and Medicaid, are especially useful. We'll talk about those programs later. But for now, the important thing is that Jolene—like other people who want to participate in those programs—must be not just disabled, but relatively poor, too. You see, the government's policy is to help people who can't help themselves because they have no money and no way to earn enough. So, the small Trust that you can create can provide Jolene additional money, and still not get drawn down to the level that the government requires in order to let her participate in the programs. But the Trust has to be drawn up properly, and that's a lawyer's job."

To Give the Trustee Maximum Flexibility in Financial Decision-Making

The Trust can and should allow the Trustee maximum flexibility. This is because your son's or daughter's needs cannot always be anticipated; events may occur that will change circumstances. For example, government benefits might be changed; your son or daughter could move into a new residence or need surgery; another family member could decide to bring your son or daughter into his or her home; your son or daughter may need expensive therapy or specialized equipment. In addition, the Trust should provide maximum flexibility in order for it to accomplish the purposes described above: preserve assets from waste, supplement government benefits, prevent cost-of-services charges, and prevent disqualification from benefits.

How can the Levines anticipate the future, help Anna, and still guide the Trustee?

* * *

"Arnold," his mother said, "your father and I appreciate your help in preparing this draft of a Trust. But, frankly, it seems to us that the Trustee has the final word on everything. We told you what we wanted for Anna, but you—and maybe it wasn't you, maybe it was your partner—have given the Trustee practically no direction whatsoever. Is that the way it should be? Don't mind our asking, but we have to know. All this language about pure and absolute sole discretion—is it really necessary, or should we be clearer and tell the Trustee just what we want done?"

"Mom," Arnold replied, "and you, too, dad, it's a complicated matter of law. And it's a reality, too. Let's talk about the reality now; we'll talk about the law later. The fact of the matter is that we can make plans, but we can't tell from one day to another what the future will hold. My senior partner tells me, 'Arnold, in practicing law, take nothing for granted, assume nothing, plan for everything, and don't rely on history to be a guide to the future in the lives of your clients. There is so much about life that is unpredictable.' Frankly, that advice is awfully good. No one in this room, or even in this world, knows what will happen to any of us, much less to Anna. So the more flexibility we give the Trustee, the better the Trustee can deal with the unanticipated events of the future."

To Provide for Expert Management of Property

Under the law, the Trustee must:

> Collect all assets put into the Trust (e.g., money, insurance proceeds, and personal and real property), sell those that should be liquidated, and collect income from income-producing assets (e.g., stocks, bonds, and real property).
> Invest assets to secure maximum income consistent with the preservation of capital and the needs of the beneficiary.
> Spend income and principal, when necessary or desirable, for the beneficiary.
> Account to the beneficiary, guardian, and other interested people (e.g., *remaindermen*, people who will benefit from the Trust on death of the first beneficiary) or courts with jurisdiction over the Trust or the beneficiary.
> File necessary tax returns or furnish necessary information to the beneficiary or guardian, if one is appointed, so that tax returns can be filed.

*   *   *

"Arnold," Ben said, "I want a good Trustee, someone who knows all about money. That way, the Trustee can be the money manager and you, Saundra, and Anna, won't need to be bothered. Let's get the bank to do the job. Mr. Mathias is a great trust officer, and that new woman in the Trust department, Ruth White, is super sharp. They can save us the trouble of doing the accounting."

To Preserve the Interests of Remaindermen

Remember that Ben and Ruth are giving money to a Trustee for Anna's benefit. They do this through inter vivos and testamentary Trusts. They also have provided that, after Anna dies, the property in her Trusts will go to Arnold's and Saundra's children. In making a gift to Anna through the two Trusts, Ben and Ruth have created a *life estate*, that is, a right of Anna to have the use of the Trust property for the duration of her life. In providing that the property will go to their grandchildren after Anna dies, Ben and Ruth have created a *remainder interest:* whatever remains in the Trust after Anna dies is the property of the *remaindermen,* namely, the grandchildren.

More than this, Ben and Ruth each have left the bulk of their other property to each other, with a remainder to Anna and then to Arnold's and Saundra's children. Thus, each of them has a life estate in the other's property, and Anna, and then Arnold and Saundra's children, are the remaindermen—the people who inherit after the last of the owners of the two life estates (each spouse and Anna) dies.

The Trustee has responsibilities to the spouse, who is the *primary beneficiary* with an interest (*estate*) during life (hence, life estate), and to the remaindermen. This is significant in terms of your planning for your son or daughter to have government benefits, because the interest of a remainderman justifies not spending down the Trust assets to enable the beneficiary to meet the needs test.

To Minimize Taxes

Generally, taxes on your estate can be minimized by putting assets into Trust (in which case, the assets are taxed later as the property of someone else). You need to decide just how important it is to minimize taxes. Then, you should compare that purpose of a Trust to its other purposes, which are concerned with the care and welfare of the beneficiaries.

WHOM SHOULD YOU SELECT AS TRUSTEE?

Ben and Ruth Levine, having decided to create a Trust for their daughter Anna, face the same two questions that confront Luis and Eloisa Rodriguez (Maria's parents), and Steven's parents, Jack and Rose Stuart. Who should the Trustee be, and should there be more than one Trustee?

Selecting a Trustee can be as important as deciding to create a Trust or designating the assets to be put into the Trust. This is because the Trustee is the person who will decide, consistent with the Trust's provisions, how its assets will be allocated to your son or daughter.

Ordinarily, it is wise to consider having two Trustees—a *corporate Trustee* and an *individual Trustee*. The corporate Trustee should be an institution (such as a bank) that can offer skill and experience concerning the duties of a financial fiduciary—managing a Trust, investing and collecting assets, preparing accounts, filing tax returns, etc. You should ask your local bank or Trust company if it will agree to serve as Trustee. You should also inquire about its fees, its experience (if any) with beneficiaries who have disabilities, and what size Trust it will agree to manage. Ben and Ruth have designated the First National Bank of Chicago as a Trustee; Luis and Eloisa have asked their local savings bank, as have Jack and Rose.

The individual Trustee should be someone who is familiar with your son or daughter, understands and supports the type of consent he or she is able to give, is cognizant of and respectful of his or her preferences, takes a personal interest in his or her well-being, is able and willing to visit with him or her, and can reasonably and fairly determine whether Trust funds should be spent. This trustee's duties are very different from those of the other Trustee. The individual Trustee is not so much a manager of the Trust's assets. He or she is more of an advocate for the beneficiary, and must also see to it that the intentions of the Trust (as expressed in a separate Letter of Intent) are carried out to the greatest extent possible.

To this end, Ben and Ruth have asked their son Arnold to be the personal Trustee for Anna. Luis and Eloisa have asked their son Geraldo to be the Trustee for Maria. Jack and Rose, however, feel that their daughters Sally and Theresa are presently too young for such a responsibility. Jack and Rose also feel that their daughters should not be asked, when they are adults, to become so involved with Steven that they may be unable to develop their own lives. ("I don't want them to be 'shipwrecked sisters,' unable to make their own way because of Steven," Rose said.) Therefore, they have asked their close friends, the Wilsons, to be Steven's personal Trustees.

You may decide that your child needs an individual Trustee for the purposes of managing the acquisition and dispersion of funds. This is the decision made by the Levines, the Rodriguezes, the Stuarts, and Odessa Harris and her brother Owen Weeks. Other grantors may decide that the beneficiary does not need an individual Trustee and may rely solely on a corporate Trustee.

If the corporate Trustee has experience with the grantor, the grantor's family, the beneficiary, or other beneficiaries with disabilities, a decision to use only a corporate Trustee may be valid. Usually, however, the representatives of a corporate Trustee do not have that experience, and will decline to visit the beneficiary or make other efforts to determine individual preferences about how funds should be dispersed. There may be an exception to this general rule in the case of "Congregate/Pooled Trusts" that are set up by state or local disability organizations for the express purpose of taking on both the corporate role of fund management and the individual Trustee's role of visiting and deciding about dispersement.

Take, for example, the Harris family. Odessa's concern for her daughter has prompted Odessa to put a small amount of money into a Trust for Jolene, the Trustee being the Chattahoochee Valley Association for Retarded Citizens (ARC). Odessa recognizes that Owen, who lives an hour's drive away from Jolene, would be happy to be the Trustee if he were closer. But, distance and the fact that the ARC is set up to be a Trustee and to handle small Trusts makes it wise for her to choose the ARC. Indeed, like many parents who want to establish Trusts with small amounts of money, you may find that these types of congregate Trusts are very useful, in part because banks will often handle only large Trusts (e.g., over $50,000), and will not agree to serve as both corporate and personal Trustee. In the case of congregate Trusts, however, the trustee will handle small Trusts (e.g., $5,000), and will also serve as a personal Trustee.

Trustees and Guardians

You may be experiencing a situation in which your child has been adjudicated as having partial competence or complete incompetence and has been placed under financial guardianship, with a financial guardian appointed by a court. In this case, you have two choices:

1. Ask the financial guardian to serve also as individual Trustee. This decision expresses confidence in a single person to serve as both guardian and Trustee.
2. Appoint an individual Trustee who is someone other than the financial guardian. You may want to do this to assure an additional perspective on your son's or daughter's need for funds from the Trust, to provide a checks-and-balances system of financial assistance, or to place the Trust in a person who may be more reliable or knowledgeable than the financial guardian.

You may face still another possibility, namely a situation in which your son or daughter has been adjudicated as having partial competence or complete incompetence and has been placed under personal guardianship, but not under financial guardianship. In such a situation, your son or daughter has a personal guardian, but not a financial guardian. Your options include using an individual Trustee as a supplement to the corporate Trustee and as a supplement to the personal guardian. This can be done in two ways:

1. Ask the personal guardian to be the individual Trustee, thus having the same person fill two similar roles.
2. Appoint someone other than the personal guardian to be the individual Trustee. This decision assures additional perspectives concerning your son's or daughter's needs for funds from the Trust, provides a checks-and-balances system of personal and financial assistance, and places authority over the Trust in a person who may be more reliable or knowledgeable than the personal guardian.

Another option, instead of using an individual Trustee, is to allow the corporate Trustee to pay funds directly to your son or daughter. This judgment reflects your belief that your son or daughter has sufficient competence to manage the money from the Trust. (However, as we point out in Chapters 14–16, this decision may make your son or daughter ineligible for government benefits.)

The Trust will be required to reimburse the individual Trustee, just as it reimburses the corporate Trustee, for services rendered and expenses incurred. However, the individual Trustee may waive (i.e., not claim) the fees and expenses.

Selecting an Individual Trustee

Selecting the individual Trustee requires that you be very careful about that person's concern for your son or daughter and ability to carry out the duties of individual Trustee. Accordingly, you may want to review the considerations outlined in pp. 136–138 to determine who is qualified and available to be the individual Trustee. You can determine if you and a prospective individual Trustee have consistent views by having him or her fill out "Things That Are Important about My Job," included in Section 5 of the Preference Checklist, and then deciding if there is sufficient agreement between your child, yourself, and the prospective Trustee to justify appointing him or her as Trustee.

Table 14.1.   Who should be involved in future planning?

A. Consider your son or daughter with the disability

1. How old is your son or daughter? What is his or her life expectancy?
2. Does your son or daughter have serious medical problems that may result in a shortened life expectancy?
3. Is your son or daughter now living at home?
4. Will your son or daughter eventually move from home?
5. When will your son or daughter move?
6. Where will your son or daughter live?
7. What are your son's or daughter's financial needs now?
8. How will your son's or daughter's financial needs change?
9. Does your son or daughter now work?
10. Will the work change?
11. How might health, residential, or employment changes affect financial needs?
12. What are your son's or daughter's abilities?
13. Can your son or daughter make simple, medium-level, or difficult decisions related to acquiring money? Can your son or daughter make simple, medium-level, or difficult decisions related to spending money?
14. What type of consent is appropriate for financial decisions?
15. How much money can your son or daughter prudently handle?
16. Has your son or daughter been adjudiated as having partial competence or complete incompetence?
17. Does your son or daughter understand that you are considering financial and other arrangements?
18. Does your son or daughter understand the effects such arrangements may have on his or her life?
19. To what extent can your son or daughter be actively involved in financial planning?
20. Does your son or daughter want to be involved?
21. What might be your son's or daughter's reaction to not being involved?

Anger?	Feeling no control
Resentment?	over his or her life?
Feeling unimportant?	Relief?
Feeling unloved?	Feeling protected?
Really doesn't care?	

22. Does your son or daughter agree with your choice of a guardian?
23. Have you talked about this with him or her?
24. What might be the effects of financial guardianship on your son or daughter?

B. Consider other family members

1. Who else in the family should be involved in financial planning?

Siblings?	Aunts?	Uncles?
Grandparents?	Cousins?	Others?

2. What are the ages of these people?
3. Do they understand the complexity of financial planning?
4. Do they understand the extent of your son's or daughter's disability?
5. Do they understand how this disability limits your son or daughter?
6. Do they understand the strengths your son or daughter has?
7. What are the abilities and strengths of these family members?
8. What could they add to the financial planning process?
9. What might be some negative aspects of involving certain family members?
10. Would you feel more comfortable working with certain people than with others?
11. What is the personal relationship between the family member and your son or daughter?
12. Do the other family members share your son's or daughter's values, ideas, preferences, and aspirations?
13. Do these family members share your values, ideas, preferences, and aspirations concerning your son or daughter?

(continued)

Table 14.1. *(continued)*

14. Do these other family members want to be involved?
15. Are there ways you could convince them of the importance of their involvement?
16. Do you value their input?
17. If there are disagreements between you and the other family members whom you involved in planning, how might you resolve them?
18. What might be the reactions of other family members if you do not involve them in planning?
19. What might the long-term effects of these reactions be on the family unit?

C. **Consider the family's future**
1. Changes are bound to occur to other family members:
   Other sons or daughters marry.
   Other sons or daughters have their own children.
   Members divorce.
   Members retire.
   Members' financial situations change.
   Members experience severe illnesses.
   Members move away.
   Members die.
   How might these changes affect your son's or daughter's financial needs?
2. What might other family members expect of you and your potential estate?
3. What do you feel about these expectations?
4. How do these expectations affect your son or daughter?
5. What are the goals and aspirations for the future of each family member (e.g., college, career, family life)?
6. What would the ideal future situation be for your son or daughter?

D. **Consider other people**
1. Are there close friends who should be involved in the planning?
2. Who are they?
3. How might they be involved?
4. Do you want them to be involved?
5. You will be discussing your own and your family's finances; are you comfortable doing so with friends?
6. What positive contributions might a person outside the family offer to the financial planning process?
7. What might be some drawbacks of involving friends?
8. Do you still want to involve friends?
9. Do your friends share your son's or daughter's values, ideas, preferences, and aspirations?
10. Do your friends share your values, ideas, desires, and aspirations concerning your son or daughter?
11. What is the personal relationship between your friends and your son or daughter?
12. Might your friends want to participate out of a feeling of obligation?
13. How will a friend's participation affect your friendship?
14. How will it affect your friend's family?
15. Will other friends resent not being invited to participate?
16. Do you have friends in mind who may want to be the guardian or trustee?
17. Have you discussed guardianship or Trusts with these people?
18. Do these people understand the duties a guardian or trustee must perform?
19. Are these people likely to change their minds in the future?
20. What will be the effects of being a guardian or trustee on their personal lives and those of their families?
21. What will happen if the guardian or trustee becomes severely ill, moves away, or otherwise becomes unable to fulfill responsibilities?
22. What if he or she dies?

(continued)

Table 14.1.   *(continued)*

23. Do you have a back-up person who might serve as a guardian or trustee?
24. Might some person resent the fact that you did not ask him or her to be a guardian or trustee?
25. How might you resolve any problems involving guardianship or Trusts?
26. Guardians can be appointed by the courts; what are your feelings about possibly having no control over who might be the guardian?
27. How might other family members feel about this possibility?

Last, you may want to consider whether the criteria you used to select a financial guardian are helpful guidelines for selecting an individual trustee. Both the financial guardian and the Trustee perform essentially similar jobs—they help your son or daughter with financial matters.

The 'Whole Family-Whole Life' Approach

When planning for your son's or daughter's future, you may have to take a close look at some hard facts. The process may not be pleasant. It may even be emotionally draining. Yet, this may be the most effective way to make decisions.

A basic assumption of this method (we call it the *whole family-whole life* approach) is that the way you and your family make decisions will be unique. What is right for another family may not be your style of doing things.

Table 14.1 includes a checklist that may help you think through the issues involved in financial planning for the future. Some items on the list may help you identify others who should be involved in the planning process. They are only suggestions to prompt you.

The considerations addressed in Table 14.1 can be overwhelming. Perhaps it would be best simply to bear in mind that the most important consideration is the match between: 1) the plans you make as the person who creates the Trust, 2) the willingness and ability of the individual Trustee to carry out those plans, and 3) the needs and preferences of the son or daughter for whom the Trust is created. If these three considerations fit well together, you should be confident that you have selected an appropriate individual Trustee.

*   *   *

In their separate and different worlds, Ben and Ruth Levine in Illinois and Henry and Lillian Weber in New York have come to the same conclusion: Their respective children with disabilities will have Trusts. The Levine Trust will be large compared to the Weber Trust, and Anna Levine, unlike David Weber, will not have a financial guardian. Notwithstanding these differences, each family has to face the same problem, now that each has decided to use a Trust: How can they use a Trust and at the same time avoid the spend-down rule, avoid cost-of-care charges, and still protect their children's eligibility for SSI, Medicaid, housing, and food stamp programs that require the recipient to be financially needy? To answer that question, each family has to learn how to make Trusts and programs based on need, especially SSI, work together.

15 HOW CAN TRUSTS AND SUPPLEMENTAL SECURITY INCOME BE PACKAGED?

As we pointed out in Chapter 9, a properly written Trust serves some important purposes. It provides for financial arrangements to be carried out by allocating funds to your son or daughter, passing along your estate, and packaging your private resources (money or other assets in the Trust) with the government benefits available under Social Security Disability Income (SSDI) or Supplemental Security Income (SSI):

> By packaging private and public benefits and avoiding spend-down and cost-of-care expenses, the Trust essentially serves as a source of private funds to supplement government benefits.
>
> By ensuring that the Trust assets do not belong to the beneficiary (are not assets), and that the Trust income is distributed in a special way, the Trust protects the beneficiary's eligibility for government aid based on need.

To accomplish these purposes, it is always best to create a *pure discretionary Trust*, avoiding any *mandatory Trust*. A mandatory Trust might be useful if the beneficiary did not have a disability, but it should be avoided in your child's case.

WHAT IS A MANDATORY TRUST?

A mandatory Trust typically requires the Trustee to make payments on behalf of the beneficiary. It also normally specifies when the distributions should be made (for example, quarterly) and the amount of the distributions (e.g., "all earned income" or "$1,000," or some other fixed sum). Because the mandatory Trust renders the Trustee powerless to withhold payment, it creates the potential for a government to assess a spend-down or cost-of-care charge against the distributions. The government would argue that the Trustee must make the payment to the beneficiary, because the mandatory trust, by its very nature, requires that payments be made. Once the Trustee makes the payment, the government will assess spend-down or cost-of-care charges against the beneficiary. Alternatively, it will assess those charges against the Trustee, who cannot withhold payment and therefore must pay a legitimate spend-down or cost-of-care charge.

A mandatory Trust also requires the Trustee to make the distribution if the Trust requires it for certain purposes (for example, for maintenance, room, board, or medical or other health and psychological care), even if government assistance is available for that purpose. That is, the Trustee of a mandatory Trust must spend the Trust assets for these purposes, and may not use the Trust assets to supplement the government benefits. The mandatory Trust, therefore, assists not only the beneficiary but also federal and state governments. This is so because the mandatory Trust makes the Trust assets available to the beneficiary for purposes that otherwise might be satisfied by the government programs.

The mandatory Trust can be used to prohibit the Trustee from spending for certain purposes, usually for purposes that can be paid for with government funds. This type of provision, however, is more typical in discretionary Trusts, and is discussed later in this chapter. Generally, it is a good idea to prohibit expenditures to cover charges that are reimbursable by government funds. For these reasons, mandatory Trusts generally are not favored by lawyers or Trust officers when the beneficiary has a disability. Instead, these experts favor pure discretionary Trusts.

WHAT IS A PURE DISCRETIONARY TRUST?

The *pure discretionary Trust* gives full discretion to the Trustee (who has "sole and absolute discretion"), with no payment amounts or standards specified by the terms of the Trust. As much as possible, it also insulates the Trust from spend-down and cost-of-care claims. This is because the beneficiary cannot compel the Trustee to spend any money; the Trustee's discretion is sole (belonging only to the Trustee) and absolute (unrestricted by specified payment amounts or standards).

On pages 143–145 of this chapter, we provide three illustrations of pure discretionary Trusts. As you read them, note how the language permits the Trustee to make whatever decisions are necessary or appropriate, including decisions to withhold payment on any or all occasions and for any or all reasons. Thus, the Trustee may refuse to make any payment to a government for spend-down or cost-of-care claims. With these powers, the Trustee can withhold the Trust assets from the government.

The grantor's intention as stated in the Trust determines whether Trust assets can be *reached* by government agencies, (i.e., whether spend-down or cost-of-care claims will be successful). So, language (i.e., the "drafting" of the Trust) is important. Consider two common types of language, *mandatory* and *precatory*. When the grantor uses words such as *hope, expect, wish,* and *desire,* he or she is using precatory language. Words like *direct* and *command* are mandatory language.

The best practice is to use language similar to that in the illustrative Trusts on pages 143–145. The key is to use precisely the right language, according to state law. This is so because in many states, 1) language that calls on the Trustee by command or wish to support the beneficiary may allow claims by governments to succeed, and 2) if another purpose is stated (e.g., "to supplement available governmental benefits"), those claims may not be successful, but the possibility still exists that they will be. Some states allow Trust assets to be totally insulated from state government cost-of-care or spend-down claims. You should check your state's law on that matter. Other states regard Trust assets as available to the beneficiary for spend-down and cost-of-care claims.

The best wording avoids the use of any standards that can be interpreted as creating a "Trust for support." Thus, you will want to avoid mandatory language, and even precatory language. This is because no claims by a government will be allowed if the beneficiary also cannot compel payment. Likewise, the best practice is to use "absolute discretion" language. For example, if a mandatory Trust requires the Trustee to make payments for the support and maintenance of the beneficiary, a government cost-of-care claim most likely will be successful. This is because the Trustee must pay the government for support and maintenance. The same result applies to other types of expenses, such as for medical care, education, training, recreation, or transportation. On the other hand, a Trust that includes "absolute discretion" language allows the Trustee to spend Trust funds for any purpose, or for no purpose. The Trustee therefore may refuse to pay spend-down or cost-of-care claims.

How can you give direction to the Trustee if you have to be so careful about the language in the Trust? First, you can speak to the Trustee about your plans and be careful to select a Trustee who understands what they are. Second, you may consider putting such information in a separate document, such as a Letter of Intent. The risk of putting any instructions—or even requests—into any written document is that a court may treat the Trust and written document, which physically are two documents, as one. Then, the court would read the two together and might interpret them as authorizing payment of spend-down or cost-of-care claims. Consult the illustrations on pages 143–145 to see how to draft a Trust so that (under present law) it can most successfully avoid spend-down and cost-of-care claims.

Some people think it is wise to add precatory language, stating the grantor's hopes and intentions, factors to be considered in deciding whether to make distributions, and general attitudes expected from the trustee. Those who like to use precatory language argue that it places a buffer between the Trustee and a government that wants the Trust to be spent down or wants it to pay cost-of-care charges. But, as a rule, this buffer will exist only when the grantor says that the intent of the Trust is to avoid spend-down and cost-of-care claims.

In that case, the Trustee who refuses to make distributions on the ground that government benefits are available and that the Trust should not be used to pay spend-down or cost-of-care claims is in a stronger position to resist a government claimant if the grantor states that the intention is to allow the Trustee to take that position. In the illustrations you will see language that suits this purpose. Whether to use precatory language is a technical and legal decision based on state law. The general rule is: Don't! It is very important to check state law and consult an attorney.

Whether or not precatory language is used, other provisions in a discretionary Trust are most useful. We advise that the following guidelines be observed when you draw up a discretionary Trust:

1. State the grantor's intention that: a) absolute discretion reside in the Trustee, b) the Trust is not to be the primary means of support of the beneficiary, and c) the Trust be used to provide supplementary benefits, beyond those provided by government programs.

2. Do not establish standards for the Trustee to follow (e.g., "support, care, maintenance, habilitation, rehabilitation, education, training, well-being") because those standards may provide an opening for a government that provided those services to sue for their costs. That kind of language also may create a right ("beneficial interest") in the beneficiary to enforce payments for those purposes. In that case, a government that is a creditor also can enforce them for the same purposes. This is so because if the beneficiary can require the Trustee to pay the beneficiary or another person for the costs of support or other costs, then the government also may sue the

Trustee to recover the costs of providing its services. Again, look at the illustrations on pages 143–145.

3. Include a *defeasibility* or *termination* clause authorizing the Trustee to terminate all or part of the Trust if any income or principal is required to be paid to a government creditor. If a defeasibility clause is used, the Trust also should contain instructions to the Trustee to distribute the Trust's assets to others when the Trust terminates. Typically, a Trust instructs the Trustee how to distribute the assets when the beneficiary dies. But the point is that the Trust should contain a clause that says that the Trust for the beneficiary with a disability automatically terminates (is defeasible) if a government successfully brings a spend-down or cost-of-care claim against the Trustee.

4. Include a provision allowing the Trustee to "accumulate income," thereby authorizing the Trustee not to pay out income and thereby help the Trust last as long as possible.

5. Consider giving the Trustee power to *invade principal* (i.e., to spend capital). This makes allowances for unforeseen circumstances in the beneficiary's life that require extra money. But there are disadvantages: a court may say that an invasion clause shows the grantor intended to provide support for the beneficiary and thus that a spend-down or cost-of-care should be paid by the Trustee; and therefore, the clause may create a "beneficial interest" in the beneficiary, which in turn may allow a government creditor to require reimbursement or spend-down. Again, the best practice is to avoid any standards for invasion of the Trust.

6. Require the Trustee to look into government benefits annually (and any amendments made to laws over the past year) and to apply for, collect, and use the appropriate ones.

7. If there is more than one Trustee, provide for how any conflict will be resolved.

8. Require the Trustee to visit the beneficiary and to obtain and pay for medical and other habilitation services, for necessary legal services, and for other types of services (e.g., recreation) that are not paid for by government benefit programs.

9. Name remaindermen (e.g., individuals or charitable organizations). The remaindermen clause may prevent a government from requiring the Trustee to spend down the Trust assets or pay cost-of-care charges. This is so because the Trustee has a duty not only to the primary beneficiary (the person with a disability), but also to the remaindermen. If the government creditor seeks to have the Trustee spend down the Trust or pay cost-of-care charges, the Trustee will argue that the Trust is established not just for the person with a disability, but also for others (the remaindermen), and that a spend-down or payment for cost-of-care charges will impair the interests of the remaindermen. In some states, this argument may convince a court to protect the Trust from a spend-down or cost-of-care claim.

MODEL LANGUAGE

As we discussed earlier, many technical problems can arise when you draft a Trust for your son's or daughter's financial support. The most important consideration is to draft a Trust in connection with government claims and in light of your son's or daughter's future financial needs. You should consult a lawyer. When you do, you and your lawyer may find the three following models helpful. Using the sample language below and following the warnings set out above will help protect the Trust from state and federal spend-down and cost-of-care claims, and help assure that your private funds supplement government benefits.

The Lawrence Trust

The following Trust language was used in Lawrence, Kansas, by the senior authors:

> The property identified in paragraph B hereof shall be held as a separate Trust, identified as the Family Discretionary Trust, and administered and distributed as follows:
> 1)   The Trustees shall utilize such portions of the income and principal of said Trust as, in their sole discretion, may be appropriate for the care and welfare of _____. In making such determination or determinations, the Trustees shall be guided in their sole and absolute discretion by their determination of what is in the best interest of said beneficiary and, in so doing, the Trustees may take into consideration all other resources which may be available for his support and maintenance.

The above paragraph has the following useful features:

1.   The Trustees are a bank and a relative of the beneficiary, but not his parents.
2.   The Trustees have "sole and absolute discretion" and "may," but are not required to, make any payments.
3.   The only "standard" for the Trustees is the beneficiary's "best interests," and that standard probably is too broad to create a trust for education, maintenance, habilitation, medical care, or other purposes for which government benefits are or may become available.
4.   The Trustees "may take into consideration all other resources available" for the beneficiary's maintenance and support and thus may decide whether to make or not make a distribution on the basis of available or unavailable government benefits, such as under Social Security or Vocational Rehabilitation.

The provisions in paragraph 1 of the Lawrence Trust will help keep the private funds in the Trust as supplements to government benefits, protect the beneficiary's eligibility for government benefits, and prevent spend-down and cost-of-care charges.

Paragraph 2 of the Lawrence Trust provides for further controls over how Trust money is spent:

> 2)   The Trustees shall not be required to make any distribution or distributions hereunder during the lifetime of _____, and may, in their sole and absolute discretion, accumulate and add to the Trust corpus all income earned during this period. The Trustees are specifically directed to make no payments in reimbursement to or for any governmental authority which may have incurred expense for the benefit of _____, nor shall the Trustees pay any obligation of said beneficiary where such obligation is otherwise payable by any governmental entity or pursuant to any governmental program of reimbursement or payment.

The above paragraph has the following useful features:

1.   The Trustees are never required to make any payments.
2.   The Trustees may accumulate—that is, save and not distribute—all Trust earnings.

3. These powers over Trust earnings are exercised at the Trustees' sole and absolute discretion.
4. The Trust commands the Trustees to make *no* distribution for spend-down, cost-of-care, or other government charges.
5. The Trust commands the Trustees to make *no* distribution for any purpose if government benefits are available for that same purpose.

All these provisions have the same effect as those in paragraph 1 of the Lawrence Trust.

The Wichita Trust

The Wichita Trust was developed by lawyers, trust officers, and disability specialists in Wichita, Kansas. Following are some excerpts from this model Trust:

> The remaining three-fourths (of my estate) thereof I direct that my Executor pay over to the (*bank's name*) in (*city*), and (*Trustee's name*) and (*Trustee's name*), as co-Trustees, to have and to hold the same in Trust, nevertheless for the benefit of my daughter, (*her name*), upon the following terms and conditions:
>
> 1. During the lifetime of my daughter, (*her name*), the Trustees shall pay so much of the net income and principal of the Trust to my daughter, (*her name*), as the Trustees in their absolute discretion deem necessary or advisable for the welfare of (*daughter's name*), after taking into consideration any other resources available to her including any benefits to which she is entitled through public assistance. Due to the anticipated size of the Trust corpus, it is contemplated that the Trust income and principal will not be available to provide primary support for my child. However, this Trust is for the benefit of my daughter, (*her name*), and I intend in no way to restrict the Trustees' absolute discretion in expending income and principal on (*daughter's name*)'s behalf. (*Daughter's name*) shall have no right in the income or principal of the Trust, other than those amounts distributed to her, in the exercise of the sole discretion of the Trustees. In the event my daughter, (*her name*), is unable to personally manage any payments of income and principal made to her by Trustees, then the Trustees shall make such payments of income and principal for the benefit of my daughter, (*her name*), as the Trustees in their absolute discretion deem necessary or advisable for (*daughter's name*)'s welfare.

The above excerpt includes some provisions similar to those found in the Lawrence Trust:

1. The Trustees have sole and absolute discretion, and the Trust is a *pure discretionary Trust.*
2. The Trustees must take into consideration the beneficiary's entitlement to government benefits.
3. The beneficiary has no right of ownership. Thus, the Trust assets cannot be regarded as belonging to the beneficiary, and the Social Security Administration cannot require her to spend them down or pay cost-of-care charges.

The purposes of the preceding provisions are the same as those of the Lawrence Trust.

The following provision divides responsibility between the corporate Trustee, which has financial duties, and the individual Trustee, who has personal duties to the beneficiary. This is the usual, prudent practice when there is more than one Trustee.

> 2. (a) In the administration and management of this Trust for the benefit of my daughter, (*her name*), the corporate co-Trustee shall have the primary responsibility of managing and investing the property and funds comprising the Trust estate while the individual co-Trustee, being sensitive to the problems, needs, and concerns of (*daugh-*

ter's name), shall have the primary responsibility of ascertaining and providing for her care and needs and directing such expenditures from the Trust fund as will best fulfill and attend to (*daughter's name*)'s care and personal welfare.

The following provision imposes a *visitation duty* (that is, a duty to accept personal accountability) on the individual Trustee, and imposes a similar duty on the corporate Trustee if the individual Trustee defaults. This is usual and prudent when there is more than one trustee (for example, when there is one corporate Trustee and one individual Trustee, or when there are two individual Trustees):

> (b) During the time this Trust is in existence for my daughter, (*her name*), I direct that the individual Trustee (and the corporate Trustee also, should the individual Trustee cease to act or serve for any reason) shall frequently and regularly make contact with (*daughter's name*), shall annually evaluate (*daughter's name*)'s current status, the services being provided to her and the prognosis for her development, and the suitability of her environment.

The following paragraph directs that potential disputes between the Trustees be resolved by the individual Trustee. This is usual and prudent when there is more than one Trustee.

> (c) In the event there should be any disagreement between the Trustees as to expenditures from the Trust for the benefit of (*daughter's name*), the view of the individual Trustee shall control.

The Maryland Trust

The Maryland Trust has been reviewed by staff at a Social Security Administration office. The beneficiary has been ruled eligible for SSI benefits, but payments by the trustees are made to his parents, not to him, so that he does not have assets or income. Following is an excerpt:

> The Trustees shall hold, receive, manage, invest, and reinvest the Trust estate and collect the rents, profits, revenues, income, and interest arising therefrom, and after first paying therefrom all taxes, charges, and expenses incident to the Trust, including full commissions to the Trustees, the Trustees shall pay so much of the net income and if necessary, so much of the principal, as the individual Trustee may deem advisable to or for (*son's name*) for and during the term of his natural life, any income not paid out to be accumulated and added to the principal.

These are some useful features of the Maryland Trust:

1. The Trustees have unlimited discretion to make or not make distributions.
2. The Trustees have the power to accumulate income.
3. The Trust is for the beneficiary's lifetime, and there are therefore remaindermen whose interests must be asserted by the Trustees against any claims of government agencies for spend-down or cost-of-care reimbursement.

These provisions are helpful for the purposes of supplementing public benefits and avoiding spend-down and cost-of-care charges.

* * *

After the Levine and Weber family attorneys studied the Trust issues discussed in this chapter, they prepared a Trust that fit the bill—one that allows the beneficiary to avoid spend-down and cost-of-care charges, but also allows the Trustee to supplement the government benefits payable to the beneficiary.

"Now," Arnold said to his parents, "it is one thing to get the language of the Trust into the proper form. But that is only one part of the problem of using a Trust and SSI and other need-based government programs."

"You mean there's more?," Ben asked. "How complicated can this be?"

Arnold answered patiently, "Yes, dad, there is more, and it gets pretty complicated. The next issue is this: How much money should the Trustee pay, and when? You see, Anna, or any SSI recipient who has a Trust, has to be 'needy,' and that means she has to limit her income and assets. The Trustee can do that for her, but it's complicated. Ready for an explanation?"

Ben answered, with resignation, "Yes, but first let's take a break . . . a long one!"

16 HOW CAN TRUST ASSETS AND INCOME BE PROTECTED?

We pointed out in Chapter 9 that government benefits based on need raise two initial problems for your financial planning and use of a Trust: 1) The government may seek to have the Trustee spend-down the Trust to the point where it is not an asset, that point being $1,900 according to current law; and 2) The government may seek to require the Trustee to pay cost-of-care charges from the Trust's income or principal. To resolve these two problems, we advised you to have a Trust with pure discretionary power in the Trustee and with other provisions.

To complicate matters even further, you must arrange the Trust and the payments from it in such a way that your son or daughter (the beneficiary of the Trust) does not have assets or income that disqualify him or her on the basis of financial need. In this chapter we show you how you can do this, using Anna Levine as our example and assuming that she is "disabled" for SSI purposes even though she is not adjudicated (or able to be adjudicated) to be mentally incompetent.

HOW DOES A TRUSTEE COMPLY WITH THE 'NEED' REQUIREMENT?

The general rule is that Anna is not eligible for Supplemental Security Income (SSI) unless she is financially needy. This means that Anna may not have assets in excess of $1,900 at any one time. It also means she may not have income of a certain kind and in certain amounts. To make sure that the asset limitation is not exceeded and that a Trust payment is not income, her Trustee must take certain steps. We will discuss the income rules first, and the assets rules later.

Income Rules

As we mentioned earlier, the Social Security Administration allows your son or daughter to have $65 per month earned income before it begins to reduce the amount of the SSI payment; it also allows $20 per month of unearned income before it begins to reduce the size of the SSI payment. Thus, your son or daughter may have $85 per month of income and still get the full SSI payment. After your son or daughter earns more than $65 per month, however, SSI payments are reduced by $1 for every $2 earned. For example, if your son or daughter has qualified for SSI payments and earns $90 per month, the first $65 is disregarded and the other $25 reduces the SSI payment by $12.50 (from $354 to $341.50).

Keep in mind that Anna's family has created two Trusts for her benefit and that they have set them up properly—that is, the Trusts are pure discretionary Trusts and do not constitute assets that the government may require the Trustee to spend down to the $1,900 limit. The Trusts have combined principal amounts (*corpus, capital,* or *res*) of $250,000, and the yield on that principal, at the rate of 8%, is $20,000 per year. If the Trustee pays the $20,000 to Anna, the payment will disqualify her from SSI. Since Ben and Ruth set the Trusts up to supplement the SSI benefits, the Trustee must be careful about how to make payments from the $20,000. The Trustee may even want to consider making no payments to Anna. The Trustee has four options:

Option One   The Trustee may make quarterly payments to Anna or for her benefit. Assuming that the quarterly payments are in equal amounts, Anna will receive $5,000 every 3 months. Because those payments will exceed the $1,900 asset limit, the Trustee may want to make smaller payments, say $1,500 every quarter. That $1,500 will be $400 below the $1,900 asset limit, assuming Anna does not have other assets, such as wage earnings. Anna should make sure to spend her SSI and wages, plus the $1,500 Trust payments, to a level below $1,900 on the first day of each month.

Whatever amount the Trustee pays, it will mean that Anna will have income in the month that she receives payment. In that month, she will be completely disqualified for SSI because the Trust payment will exceed $354 and because, under SSI rules, the SSI payment of $354 is reduced dollar for dollar for unearned income. In the next month, however, Anna may again be eligible for SSI payments if she does not exceed the $1,900 asset limit and has only her wages as income. Thus, if the Trustee chooses the option of quarterly payments, Anna will be disqualified only in the month that she receives the trust income. She will have to account for this income, and will be required to forego a payment for that month; but she does not have to reapply for SSI after each such month.

Option Two   The Trustee may make monthly payments to Anna or for her benefit. Assuming that the monthly payments are in equal amounts, Anna will receive either $1,666 or $500 each month, depending on whether the Trustee distributes $5,000 or $1,500 each quarter. Although the $1,500 will keep her below the $1,900 asset limit, it will put her above the $354 income limit. So, too, would the $5,000. Thus, if the Trustee chooses the option of monthly payments, Anna will be disqualified every month. In effect, Anna will completely lose SSI benefits.

Option Three   The trustee may make monthly payments of less than $354 per month, such as $100 per month. Although this choice will keep Anna below the $1,900 asset limit and below the $354 income limit, it will reduce her SSI benefit dollar for dollar, from $354 to $244 (since she receives $100 per month). Still, Anna will qualify for SSI (albeit for a reduced amount). Note that the Trust must allow the Trustee to accumulate income and to make only partial payments. Also note that any Trust income that is not paid out is "accumulated" and added to the principal of the Trust. Thus, the $250,000 trust is increased annually since only part of the annual income of the Trust is paid to Anna.

Up to this point, there seem to be no good choices for the Trustee. Whatever the Trustee does, the payment will affect Anna's SSI eligibility in one way or another. It will always reduce the full amount she might receive if there were not a Trust payment. There is, however, a fourth option, which can enable Anna to receive the full SSI payment and still benefit fully from the Trust.

Option Four   The Trustee may make no payments to Anna (or, in the case of someone under guardianship, to a financial guardian), but instead may make payments to her creditors for expenses other than food, shelter, and clothing. This choice will keep Anna below the $1,900 asset limit and below the $354 income limit, since she herself will receive no Trust payments. As a result, Anna will continue to receive the full $354 monthly SSI payment. In addition, her creditors can still be paid by Trust income for expenses other than food, shelter, and clothing. For example, the costs of redecorating Anna's home or room, buying new furniture (up to $500 in value), making contributions to her religious group or to other tax-exempt organizations such as the Association for Retarded Citizens, traveling to visit her family, going on vacations, attending summer camp, entertaining family and friends, obtaining legal advice and engaging in lawsuits (e.g., concerning guardianship or sterilization), obtaining medical or habilitative care that is not covered by Medicaid or any other third party, owning or leasing and operating a personal telephone, or otherwise carrying out her daily life, can be paid by the Trustee. The Trustee would make payment directly to Anna's creditor (e.g., the painter, travel agency, or telephone company). This means that Anna herself would not have the payment treated as her income (because she does not receive it), and that her SSI payment would not be reduced in the amount that the Trustee pays to her creditor.

Considerations for the Trustee   The Trustee must make several considerations when choosing which option to pursue. First, does the Trustee have power to exercise any of these options (quarterly or monthly payments, accumulation of income, or payment to Anna's creditors)? If not, then the Trust has not been set up properly.

Second, is the Trust intended to supplement government benefits? If so, all four options are appropriate because they are consistent with the intention of the people who created the Trust. If not, they are still not necessarily inappropriate and still legitimately may be chosen. After all, the Trustee may use the Trust to maximize government benefits, even though the Trust itself does not indicate that the Trustee may use the funds in these ways (to supplement government benefits by electing one of the four options). If, however, the Trust prohibits this, it is not an option.

Third, is there a *remainder interest*? A remainder interest is a person or organization that becomes the beneficiary of the trust after Anna dies or after another designated event (e.g., after she marries). Remember that Ben and Ruth created the Trusts for Anna's primary benefit and designated her brother's children to be the remaindermen. Under these circumstances, the Trustee must consider both Anna's interests and those of the remaindermen. Accordingly, the Trustee may want to accumulate income for Anna's and the remaindermen's interests. In that case, the Trustee would want to make payments for Anna's benefit, but the Trustee would not oppose accumulating income into the principal of the Trust, thereby enlarging it for her benefit as well as for the remaindermen.

In the Levines' case, Ben and Ruth have named the children of Arnold and Saundra to be the remaindermen. What if Arnold and Saundra do not have children? Arnold, ever aware of all the possibilities, points out to his parents that they may not have grandchildren, that there may not be remaindermen.

"Dad and mom," Arnold adds cautiously, "one thing I learned at law school is a good lesson here: Never make assumptions. You've assumed that Saundra and I will have children, that you will be grandparents, and that our children and your grandchildren will be the remaindermen, as we lawyers say. That assumption may not be correct. What do you do then? Who gets the Trust money?"

Saundra, sensitive to the nuances Arnold sometimes misses, interjects, "Of course, Arnold and I want children. We've talked about it, and now that we have our degrees and once we're a bit further into our careers, we hope to have a baby, or two, or more. So, even though your lawyer son is right about assumptions, you have made one that we hope comes true. Haven't they, Arnold?"

"Yes, of course," Arnold replies. "Still," he asks his parents, "who will be the remaindermen if we don't have children?"

Arnold is right to ask that question. Any financial plan that creates a life estate (e.g., Anna's right to the Trust income and principal during her life) must also create a remaindermen interest (e.g., to Ben and Ruth's grandchildren). But if there are no grandchildren? Ben and Ruth make the decision to leave the remainder interest to the Johns Hopkins University.

"Arnold, you don't know this, but when your grandfather came to America, he lived for a while in Baltimore, before he came to Chicago and married your grandmother and started a family. During those early years he did very well at City College, that great old Baltimore high school, and then he got a scholarship to Johns Hopkins University. Your grandfather always told me that if I ever had a chance to make up that scholarship, in current dollars, I should. Now, I want to take care of you and Saundra and Anna, first, but then I want to remember what my father told me. By the way, I am sending a check this week to Hopkins, in your grandfather's memory. Better to do it while I still remember and have the cash."

Fourth, an important question for the Trustee relates to timing. Is it appropriate to make one choice now and another choice later? For example, the Trustee may choose one option now (e.g., payment to Anna's creditors), but later may choose another option (e.g., accumulation of income). Of course, the Trust must allow the Trustee to make the choices, but the Trustee may want to select one or another depending on the circumstances at the time. A careful Trustee will retain as much flexibility as possible, so that unforeseen events can be taken into account.

Fifth, is Anna's future so certain that the Trust can be spent down (even though it is not necessary to do so to qualify Anna for SSI or all income paid out or even though the pay-out may disqualify her from SSI benefits that month)? A careful Trustee will want to hedge against the future by conserving as much of the Trust as possible, consistent with Anna's SSI eligibility and her needs for food, shelter, clothing, and other necessary items.

In summary, it is absolutely essential that the Trust itself be a pure discretionary Trust (see Chapter 15) and that the Trustee expend the principal and income in ways that benefit Anna herself and maximize her SSI eligibility, since that is Ben and Ruth's intention. Some people who create Trusts are not concerned with maximizing the beneficiary's eligibility for SSI benefits. In those cases, the choices facing the Trustee are not nearly so complicated. If, however, the purpose of the Trust is to supplement the SSI benefits, the Trustee will have to calculate frequently and carefully how often payments will be made and to whom they will be made.

Rules Concerning Assets

Up to this point, we have been concerned mainly about the payment of Trust income and how the payment might be income to Anna that would reduce or eliminate her SSI payment. But we said earlier that there are special Social Security Administration rules concerning assets. These rules exist to assure that a person who applies for SSI is financially needy. In some situations, the rules will result in a determination that the person has assets that exceed the allowable limit of $1,900 and therefore is not financially needy. The following discussion illustrates the rules, and shows how a properly drafted Trust and a careful Trustee can help someone receive both the SSI and Trust payments.

Beneficiary's Assets—$1,900 Limit To begin with, Anna should not have assets worth more than $1,900 at the time when the Social Security Administration makes its monthly count of her assets (usually the first day of the month). Certain items of property are excluded from the definition of assets (e.g., clothing and furniture). By and large, assets include real property (e.g., land, house, farm, and buildings, but not the personal residence) and personal property (e.g., cars, trucks, boats, stocks, bonds, jewelry, life insurance with a face value of more than $1,500, savings accounts, checking accounts, savings certificates, items in safe deposit boxes, promissory notes, household or personal items valued at more than $500, prepaid contracts for burial expenses worth more than $2,000, cemetery lots or crypts, life estates or heir property, or cash). As noted in Chapter 11, there are limited circumstances in which real property is not an asset.

Anna's Trustee and family should not make gifts of cash or other assets to Anna, and they should discourage others (like Arnold and Saundra) from making gifts to her in any amount over $1,900 unless the gift is placed into just the right type of Trust or can be spent or depleted before the Social Security Administration can count it as an asset. Social Security normally will count assets as of the first day Anna applies for SSI, or, if she already has qualified for SSI, as of the first day of the next month after the last SSI payment made to her.

The 'First Day–Next Month' Rule The Trustee and Anna's family must make sure that the $1,900 asset limitation is not exceeded on the first moment of the first day of each month after Anna has qualified for SSI. If she has assets over $1,900 at that moment, her SSI payments will be reduced or eliminated altogether. Thus, everyone must be careful that enough of Anna's assets are spent before the first of each month so that they are not more than $1,900.

Property That Constitutes Assets—Avoiding the Effects of the $1,900 Rule
Next, the Trustee and her family must know that Anna's assets include the types of real and personal property noted above, plus wages; SSI payments; any other payments from pensions, annuities, unemployment compensation, workers' compensation, Veterans Administration payments for education, Veterans Administration payments based on need, Veterans Administration payments not based on need, Railroad Retirement Board payments, Civil Service benefits, and Black Lung payments; rental income; lease income; dividends; royalties; interest income; support or contributions from any person or organization (such as cash, free room, free food, clothing, and gifts); and other income of any kind (e.g., earned income tax credits).

Because many of these assets also may be income that can disqualify Anna from SSI payments, in whole or in part, the Trustee and her family must manage each of these sources so as to keep it from being an asset (e.g., they should put it into a Trust) or to keep it from being income. This means that they will want to make a careful estimate of all sources of income and, when possible, control the amount of payments so that Anna's assets do not exceed $1,900 on the first day of any month. They may do this by deferring or just not making certain contributions to assets. If the Trust allows it, Anna's Trustee also may defer, reduce in amount, or simply not make payments of income or principal.

For example, assume that Steve Stuart has qualified for SSI and receives $354 in SSI payments, is allowed $20 in personal funds, and earns $300 a month. His assets from these sources total $674 monthly. In addition, he receives payments of Trust income in the amount of $100 per month. He has not exceeded the $1,900 limit. He will, however, have problems with his eligibility for full (or any) SSI monthly payments, as we explained earlier in this chapter.

Or, assume that Anna Levine receives the same SSI ($354), is allowed the same personal allowance ($20), and earns $450 per month, for total assets of $824. She also receives income of $1,500 from a Trust every quarter. In the month that she receives the $1,500, she will exceed the $1,900 limit, and therefore will be disqualified in whole or in part from receiving SSI the next month. To avoid this, Anna's trustee should not make quarterly payments but instead should make monthly payments of $500 (one-third of $1,500). In that way, Anna will have assets of $1,324 in any one month, well below the $1,900 limit. (Like Steve Stuart, however, she will have problems with her eligibility for SSI monthly payments, as we explained earlier in this chapter.)

Avoiding the Effects of the $1,900 and 'First Day' Rules   Just because Anna has more than $1,900 at any one time, she is not automatically going to lose or experience a reduction in her next month's SSI. This is because Anna may spend some of those assets for personal purposes, e.g., rent, food, clothing, medical care, or recreation. She may thereby reduce her assets to an amount below the maximum sum and may even reduce them below $1,900 as of the first of the month.

Two important considerations are reducing the assets below $1,900 as of the first of the month, and not buying property that itself is counted as an asset (e.g., land, stocks, certificates of deposit), because doing so simply changes the nature of the assets instead of reducing them below $1,900 in value.

DOES SOCIAL SECURITY TREAT TRUSTS AS ASSETS?

It is important to remember that the Social Security Administration will treat as an asset (for purposes of the $1,900 limit) certain Trusts that name the person with a disability as a beneficiary. There are several important points we would like to make about these Trusts.

Trusts' Purposes and Pure Discretionary Trusts   As we have emphasized, the purpose of most Trusts for beneficiaries with disabilities is to supplement, not supplant (take the place of) government benefits, especially SSI. This is why Ben and Ruth, with Arnold and Saundra's advice, created Anna's Trust. For Trusts to provide additional income over and above SSI, they must be created as pure discretionary Trusts and payments must be carefully planned so that, together with all of Anna's other assets, they do not exceed $1,900 at any one time.

Trusts as Nonassets   Under the current rules and regulations of the Social Security Administration, a Trust created by someone for the benefit of someone eligible for SSI is not considered an asset of that person so long as 1) he or she is unable, under the terms of the Trust, to dispose of any of the income or principal of the Trust, and 2) the Trust's assets were not transferred from the person to the Trust.

The first qualification deals with the *power of disposition,* that is, the legal power of the beneficiary to require the Trustee to use the Trust income or principal in certain ways. Most Trusts are created by a parent or other family member (grantor) for the benefit of the person with a disability (beneficiary). Usually, the grantor will not permit the beneficiary to have any say in how the Trust's property is used, because the beneficiary has a disability and the grantor usually will not want to rely on the beneficiary's judgment in the distribution of the Trust assets. Therefore, the Trust's property is not considered the beneficiary's asset for the purposes of qualifying the beneficiary for Social Security benefits. Thus, Anna does not own as an asset any of the Trust property. She has no right (called an *equitable* or *beneficial interest*) to require the Trustee to make any distribution.

However, sometimes a grantor will deliberately or inadvertently give the beneficiary the legal power to say how the Trust's property is to be used (i.e., the power to dispose of the Trust's assets). In this case, the Social Security Administration regards the Trust as the beneficiary's property because the beneficiary in effect owns the Trust's property and Social Security will require the Trust to be spent down to the level of $1,900.

Trusts should be carefully drafted to make sure that the beneficiary does not have the legal power to dispose of the Trust's property and to avoid having the Trust become regarded as an asset of the beneficiary.

The second qualification is that the beneficiary's own property should not be used to create a Trust. There is a good reason for this rule. The property in a Trust will be regarded as the beneficiary's asset if the beneficiary's own property is used to create the Trust. For example, it is conceivable that a person with a disability (such as Anna) would create a Trust for her own benefit, putting property in the trust that she owns (e.g., her savings account). It is also conceivable that one or more grantors (Ben and Ruth) will put property into the trust held in joint or co-ownership with the beneficiary (e.g., stocks or bonds). Since joint or co-ownership means that each of the owners—in this case, Ben, Ruth, and Anna—are owners, the property put into the Trust is Anna's. In both cases, the Social Security Administration will regard the trust as having been created for the purpose of evading the $1,900 asset limit. The Social Security Administration will regard the property in the Trust as Anna's assets for a period of 24 months after the property was transferred into the Trust; this usually is enough time to have the Trust spent down.

Deeming, Parents, and Trusts   There is still another important Social Security Administration regulation to consider when you create a Trust. Social Security regards the assets of the parents (Ben and Ruth) as assets of the child (Anna) who has a disability and *deems* (attributes) the parents' assets to belong to their child until she is 18 years old. Even after Anna has reached age 18, Social Security deems payments for a place to live (rent or a mortgage), insurance, taxes, fuel, electricity, gas, water, sewage and garbage removal, food, and clothing provided by her parents to be her assets. This means, in effect, that Ben and Ruth, as parents, may not provide these items to Anna after she becomes 18 without her being regarded as having them as assets and therefore losing all or part of her benefits. Ben and Ruth therefore should plan carefully before adding their own funds to supplement Trust payments. (Remember the earlier discussion of the considerations relevant to where an SSI-eligible child lives. Parents who want to obtain maximum financial benefits for their son or daughter will also have to take this factor into consideration.)

Parents As Trustees and Grantors—A Bad Practice   Finally, the Social Security Administration deems the property in a Trust to be the assets of the individual with a disability (Anna) if the parents (Ben and Ruth) create the Trust, name themselves (and not the bank) as Trustees, maintain control over the Trust, and name their child (Anna) as the beneficiary. Social Security takes this position for the reason that the parents are presumed to be evading the deeming regulations—essentially, transferring assets from themselves to the Trust so that the assets will not be counted as their own and thereby deemed to the child. Because the parents retain control over the assets as Trustees, however, Social Security treats the Trust as a sham and deems its property to the parents and thence to the child.

"Well, Arnold," says Ben, "I thought the rules would be so complicated that no one could follow them. But it seems that there are only a few, and that there are some simple guidelines. It's not too terrible."

"We agree," Ruth says, "don't we, Saundra?"

"Folks," says Arnold, "it's not exactly easy, either. But these rules are easy to understand, if you know the reasons for them. The same is true of the guidelines for a trustee. A well-drafted Trust, a careful Trustee, and a lot of faith and our share of good luck—all of that will get Anna as well prepared as your money can make her. Now, let's think about her life in the community."

*   *   *

At the same time the Levines are having their discussion, Lillian and Henry Weber are concluding their conversations.

"Henry," says Lillian, "I can't tell you how much I appreciate your listening to me. I know it's hard for you, and I'm grateful."

"Hard? for me?," exclaims Henry. "Why Lil, it's a piece of cake! Or, should I say, like chain-link fences, lap rugs, and new trees. You made it so simple . . . The hard part was your learning it and telling it all to me."

Pausing for effect, and getting only an agreeing nod from Lillian, Henry adds, "All the government benefits are like chain links or lap-rug squares. They connect to each other, and our careful planning is the thread, coupled with David's disability and being financially needy, that ties each to the other. Now, about those trees. The government benefits are the dry fertilizer. Our private money can be the rain. Together, they can help David grow . . . from unsteady sapling to a strong, mature tree. You know, Lil, he may have his disabilities, but if we use the right combination of fertilizer and water, there will be enough sunlight to show him how to grow. The more I think about it, the more I think David will see the sunshine in this little town. Next week, after we go down to the lawyer's, let's talk about the kind of sunshine he wants for his life. Let's talk about what he wants, where he will live, work, play, and so on. Let's talk about his future. I'm a lot more optimistic, now, thanks to you and our government."

"Henry," replies Lil, knowing she has won her battle to have her husband face the future with all his loyal courage and faith, "That's a wonderful idea. You sure do come up with good ones!"

section three

PLANNING FOR LIFE IN THE COMMUNITY

Sections I and II of this book were concerned with building a solid foundation for your son's or daughter's adult life. One of the pillars of that foundation involved making plans about who should make decisions now and in the future about your son's or daughter's life. The process of decision-making through guardianship and alternatives were addressed. The second pillar involved making plans to assure, to the greatest extent possible, that there would be adequate financial resources to support a quality life for your son or daughter.

With these two pillars firmly in place, it is now time to think about the structure that will rest on them. That is, what will the nature of your son's or daughter's life be? In the chapters that follow we explore adult needs in four broad areas: 1) life in the community, 2) relationships with other people, 3) the place one lives, and 4) the job one will have.

Throughout this section (Chapters 17–35) there is a strong emphasis on addressing your son's or daughter's personal preferences in all aspects of daily life. Your son or daughter may lack the mental competence to choose the actual place where he or she will live, but preferences can and should be realized in this setting. The same holds true for the employment, leisure, and social-interpersonal areas. Finances may rule out certain types of residential options, but a preference for a room color, a waterbed, certain foods and other aspects of life should be satisfied.

To help you identify your son's or daughter's preferences and choices, a tool called the *Preference Checklist*[1] is introduced in this section. This tool will become an invaluable aid when you evaluate programs and services for your son or daughter. The Preference Checklist can also help you and your son or daughter identify problems that may exist in programs and services. Identifying the problem is the first step in the decision-making process. This process can resolve shortcomings, and thus improve the quality of life.

---

[1]*The Preference Checklist: What's Important in Planning a Quality Life in the Community for People with Developmental Disabilities*, G.J. Bronicki, S. Ruben, J.A. Summers, C. Roeder-Gordon, A.P. Turnbull, and H.R. Turnbull, III. Development was partially funded by grant no. G008302983 from the U.S. Department of Education, and grant no. HD-01090 from the Mental Retardation Research Center, University of Kansas, Lawrence.

In this section, we describe various models of residential, vocational, and community services. Recommendations for finding, initially evaluating, and securing the services will be offered, as well as recommendations on how to conduct ongoing evaluations. Because your son's or daughter's needs and preferences are unique, this section has been developed to indicate the many options that will secure the types of programs and services that will provide for a high-quality life. We strongly adhere to the position that choice is the basis of happiness in all people's lives.

17 WHAT IS THE PREFERENCE CHECKLIST, AND HOW IS IT USED?

Werner Bismark walked gingerly across the snow-swept, frozen ground, his shoulders hunched and chin tucked in, trying to protect himself from the bitter cold February evening. The wind howled across the barren, brown fields that last summer had yielded an above-average corn crop. As Werner glanced over his right shoulder at the stark landscape, a blast of arctic air caused him to wobble slightly. He immediately straightened, and doggedly continued his purposeful walk toward the machinery shed. With each step, the meticulous old farmer reproached himself for his forgetfulness. Earlier in the day, he had meant to stop by the shed to pick up some tools he needed to repair a cantankerous gas heater. But the errand had slipped his mind until long after dinner.

Reaching the shed, he flung open the door, scooted inside, and pulled the door shut behind him. He yanked the light chain and, in the dim light, walked toward an old chair next to a sturdy workbench and wearily sat down. His breathing was rapid and his thoughts were focused on the experience of walking from the big farmhouse to the shed. The thought that he had almost fallen on the icy ground terrified him. Two years earlier he had slipped and badly bruised his hip. It had taken months to recover from that fall. "*Ach, mein liebe Gott!,*" he thought, "what if I fell and broke my hip?"

Werner was now 74 years old and clearly understood that a serious accident could end his days as a farmer. But the need to be careful critically limited the work he could do, and his farm was slowly deteriorating from lack of maintenance. The farm was his life. Although it encompassed only 380 acres, he was intensely proud of it. His father, Manfred, had fled Europe when Werner was 11 years old, determined to free the Bismark family from the incessant warfare in which old Prussia seemed to be mired. Manfred brought his family to settle among other German immigrants in northeast Iowa corn country.

Manfred bought 80 fertile acres and through frugal living and backbreaking hours added more acres to his dream. His intention from the beginning was to pass his land on to his sons, Werner and Otto. Land, the siren's burning call—the dream born deep within the soul. Many Americans far removed from their roots will never understand the ache within many recent immigrants to own land. Land that may be worked to produce food, be it a garden or a farm. Land that is yours, not that of an aristocrat, but yours. You may build on it, you may make a living from it. You sink roots deep into your land. Your family is raised on it and protected by it. It becomes your legacy to your children, perhaps a means to immortality itself.

When Manfred died at age 64, his homeland, now called Germany, was involved in yet another war. The last vestiges of the evil Third Reich were being battered. Berlin, bombed almost daily, was a crumbling mass of despair. All of Europe lay prostrate, ravaged by the consequences of human greed, nationalistic pride, and false doctrines. But in Iowa, the farm protected the Bismark family. The land sheltered Werner and his family in its warm bosom and allowed no harm to enter.

Werner inherited the land and added to it. He inherited other things from his father—a love of the land, and the desire to pass it on to his sons so that people could see that here in Iowa the Bismarks had found a safe harbor, freedom, and dignity. On the Bismark farm generations would grow and prosper.

As Werner sat in a dark corner of the machinery shed he shivered, as much from his thoughts as from the cold that boldly entered through the many cracks between the old boards. He assessed his life. He was 74 years old and in rapidly failing health. His wife, Maya, though 4 years younger, was also experiencing health problems. His oldest son, Herman, was 49 and had left the homestead many years ago to work for and eventually become partners in his Uncle Otto's hardware and feed store in town. Otto, Werner's only brother, had severed his ties with the land, preferring life in the small farming town of Himshoot. Werner felt a pang of remorse, knowing as he had for so many years that Herman, like Otto, would never return to the land.

Werner's daughter Uta, 45 years old, was married and was finishing the task of raising her own family. Her husband worked for the grain elevator in Himshoot and neither he nor Uta had any desire to become farmers. Werner's dream of passing on the legacy was firmly bound now to his remaining child, Ludwig, age 40. Ludwig was born after a very difficult labor and from his first day in this world it was apparent that he had problems. Ludwig developed very slowly and Werner was forced to admit on the boy's sixth birthday that his son was mentally retarded.

Ludwig never attended school, which was very common in the days before mandatory education for all children regardless of the disabilities some might have. Ludwig lived a protected life on the farm. He did a variety of daily chores but was never allowed to take risks or to express his personal feelings. After Uta and Herman left, Werner found that he depended greatly on Ludwig's help on the farm. Until he retired at age 65, Werner had worked as a mechanic at the farm implement dealer's store in Himshoot. A farm of only 380 acres could not support a family no matter how fertile the soil. Working long hours each day after his town job with Ludwig's help and the help of occasional hired hands, Werner was able to keep a firm grasp on his farm—his dream.

That dream, however, was slowly fading. The firm grasp had become precarious. Uta and Herman had recently begun to drop hints that they felt their father should consider selling the farm. Werner bristled at the thought. Herman had questioned Ludwig's mental capacity to own property and run a farm. Ludwig had problems, Werner thought, but his retardation was not that great. *No*, Ludwig would inherit the land and would sustain the legacy no matter what anyone else thought. Werner himself, and no one else, would direct the course of Ludwig's life.

"It's only fair," he thought. "Otto, Herman, Uta, they all left, they all quit. They have no right now to tell me what is best for Ludwig. They talk of Ludwig living in town and getting government benefits. Haven't I taught them about governments? Who would want to trust such things? Never—Ludwig does not need government money. Mein Gott, no Bismark accepts a handout. They talk of Ludwig getting training so he can work at a job. He doesn't need a job—he has one right here on *his* farm."

He hated the feeling but found himself powerless to force the bitterness from his mind. "Sell the farm, move to town and live on a tiny patch of dirt called a lot—worse yet, maybe be forced to rent." The thought of renting revolted him, it brought back visions of the disgrace and helplessness his father had felt living under the thumb of a powerful landowner in old Prussia. "No, by the last of my strength and will I shall never live such a life," he protested out loud. There was no one in the cold shed to hear his words.

He pulled himself up from the chair and shuffled toward the door, a battered toolbox cradled stiffly in one arm. The frigid wind slapped at his wrinkled face as he began the arduous walk back to the house. Bitterness shared room in his thoughts with fear as he slowly, painfully inched toward the back door of the deteriorating farmhouse that his father had built. The cold enveloped his now frail frame, which once had been that of a robust young farmer—a landowner. He must paint the house; the barn needed repairs; his hog pens needed attention; he wouldn't sell the farm. Ludwig will help; Ludwig will stay; spring would soon come; it would be warm and his body would gain strength from the sun; his other children, they wanted only the money from a farm sale; he must get a new tire for the tractor, in the spring, yes, in the spring a new tire; corn and soybeans, that's what he would plant this year—in the spring, yes, spring, the spring. . . These and other scraps of ideas first creeped, then raced through his mind.

The 30 yards between the shed and the house took Werner almost three-quarters of an hour to cover. He finally entered the house, but the warmth of the spotless, cozy kitchen did nothing to loosen the icy grip that possessed him. His hands and feet were numb from the walk and he felt a deep chill throughout his body. Maya walked into the kitchen and saw him slumped against the wall next to the door. He looked so old. She hurried to help him move closer to the woodstove in one corner of the room. Ludwig walked in and cheerfully addressed his father; "Oh, papa, you're back. Can we play dominoes now?"

"No Luddy," said Werner, "It is 9 o'clock, your bedtime—go, go to bed Luddy." "But papa . . . ," Ludwig tried to protest. "Luddy, you are tired, go to bed," Werner said, ending the conversation. After Ludwig left the room, Maya and Werner were alone with only the sounds of Ludwig trudging up the stairs to break the silence. "Some tea, my husband, I'll get some tea for you and you will feel better. Sit, get warm, I will get the tea," Maya said, moving toward the cupboards.

"This old horse, Maya, will not die, not yet. This old horse will not quit. This farm will remain the land of the Bismarks!," Werner proclaimed loudly, although his voice seemed to lack the resolve of years past.

* * *

Like your family and others, the Bismarks have been through many transitions. Werner and his wife are aging parents who have chosen to keep their son at home. Many other parents with a son or daughter with a disability have made the same decision; it remains a popular option for families today. Ludwig's brother and sister undoubtedly left home at a time that some would say was "on schedule." That is, they finished school and, perhaps went on to college. It is possible, given his age, that Herman was drafted, completed his military service, and returned to his home community, although not to his parents' home. Uta left home, perhaps after finding a job, and soon after married and began raising her own family, as did Herman. Uta and Herman made lives for themselves, most likely with minimal help and planning from their parents. This is the case of most children in most families.

Children grow up, mature, find jobs, rent apartments, find spouses, raise families, pursue personal interests, find jobs and change them, divorce, and remarry. They generally do these and other things "on schedule." However, the schedule for those with disabilities is often delayed. To succeed as adults, in adult roles, such individuals require considerable help and intensive planning.

Let's continue our comparison between the Bismarks and other families, perhaps, your family. Werner's older children developed their own interests and careers, and have no interest in following in their father's footsteps. While they love their parents and each other deeply, Uta and Herman are not part of what some would call a very close or tight family. That is not a criticism, all families are unique—what works for one does not work for another. Uta and Herman have recently started talking about their brother's future. Many people with brothers or sisters with disabilities have told us this is often the situation in their families. Although their reasons differ, they open the door. They see their parents growing old; they wonder what will happen to their brother or sister; they wonder what their role will be; they are often unsure of what is expected of them; they worry about finances; they ponder their own mortality, needs, and preferences; they seek closure, perhaps the security that comes from knowing a plan exists; they try to run, to hide; they fear; they hate the uncertainty; they love.

Werner is semi-retired, and although not poor, he and his wife face a precarious future, as does Ludwig. Werner has not drawn up a Will. He has life insurance, but has not had his policies reviewed in decades. He has an idea of what he and his wife can fall back on in an emergency—but only an idea. There exists a vast unknown down the road. Will Ludwig inherit the farm? Can he manage it? If not, who will help him? Should the farm be sold? If it is sold, what will Werner do? What will Ludwig do? If Werner dies, what will happen to Maya? To Ludwig? To the rest of the family? What if Maya dies first? Too many other families face a similar future of doubt. The importance of the issues discussed in Sections I and II of this book is now re-emphasized.

At age 40, "Luddy" Bismark is representative of many people. He never went to school, because in his youth there were no laws to guarantee what we now consider the absolute right to an education for people with disabilities. He missed out on the growth that accompanies the institution we call school—growth in academic and self-help skills; in friendships; in self-concept and feelings of personal worth. But, Luddy has grown and matured. We really are not sure of his tested and documented level of functioning, and frankly we don't care, because quality-of-life will not be found in test results nor in an IQ score.

Ludwig has deficits, but he has tremendous abilities. He can handle all the machinery on his family's farm. He has patience and compassion from which all the farm animals have benefited. He can read because his mother taught him. He knows what money is and like his father is frugal with his meager funds. He has friends—people from his church, people he's met and dealt with in town, and members of other farm families. His best friend is Gustar Ritter Von Kahn, the farmhand on the Heidelmanns' place just down the road. Gus is about Ludwig's age and they have much in common. They fish farm ponds together, they talk about crops, they help each other do their assigned chores, they share their pasts and talk about their hopes for the future. They are friends.

Oh, one more thing—Gus introduced Luddy to Helena Notsula. Holly, as her friends call her, and her older sister Paulina inherited their homestead when their father died. The sisters are making a go of their farm, but only because Gus and Luddy often lend a hand. The Notsulas raise chickens and eggs on a small, intense operation very different from the Bismark farm. Gus and Paulina consider themselves engaged and are planning for a combined future—hopefully soon. Holly calls Luddy her boy-friend—she cares deeply about him and the feeling is mutual.

Luddy's father does not believe his son has social and sexual needs and desires, and is very opposed to Luddy's interest in Holly. He refers to Holly as "that pushy Pole, pretty, but she should leave Luddy alone." It's not what you think—Werner harbors no prejudice, his own life found him the butt of crude, cruel treatment because of his background. Yes, he is set in his ways, but the pains of youth do not allow a mind that hates color, religion, or ethnicity. Werner's best friend is Chaim Moss, a remarkable man of Polish-Lithuanian and Jewish ancestry who farms the land next to Werner's holdings. Chaim's family fled the Old Country for reasons very similar to those of Man-fred Bismark, and Chaim happens to have a nephew with mental retardation who lives, on his own, in Des Moines.

Werner, in an attempt to protect his son, has allowed Luddy few opportunities to be independent. When Chaim questions Werner's reasoning, his answer is always the same—"Luddy is different, I will take care of him." Werner has tried to stop his son from seeing Holly—he fears what may happen. This has forced Ludwig into a situation he hates—seeing Holly on the sly. Ludwig has many aspirations in life and often finds the restrictions imposed by his loving parents troublesome. Ludwig also has fears—he knows that his parents and the farm—his life as it now is—will not always be there. Often he wonders, "Why can't I be what I want to be, why won't they let me?" Who are *they*? The answer is complex. Family, society, laws, fears, old wives' tales. Luddy has preferences and wants to make choices. He wants a say in his life, but he faces a wall of doubt, confusion, and denial: How far to let go? When to pull in? When and how to protect? How to determine what is best?

There are other similarities between the Bismarks and other families. The Bismarks are a first generation American family, a characteristic they share with the Rodriguezes and many other families. The American system may ignore cultural val-ues and appear distant and aloof. Government benefits may go unused, to the detri-ment of people who need them. Figuring out the American system can be difficult, so the information in Sections I and II of this book should be especially helpful.

First-generation American families such as the Bismarks are often deeply re-ligious—their faith sustains them through many a trial. Professionals in the field have been slow to recognize the incredible strength that accrues to families from the reser-voir of religious belief. That is changing, and the change is long overdue.

The Bismark family is not alone. Many families must deal with the conflicts of adulthood that face sons and daughters with disabilities. Personal preferences often clash with "the reality of the world." Yet, too often, preferences are sacrificed because they are not properly identified. This is often the case for people with disabilities, and it need not and must not continue. Personal preferences can be and should be the driving force behind any plan for the future. In this chapter, we explore some ways you can guarantee personal preference—the most important component of quality-of-life.

Who could best describe your personal preferences? The answer is obvious—if someone wanted to know your desires in life they would ask you to detail them. If for some reason you were unavailable, there are undoubtedly other people in your life who could provide some accurate insights into your preferences. Your husband or wife, a close friend, or a relative may be able to identify important issues in your life.

What of your son's or daughter's preferences? Who can best provide this information? In your planning for the future, you have been and will continue to be confronted with questions concerning your son's or daughter's preferences:

> Where would he want to live?
> What kind of job would she want?
> What sort of activities would she want to do in her free time?
> What does he like?

We are steadfast in our belief that any plans made for the future of a person with a disability must take into account that person's preferences and choices. If your son or daughter has a mild disability, he or she should be an active participant in your planning process. The situation becomes less clear as the degree of disability becomes more pronounced. Maria Rodriguez, for example, knows what she wants and can thoroughly describe her preferences. Jolene Harris has firm preferences, but may be less capable of making them clearly understood by others.

The manner in which you determine your son's or daughter's preferences will depend on the severity of his or her disability. You may find yourself in the position of being the person who must speak for your son or daughter or must interpret what your son or daughter says. You may be wondering, "What do they mean by 'interpreting'?" This can be answered with a real-life example:

A family was planning for a residential placement for their son, Jesse. Jesse has moderate mental retardation, but has only mild communication problems. Jesse's parents considered his preferences to be very important and wanted any future residential arrangements to be consistent with what he would want. One evening Jesse's parents were determined to pinpoint exactly what he wanted. His father asked in a straightforward manner, "Jesse, where do you want to live?" Jesse quickly replied, "In Massachusetts."

To many the response would appear senseless. The family had lived for years in Kansas, and before that they had lived in North Carolina. Why would Jesse want to live in Massachusetts? His parents, at first, were also confused, thinking that perhaps he could not comprehend the concept. Following some discussion, the picture became clear. As a youngster, Jesse had lived in a group home in Massachusetts during a period when his father and mother were experiencing personal difficulties and felt his needs could best be met in a group home setting. Jesse had returned to his natural home more than 10 years ago.

For Jesse, Massachusetts was not a state, but rather a statement of his preferences. The home in Massachusetts was a small, family-style setting where Jesse had lived with three other youngsters. The staff were well-trained and caring. Jesse lived in an environment where his dignity was respected. He learned new skills and had room for personal growth. The group home stressed individuality within a structured learning environment. Jesse made friends during his stay and over the years they were still remembered in his bedtime prayers.

Jesse's parents interpreted the meaning of "Massachusetts" for their son. Jesse wanted to move into his own home and into his own life as an autonomous adult, but he was not interested in just any home or the first available placement. He wanted to live in a place where he could have personal possessions, learn new skills, be respected, have friends, continue to go about his community freely, express his preferences, make choices, and continue to grow personally. Those were his preferences.

WHAT IS THE 'SHOES TEST' AND HOW CAN I IMPLEMENT IT?

In other cases, parents and family members must go beyond interpreting statements; they need to interpret meaning from behavior and from a person's past history. The *Shoes Test*[1] requires that a person view the world from the perspective of another, that is, place himself or herself in another person's shoes. If your son or daughter were able to express his or her feelings fully, what would be his or her preferences for the life he or she would want? We introduce the Hughes family in the next chapter, but for now, let's look at how they used the Shoes Test in their planning for their son Brian, 17, who has severe brain damage, limited mental capacity, and a limited ability to communicate.

Brian has severe and multiple handicaps, among which is the absence of speech. He has not yet learned to use an alternative mode of communication such as signing to make his wishes consistently known. There are, however, many behaviors that his parents have identified that indicate definite preferences. Throughout his life, Brian has shown on unusually strong dislike of confusion and noise. Whenever the Hugheses are entertaining friends, Brian fusses and cries until he is taken from the area of conversation and activity. He prefers music that does not include the harsh banging of drums, the sharp tones associated with reed instruments, or the tinny sounds of brass. In school, his teachers have long known that he does better in small groups.

When placements for Brian are considered, his preference for low-key environments should be kept in mind. It is unrealistic, and unfair to Brian, to expect him to adapt suddenly to things he has disliked his entire life. Some years ago, an attitude pervaded the service system that people with disabilities "need to adjust to situations around them because that is the real world." We now know that this attitude was only an excuse for a system that did not adapt to people. The adult service system must create a wide range of options to meet the individual preferences and needs of people such as your son or daughter.

Starting with this chapter, we introduce a *Preference Checklist* designed to help you and your son or daughter identify his or her preferences and choices in four major areas of daily life: *social-interpersonal concerns, community and leisure participation, residential placement,* and the *vocational area.* The checklist also contains an introductory section called the *Preference and Choice Questionnaire.* This section is designed to help you and your son or daughter identify general likes and dislikes, as well as to note the manner in which preferences are expressed.

Checklist Development

The development of the Preference Checklist was based on information collected during a 3-year investigation into the transition from school-based services to community-based adult services for people with disabilities. Working with 20 Kansas families, project staff identified a range of issues that were of primary concern in transition. More than 200 specific items were identified in the first phase. An early draft of the checklist was sent to more than 400 families throughout the United States that had

---

[1]The Shoes Test is described in detail in Hazel et al.'s 1988 book, *A Community Approach to an Integrated Service System for Children with Special Needs* (Baltimore: Paul H. Brookes Publishing Co.). Robin Hazel, in turn, acknowledges Elizabeth M. Boggs's essay, "Who Is Putting Whose Head in the Sand or in the Clouds as the Case May Be?," as an inspiration for the Shoes Test. Boggs's essay appears in the 1986 book, *Parents Speak Out: Then and Now,* H. Rutherford Turnbull III and Ann P. Turnbull, editors (Columbus, OH: Charles E. Merrill).

members with a disability. More than 200 completed checklists were returned and analyzed. Many new items were mentioned, but most of the original items were consistently rated as important by the families that participated. Items that were generally rated as having low or no importance were removed from the survey.

The checklist has been further reviewed by professionals in the human services field and their suggestions have been incorporated. It has been widely field-tested, and portions have been presented before several professional workshops and conferences across the United States.

WHO SHOULD PARTICIPATE IN
COMPLETING THE PREFERENCE CHECKLIST?

People with disabilities can and do express their preferences in one way or another about what is important to them. Certainly, those people who can speak or communicate through other means (such as voice synthesizers and Speak and Spell) can tell how they feel about things, places, and people in their lives.

It is imperative that your son or daughter be involved to the maximum extent possible in completing the Preference Checklist. You may also want to involve other family members and friends who are helping you plan, or who may be affected by any planning decisions. For example, if you were to determine that your son or daughter wants a job in an industrial park across town, the issue of transportation would certainly be a consideration. The decision that another son or daughter could provide the necessary transportation should be made only with the involvement of the affected person.

Given your unique circumstances, you may need to interpret for your son or daughter, or use the Shoes Test approach. If this is the case, you may find it useful to get input from other people who know your son or daughter. Knowing that other people agree with your interpretations and observations can provide peace of mind. If you encounter areas of major disagreement, discussing relevant issues can result in a clearer understanding of your son's or daughter's preferences.

HOW DO I COMPLETE THE
PREFERENCE AND CHOICE QUESTIONNAIRE?

Section I of the Preference Checklist (The Preference and Choice Questionnaire) is self-explanatory. It is designed to direct your attention to the general concepts associated with expressing preferences and making choices. It should also help you identify the many subtle ways in which your son or daughter indicates his or her preferences. View this section as a primer for the checklist itself. The Preference and Choice Questionnaire appears at the end of this chapter as well as in Appendix 3. You will also find the complete Preference Checklist in Appendix 3. As we proceed through this chapter offering suggestions for using the Preference Checklist, you may find it useful to refer periodically to the complete checklist. In this chapter, we use items from the checklist to help explain its use. We always identify the items so you can easily find them in the checklist provided in Appendix 3. We identify the items as follows:

Section _____ refers to one of the five sections of the checklist numbered 1 to 5.
Part _____ refers to one of the parts within each section lettered A, B, C, etc.
Item _____ refers to an item within a part, numbered 1, 2, etc., to the end of the
particular part.

Before proceeding with suggestions for completing the actual checklist, we
need to tie preferences and choices into the big picture of mental competence. Think
back to the material presented in Chapter 4. Some of the tables in Chapter 4 are referred to in this chapter to clarify the issue of preference and its relationship to competence (that is, the mental capacity to make decisions).

Now, turn back to Figure 4.1, on p. 32 in Chapter 4. Notice the first four columns relating to decisions your son or daughter will face as an adult. The chapters in
this section of the book deal with the areas listed in the first four columns of Figure 4.1:
life in the community, relationships with other people, the place one lives, and one's
job. In Chapter 4, we discussed the concept of the complexity of a decision and the
effect of complexity on the ability of your son or daughter to make reasoned decisions.
We said there were three levels of complexity: simple, medium, and difficult. We
noted that some people could make reasoned decisions at some levels of complexity,
for example simple or medium, but not at another level, such as difficult. Now, look at
Figure 4.2, on p. 34. This figure includes the concept of complexity in the decision-
making process.

The sections of the Preference Checklist that correspond to the areas listed in
the first four columns in Figure 4.2 contain items that correspond to the three levels of
complexity (simple, medium, difficult). In determining the extent to which your son or
daughter will indicate a preference for an item, you need to consider the complexity of
the item.

An example follows from Section 2, Part A. The purpose of the range of numbers from +3 to −3 is to indicate each item's degree of importance to your son or
daughter. For example, +3 indicates "Absolutely yes," a zero indicates "Don't care,"
and −3 indicates "Absolutely no."

9) I may vote.   +3   +2   +1   0   −1   −2   −3

Most people would agree that voting is a decision of at least medium complexity—many would put it at the difficult level. For Steve Stuart, this item would be
nonapplicable because his mental competence is such that he would not be able to
make a reasoned decision at the complexity level required for voting. Maria Rodriguez, however, could easily handle the complexities of voting. If she indicates a strong
preference to vote (a +3), her preferences should be respected. Of course, she may
indicate little interest in voting (a 0). Either way, she determines the importance and
should have complete freedom to act on her preference. Jolene Harris presents a different situation. Let's say Jolene indicates a strong preference (a +3) to be in an adult
environment where she can express her preference and vote. She can handle some
aspects of voting, such as the concept of casting a ballot, reading the list of candidates,
and actually checking the ballot or working a voting machine. But she may require
some help to express her preference fully. Someone may need to help her identify the
issues in an election, determine her own position on the issues, and identify the candidate who most closely supports that position. Given this information, when Jolene and
her mother are evaluating a residential option, one question they might ask of the pro-

gram or agency directing the residence would be, "Are there people on your staff who would help Jolene identify election issues so she can vote as she wants?"

Here's another example, from Section 2, Part A:

15) I may go to classes or get advice about my voting rights and responsibilities.
$$+3 \quad +2 \quad +1 \quad 0 \quad -1 \quad -2 \quad -3$$

Jolene might indicate a strong preference (a $+3$) on this item, and the residential program's ability to provide the help or advice would answer the question we raised.

Here's one more example, from Section 2, Part A:

9) Someone acts as my advocate regarding my human rights.
$$+3 \quad +2 \quad +1 \quad 0 \quad -1 \quad -2 \quad -3$$

Understanding the scope of human rights within a philosophical and legal framework clearly represents a difficult level of complexity. Add to this the full implications of what it means to be an advocate and we are presented with an item most of us would agree represents difficult complexity. The responses to this item from some of our family members may be surprising. Steve Stuart may not be able to comprehend the complexities involved, but he's always had someone in his life who protected his rights. In any future situation, it is reasonable to expect he would want an advocate. His response might be a $+3$. His parents might decide who would serve as an advocate, thereby meeting Steve's preferences. Anna Levine, however, most certainly has a clearer understanding of the nuances involved in this item, but may rate it lower, for example, a $+1$. Her reasoning may be that she can be her own advocate, so an outside advocate is less important to her than to Steve.

We would like to make one final point concerning identification of individual preferences within the context of the decision-making process is introduced in earlier chapters. Refer again to Figure 4.2. Identifying preferences should be viewed as a means to solving problems or satisfying needs. Consider the area, *relationships with other people,* in the case of Jolene Harris:

Defining the problem: Jolene wants friends in her community who have disabilities, as well as friends without disabilities. She also wants an intimate relationship with a male.

Question: What is the level of complexity of this decision?
Answer: In Jolene's case, it is simple to medium.
Question: Can Jolene identify her needs?
Answer: Yes, with limited help.

Brainstorming
Question: Level of complexity?
Answer: Across all three levels.
Question: Can Jolene brainstorm a range of options?
Answer: Yes, the Preference Checklist actually addresses a list of options, and Jolene may add to the options. Her family and friends can add further options.

Evaluating and choosing alternatives
Question: Level of complexity?
Answer: Across all three levels.
Question: Can Jolene evaluate and choose options?
Answer: Yes, those of simple to medium complexity. For example, she certainly should make the decision regarding who her boyfriend will be, but decisions about issues such as birth control would be made by others because of the complexity of such decisions.

Communicating the decision to others
Question: Level of complexity?

Answer: Simple to medium.

Question: Can Jolene communicate her decision to others?

Answer: For the most part, yes. She may need some help setting up an appointment with a doctor to have a physical and receive a prescription for birth control pills.

Taking action

Question: Level of complexity?

Answer: Across all three levels.

Question: Can Jolene take action to implement her decision?

Answer: Again, for the most part, yes. She will need help understanding the schedule of taking birth control pills and may need regular reminders to do so.

Evaluating the outcome of the action

Question: Level of complexity?

Answer: Across all three levels.

Question: Can Jolene evaluate the outcome of her decisions?

Answer: For the most part, yes. Only she can say if she is happy, but family members and friends may offer help with looking at the total picture. Maybe she stays up so late with her boyfriend that her loss of sleep is hurting her job performance. She, along with the others, can evaluate the situation, identify the problem, and start the decision-making process anew.

Now we will discuss ways you may choose to complete the Preference Checklist. When using this checklist, remember throughout the chapters in this section that issues will always arise concerning levels of complexity, who will make decisions, to what extent certain people will make decisions, and the evaluation process.

HOW DO I COMPLETE THE CHECKLIST?

We have divided the Preference Checklist into five sections. Section 1 is a "primer" for the following sections. Section 2, "Things That Are Important in My Life in the Community," is concerned with the legal rights, personal autonomy, and leisure time issues that are discussed in Chapter 18. Section 3, "Things That Are Important in My Relationships with Other People," guides your son's or daughter's choices about family and friends, sexuality, and other social relationships, as they are described in Chapter 19. Section 4, "Things That Are Important about the Place Where I Live," is concerned with issues and choices related to residential programs, which are discussed in Chapter 24. Section 5, "Things That Are Important about My Job," considers choices about employment, which are presented in Chapter 31.

We present the sections of the checklist in each of the relevant chapters to help you and your son or daughter consider what's important in each area. However, to put it all together again, another copy of all the sections appears at the back of the book. Those pages are perforated to allow you to pull them from the book and take them along on visits to programs or to various other people who might advise you and your son or daughter. Use it in the way that is most comfortable for your family.

Each item in each section is followed by a scale to indicate the degree of importance of the item for your son or daughter. The scale works as follows:

Absolutely yes			Don't care			Absolutely no
+3	+2	+1	0	−1	−2	−3

If it were essential that a particular setting (for example, a work site or a residential setting like an apartment) provide or offer whatever option is described in an item, you or the person completing the checklist would circle the +3. If it were just as important to you or your son or daughter that the setting absolutely not provide or allow for a particular item, you would circle −3. The negative numbers (−1, −2, −3) do not indicate wrong or undesirable feelings. They are negative only in the sense that something is not wanted or that something needs to be removed from a setting to make that setting right for your son or daughter.

There are no right or wrong answers. The right answers for you and your son or daughter are the ones that you will provide. The numbers indicate the different degrees of preference or importance attached to those items by you and your son or daughter. A zero indicates that the things described in an item are totally unimportant. The presence or absence of the things described in an item have no bearing whatsoever on the appropriateness of a setting for your son or daughter.

Some items may not be applicable to your son or daughter, For example, Item 16 from Section 2, Part A ("I may get advice about my duty to register for Selective Service.") does not apply to women. You may either leave such items unanswered or you may choose to rate these as a 0 if they have no bearing on your son or daughter.

At the end of each section, space has been provided so you or your son or daughter may add items that are important to him or her, but were not addressed in the checklist. After you have added your items, they should be rated on the same scale as the other items.

Some sample items have been completed below to show how the checklist works:

Section 2, Part C
12) I may smoke cigarettes, cigars or pipes.   (+3) +2   +1   0   −1   −2   −3

Maria Rodriguez, going through the checklist with her mother, circled +3 for this item, since she smokes (and, even though she knows it isn't good for her, she doesn't want anybody else to tell her when, or if, she should quit). Odessa Harris rated this item −3, because she felt that because of her daughter's heart condition, Jolene should never smoke.

Here are two other items in the section on legal rights:

Section 2, Part A
9) I may vote.   (+3) +2   +1   0   −1   −2   −3
10) I may work for a candidate of my choice.   +3   +2 (+1) 0   −1   −2   −3

Anna Levine comes from a family in which politics is a lively topic of conversation. She knows about voting and believes she should vote, like any other citizen, so she circled +3 for the item, *I may vote.* But working for a candidate gave her a little pause. "Maybe I'd like to someday," she thought, "but right now I'm not very interested." She circled +1 for that item. Henry Weber's reaction was different. "Humph! Politicians! I wouldn't go across the street to shake one's hand." Putting himself in David's shoes, he thought, "He could care less about politics, so long as he's warm and comfortable." Henry circled the zero for both these items.

Section 4, Part A
13) I may choose to continue to use my family physician, dentist, and other specialist.
                        (+3) +2   +1   0   −1   −2   −3

In the case of David Weber, given his complicated medical condition, continuity of care is absolutely essential. The Webers would rate this item +3. Maria Rodriguez, on the other hand, might respond differently. She is in excellent health, and let's say she doesn't especially like the doctor her family has been seeing. She might rate this item 0 or maybe even -1 or -2, to indicate that she really would rather find a new doctor.

Section 2, Part B
19) I may spend large amounts of money however I want to.
$$\text{(+3)} \quad +2 \quad +1 \quad 0 \quad -1 \quad -2 \quad -3$$

Brian Hughes and his family may consider this item inapplicable to their situation. Brian may or may not have access to large amounts of money, but he has never spent money and it is doubtful that he has the mental competence to do so. In his case, an outside financial manager is indicated. However, Anna Levine presents a very different situation. She may insist that she handle all of her own finances, and respond $+3$ on this item. But what if Anna were the type of person who would spend her money quickly and foolishly if she did not have outside help with budgeting her resources? Although this is not the case with Anna, such a situation may exist in some families.

The 'Best Interest' Approach

You may find it necessary to use the *best interest* approach to resolve conflicts between expressed preferences and the reality of the situation. For example, Maria Rodriguez wanted to buy a car. Her family and friends, realizing they did not have the right to say she could never do so, dealt with the reality of the situation instead. They explained the legal and financial responsibilities of automobile ownership. Maria would need to pass a test to obtain a driver's license. Beyond this was the initial cost of purchasing a car, followed by other expenses such as insurance, maintenance costs, and the costs inherent in the daily operation of a vehicle. No one said that Maria couldn't plan for a car, but she now realized what was involved. She has started working toward her goal by studying the driver's manual and saving some money each month. Someday she will be able to buy her car and obtain her driver's license.

Personal preferences that may exceed mental abilities (as in the case of Anna Levine) or physical abilities (such as when a required skill is lacking) can lead to situations that are difficult to resolve. It might be wise for you and other family members to identify the risks associated with some preferences. For example, what about the person who wants to live in an independent apartment setting but has limited self-help skills? What about the person who wants to marry, yet has a very limited understanding of the responsibilities involved? Or the person who wants to work at a job that necessitates taking a bus trip with two transfers and who may be unable to reach the work site safely? You can, undoubtedly, add numerous other examples.

The basic question is, What is to be done that will be in the *best interest* of everyone involved? Look again at the hypothetical case of Anna Levine. She wants to handle all her own finances, but would spend her money in a way that would leave her dependent on her parents in the latter half of each month. Ben and Ruth, her parents, could just decide that someone else will take care of her money and inform their daughter of that fact. The consequences of this action may be undesirable. Anna may feel resentful and the relationship between daughter and parents may deteriorate. Anna may decide to cease confiding in her parents and this may expose her to risks in other areas of her life. A deteriorating relationship can also have an adverse effect on Ben and Ruth. Anger, regret, and confusion can affect all family members to varying degrees. Forcing the issue with Anna may not be in anyone's best interest.

A compromise between what Anna prefers and what is best for her seems the best approach. Anna may be provided assistance with her budget with the understanding that the help is aimed at teaching her the skills she will need to gradually take control over her finances. Such a program would address Anna's preferences, and she would most likely be responsive and eager to learn because she identified financial management as an important issue. Her choices, therefore, dictate the assistance she will receive in her life, leaving her in greater control.

HOW DO I USE THE PREFERENCE AND CHOICE CHECKLIST?

The Preference and Choice Checklist was developed to be flexible. Each person using it can modify the approaches it suggests to suit individual decision-making styles and individual needs. We describe three possible ways the checklist might be used, but must stress that there are probably as many different methods for using the checklist as there are people involved in future planning.

A Structured Approach

Brian's father, Lowell Hughes, has always approached life from the perspective that it is orderly and should be treated as such. He feels that a person should treat all decisions systematically. At the bank where he works, he thoroughly investigates all loan applications before approving or disapproving them. He devised a highly structured process for using the checklist. Using a portion of the checklist, let's follow Lowell's structured approach through part of Section 2, Part D (see Figure 17.1).

   1)   Lowell and his wife, Barbara, using the Shoes Test approach, completed the items and circled their responses as they thought Brian would have responded.

   2)   Lowell then concentrated on all items ranked $+3$ or -3, as these represented issues of equally great importance. In our small sections of the checklist, Lowell found five items rated $+3$ and none rated -3.

   3)   Lowell next determined the importance of the five items rated $+3$, relative to one another. That is, he understood that the issues addressed in some of the items were more important to an overall quality life for Brian than other items were. (Consider this for yourself. If you were looking for a new job, finding one that allowed you considerable freedom in scheduling your vacations might be an important consideration. Yet, there are other aspects of a job that would be considerably more important, such as social meaningfulness, working conditions, and wages.)

   Using his ranking system, Lowell determined the relative importance of all $+3$ items. Some items were of equal importance.

   4)   Lowell then ranked the importance of the $+2$ items following the same system.

   5)   When Lowell, Barbara, and Brian visited some residential options, they took the completed checklist with them. It served as a guide for them in asking specific questions. (For example, by relying on his checklist, Lowell might quickly notice that a particular residence did not have hallways wide enough to accommodate a wheelchair. The list might also prompt Lowell to ask specific questions such as: "Can Brian go downtown to shop whenever he wants to?" "What are your policies about unsupervised trips downtown?" "What sort of recreational activities are there here?" "Who takes part in them?")

   6)   Based on the answers the program staff provided, Lowell rated the extent

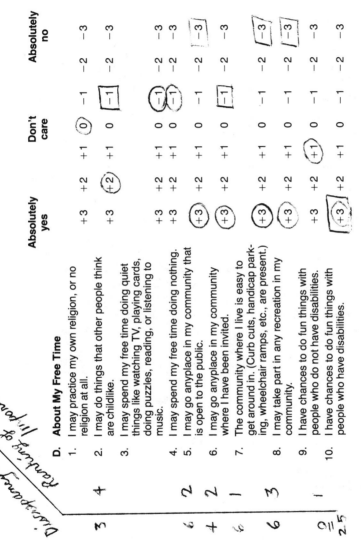

Disagreement Score | **Ranking of Importance** (handwritten, rotated)

	Ranking of Importance	**Disagreement Score**		About My Free Time	Absolutely yes			Don't care		Absolutely no	
D.											
1.	3		I may practice my own religion, or no religion at all.	+3	+2	+1	⓪	-1	-2	-3
2.	4		I may do things that other people think are childlike.	+3	(+2)	+1	0	[-1]	-2	-3
3.			I may spend my free time doing quiet things like watching TV, playing cards, doing puzzles, reading, or listening to music.	+3	+2	+1	0	(-1)	-2	-3
4.	2		I may spend my free time doing nothing.	+3	+2	+1	0	(-1)	-2	-3
5.	2		I may go anyplace in my community that is open to the public.	(+3)	+2	+1	0	-1	-2	[-3]
6.	1		I may go anyplace in my community where I have been invited.	(+3)	+2	+1	0	[-1]	-2	-3
7.	3		The community where I live is easy to get around in. (Curb cuts, handicap parking, wheelchair ramps, etc., are present.)	(+3)	+2	+1	0	-1	-2	[-3]
8.			I may take part in any recreation in my community.	(+3)	+2	+1	0	-1	-2	[-3]
9.	1		I have chances to do fun things with people who do not have disabilities.	+3	+2	(+1)	0	-1	-2	-3
10.			I have chances to do fun things with people who have disabilities.	[+3]	+2	+1	0	-1	-2	-3

9 = 25 (handwritten at bottom left)

Figure 17.1. Lowell Hughes's "structured approach" to the Preference Checklist.

to which each residential setting dealt with the issues represented by the important items. He used the same $+3$ to -3 scale, where $+3$ meant that a program definitely provided for an item or the policies were such that a program strongly encouraged or mandated that the issues addressed in an item be taken care of. A -3 meant the program did not provide for an item, or discouraged or forbade that the issues in an item be addressed. (For example, one program Lowell visited had no wheelchair ramps at the entrance of a house, and the agency that operated that residence had no intention of installing one. The agency representatives said they would simply carry Brian up the step. The program also strictly limited the residents' freedom to use community services and recreational activities. However, regarding religious life, residents were free to do as they pleased.)

Based on his visit to this particular program, Lowell's rating appeared as is shown in the sample section of the checklist above. He drew boxes to indicate how the program scored on each item of importance.

7)   Lowell then determined the *discrepancy score* of the program, that is, the difference between what was important to Brian and the extent to which the program addressed the important items. For example:

Section 2, Part D
2)   I may do things that other people think are child-like.
$$+3 \quad \boxed{+2} \quad +1 \quad 0 \quad \boxed{-1} \quad -2 \quad -3$$

It was fairly important to Brian that he be allowed to engage in such activities. The program, however, somewhat discouraged what is considered age-inappropriate behavior. This resulted in a discrepancy of 3 points between what Brian wanted and what the program allowed. Lowell determined other discrepancy scores and entered them on the checklist, and determined the total discrepancy score for the subsections of the check list applying to residential settings. (In our sample, the discrepancy score is 25.)

8)   Lowell now found himself armed with some powerful information. The

		Absolutely yes			Don't care			Absolutely no

A. About My Legal Rights and Programs

1. I may attend my own IEP, IPP, IHP, or other meetings. $+3 \quad +2 \quad +1 \quad \boxed{0} \quad -1 \quad -2 \quad -3$

2. I may refuse to have certain goals or objectives included in my IEP, IPP, IHP or other programs if I feel that they are not right for me. $+3 \quad +2 \quad +1 \quad 0 \quad -1 \quad \boxed{-2} \quad -3$

3. My own programs and goals are fully explained to me. $+3 \quad +2 \quad \boxed{+1} \quad 0 \quad -1 \quad -2 \quad -3$

4. I have a say about the times I work on my programs and goals. $\boxed{+3} \quad +2 \quad +1 \quad 0 \quad -1 \quad -2 \quad -3$

5. I may see the records on my progress in my programs. $+3 \quad +2 \quad \boxed{+1} \quad 0 \quad -1 \quad -2 \quad -3$

6. I have a say over who can see my records. $\boxed{+3} \quad +2 \quad +1 \quad 0 \quad -1 \quad -2 \quad -3$

7. Only people who really need to know may see my records or files. $\boxed{+3} \quad +2 \quad +1 \quad 0 \quad -1 \quad -2 \quad -3$

8. Someone explains my rights to me about my own records or files. $+3 \quad +2 \quad \boxed{+1} \quad 0 \quad -1 \quad -2 \quad -3$

Figure 17.2.   Jack Stuart's "less structured approach" to the Preference Checklist. (IEP = individualized education plan, IHP = individualized habilitation plan, and IPP = individualized program plan.)

particular program he had visited had a high discrepancy score. Lowell now felt he had two options. He could explore the possibility of achieving some compromise with the program over the important issues, or decide the program was inappropriate and investigate other options.

9)   As Lowell, Barbara, and Brian visited other programs, they rated them in the same manner and compared them to each other.

A Less Structured Approach

Jack Stuart views life through the eyes of the skilled carpenter that he is. "Life," he likes to say, "is like a building. There's a lot of fluff, but what really matters is a sound foundation." He incorporated his personal philosophy into completing the checklist with his wife Rose and his daughters, Sally and Theresa. He wanted the input of the entire family to ensure that Steve's true wishes would be addressed. Again using a portion of the checklist, we will look at the Stuart method (see Figure 17.2).

1)   Using the Shoes Test as the Hughes family did, Jack and the other Stuarts completed the checklist and circled their responses.

2)   The family then reviewed only those items rated +3 or −3. According to Jack, these were the bottom line items—the "foundation."

3)   They ranked the importance of the items.

4)   The Stuarts used their completed checklist as a guide when visiting residential options.

5)   They formulated specific questions based on the checklist, for example, "Will Steve's program be flexible and allow him to work on goals based on his preferred times," "What are the agency policies regarding the confidentiality of Steve's records," and "Who has access to his files?"

6)   The Stuarts noted on the checklist the extent to which the programs they visited accommodated Steve's preferences. Again, according to Jack's bottom-line philosophy, a program either met the preference, or did not.

An Even Less Formal Approach

Odessa Harris believes some people make life more difficult than it needs to be, so she used the checklist in a very informal way. Over the course of a week, she and Jolene sat on the old porch swing after supper in the relative cool of the Georgia evening. Odessa asked Jolene how she felt about specific issues addressed in the various checklist items. Mother and daughter spent those quiet evenings learning more about each other, and Odessa noted on the checklist those things that were truly important to Jolene. The conversation went something like this:

"Jolene, honey, when you grow up and have your own house, things are going to be a litttle different. Now, if you lived in a house where someone told you when you could or couldn't use the phone, how would you feel?"

"Why would someone do that?" Jolene asked, puzzled. "Mom, I don't talk on the phone too long. No, gotta be able to use the phone. Will wanna call you."

Other issues were less important to Jolene than phone access. For example:

"Jolene," Odessa asked, "would you want to have help taking care of your money or would you want to take care of your money all by yourself?"

"Don't matter to me. Why?"

"Well, money is important. Would you want to take care of it alone or have help?"

"Gee, don't know, mama. Guess somebody could help. Long as I got some to spend now and then. Don't matter to me."

The examples provided by the Hugheses, Stuarts, and Harrises show how different families used the checklist in very different ways. You may like one of these methods and adopt it for yourself, or you may have your own ideas about what is the best way for you and your son or daughter. The purpose of the checklist is to help you and your family identify your son's or daughter's preferences. The way you use the checklist matters less than the purpose for using it—to understand what is important so that you can plan accordingly.

SECTION 1:   PREFERENCE AND CHOICE QUESTIONNAIRE

What are _____'s major means of communication?

_____ Speech   _____ Gestures (pointing, gazing, etc.)
_____ Signing   _____ Gestures and vocalization
_____ Communication device   _____ Vocalization
_____ Other (specify) _____

What are some ways that _____ expresses pleasure?

_____

_____

_____

What are some ways that _____ expresses displeasure?

_____

_____

_____

What are some of _____'s particular likes?

_____

_____

_____

_____

How do you know?

_____

_____

_____

_____

What are some of _____'s particular dislikes?

_____

_____

_____

_____

How do you know?

_____

_____

_____

_____

How does _____ generally indicate preference when given a choice between two or more activities, foods, objects, and so forth?

_____

_____

What kinds of choices does _____ characteristically have the opportunity to make?

_____

_____

On the average, how many times per day does _____ have the opportunity to make choices concerning where, when, and what to eat; where, when, and how to spend leisure time; when to get up and go to bed; what to wear; with whom to associate; how to spend money, etc.?

               Never   1–5 times   5–10 times   10–15 times   15+ times

When was the last time _____ had an opportunity to make a choice?

_____

_____

Who usually decides what clothes _____ wears each day?
- ____ The person
- ____ Mother
- ____ Father
- ____ Both parents
- ____ Mother and the person
- ____ Father and the person
- ____ Both parents and the person
- ____ Other (specify) _____

Who usually decides what _____ will do at any given time of day?
- ____ The person
- ____ Mother
- ____ Father
- ____ Both parents
- ____ Mother and the person
- ____ Father and the person
- ____ Both parents and the person
- ____ Other (specify) _____

Who usually decides how _____ will spend an allowance or other money?
- ____ The person
- ____ Mother
- ____ Father
- ____ Both parents
- ____ Mother and the person
- ____ Father and the person
- ____ Both parents and the person
- ____ Other (specify) _____

What was the last choice situation?

_____

_____

What home-management activities does _____ prefer to do or assist with?
- ____ Shopping
- ____ Setting the table
- ____ Clearing the table
- ____ Washing dishes
- ____ Drying dishes
- ____ Emptying the trash
- ____ Mowing the lawn
- ____ Shoveling
- ____ Cleaning
- ____ Dusting
- ____ Sweeping
- ____ Mopping
- ____ Cooking
- ____ Ironing
- ____ Mending
- ____ Gardening
- ____ Repairs
- ____ Child care
- ____ Pet care
- ____ Farm chores
- ____ Other _____

How does _____ prefer to spend leisure time at home?

_____

_____

How often does _____ participate in recreation and leisure activities in the community, such as movies, plays, shopping, dances, video arcades, bowling, concerts, eating out, sports events, and so forth?

             Frequently   Sometimes   Seldom   Never

What are some examples of the community-based recreation and leisure activities that _____ prefers?

Activities	How often does _____ participate in this activity?
_____	_____
_____	_____
_____	_____
_____	_____

What are _____'s special needs or preferences concerning
- ____ Positioning? _____
  _____
- ____ Diet? _____
  _____

_____ Health?   _____

_____

At what time of day does _____ usually prefer to be active and productive?

_____

At what time of day does _____ usually prefer to rest and relax?

_____

Consider the following items. Which response might be most appropriate for your son, daughter, or other relative?

1. In most cases, when opportunities arise to make choices, _____ prefers to

| make choices independently | make choices with minimal help from others | make choices with moderate help from others | leave the choice completely to someone else |

2. In most cases, _____ prefers situations that offer

| unlimited choices | many choices | few choices | no choices |

3. In most cases, _____ prefers temperatures which are

| very warm | somewhat warm | somewhat cool | very cool |

4. In most cases, _____ prefers lighting which is

| very bright | somewhat bright | dim | virtually dark |

5. _____ prefers environments where there is

| lots of variety in activity from day to day | a moderate degree of change in daily activity | a low degree of change in daily activity | no change in activity from day to day |

Most of the time, _____ prefers to be

6. | alone | with one other person | with a small group | with a large group |

7. | very active | moderately active | relaxed | |

8. | independent | supervised | dependent | |

9. | with age peers | with older persons | with younger persons | |

Most of the time, _____ prefers to be

10. | the center of attention | one of the crowd | seen but not heard | |

11. in the company of

| persons of the same sex | persons of the other sex | a mixed group | no preference |

12. involved in

| fast-paced activities | moderately paced activities | slow-paced activities | |

13. engaged in

| highly repetitive activities | moderately repetitive activities | nonrepetitive activities | |

14. in environments where there is

| lots of action | a moderate degree of action | limited action | |

Most of the time, _____ prefers to be

15. | in highly competitive situations | in moderately competitive situations | in noncompetitive situations | |

16.   in highly   in moderately   in loosely
      structured   structured   structured
      situations   situations   situations

17.   in unfamiliar new   in familiar
      surroundings   surroundings

18.   in highly   in moderately   in visually
      visually   visually   unstimulating
      stimulating   stimulating   environments
      environments   environments

Most of the time, _____ prefers to be

19.   in noisy   in moderately   in quiet
      environments   noisy   environments
                               environments

20.   If you can think of any other particular preferences that _____ may have regarding everyday
      surroundings, environmental conditions, likes and dislikes, etc., please list them below.

_____

_____

_____

_____

Has _____ ever indicated a preference for a specific type of career? If yes, what?

_____

_____

_____

Has _____ ever indicated plans for the future? If yes, what are they?

_____

_____

_____

_____

18 HOW DO I DETERMINE MY SON'S OR DAUGHTER'S LEISURE AND COMMUNITY PREFERENCES?

The Hughes family lives in Indianapolis, in a fine old home that Lowell Hughes, a 45-year-old banker, inherited from his parents. Barbara Hughes, 40, is a successful real estate agent. They have a son, Brian, age 17. He was Barbara's child by a previous marriage. (The father left when Brian was 2 and hasn't been heard from since.) Lowell married Barbara about a year later and adopted Brian. The Hugheses also have a daughter, Abby, 4 years younger than Brian.

Just after Abby was born, Brian (age 4 at the time) contracted encephalitis (inflammation of the brain) and was left with brain damage. Brian is now in a class for students classified as trainably mentally handicapped. Lowell spent a great deal of time with his baby daughter in the months when Barbara was involved with Brian's hospitalization and rehabilitation. He dotes on Abby to the point that Barbara sometimes thinks he is ignoring Brian. Abby has shown what her teachers call a "promising talent" in music and dance, and Lowell serves on the board of the local community dance company. He calls it his "civic time."

For her part, Barbara tries to include Brian in most of the things she does for fun. She takes him shopping and to the racquet club, where the Hugheses have a family membership. Last year, she hired a student in recreational therapy to teach Brian how to play tennis. Brian always goes along amiably, but it's clear that his heart isn't in the game. If he had his druthers he would sit quietly watching his sister at dance practice. Abby taught Brian to play a few chords on the guitar, and now he often sits alone in his room, strumming and humming.

Barbara is active in the local Association for Retarded Citizens (she says that's *her* "civic time"). She is considered one of the strongest parent advocates in the city, and has been involved in organizing workshops on parent-professional relationships and with special committees promoting state legislation. One day Barbara came home from a meeting filled with enthusiasm for their latest project. She told Lowell about it as they sat sipping their before-dinner martinis.

"We're going to have a coffeehouse for young people with disabilities," she told him. "Isn't that great? The kids can go and socialize and participate in the entertainment. Brian could take his guitar."

But Lowell wasn't so sure. He looked over the committee report Barbara had brought home. "It says here that it'll be open from 5 to 8 on Thursday evenings. Seems

I remember from my youth," he said dryly, "that young people like to go to coffee-houses and such on the weekends."

"Oh, well," Barbara said, "it's going to be on Thursday nights because that's the time we can get volunteers to staff it. But anyway," she went on, "that's only the beginning."

"Hmmm." Lowell took a long swallow of his drink. "I don't know. What's wrong with taking three or four kids at a time to a regular coffeehouse? Or even a bar?" He knew he was annoying his wife; sometimes Barbara thought he enjoyed it.

"And what fun could they have being ignored in those places?," Barbara countered. "And who would make sure they didn't get into any trouble?"

"You're overprotective, Barb."

"Just realistic," she responded, in her usual manner.

Lowell looked at her over the top of his glass. This was an argument they'd had before, and no doubt would have again. But he didn't feel like pursuing it tonight. He leaned back in his chair and stretched his long legs. "Well, maybe so," he said noncommittally.

But Barbara wasn't ready to leave the issue behind. "And anyway, did you ask Brian what *he* wants? Maybe if you did you'd take him with you to Abby's rehearsals more often."

Lowell sighed, stood up, and walked over to the bar to mix a second pitcher of the potent drinks. It was going to be a long evening.

*   *   *

As adults, all of us are part of a community—that is, a place (neighborhood, town, or city) where people come together to meet each other's needs for shelter and protection, and to enjoy life in general. Within these communities, we all have certain responsibilities: to do the best we can to support ourselves and our families, to do something to contribute to the well-being of the community (like Barbara and Lowell's "civic time"), and in general to obey the laws and try to get along with others. In return for fulfilling these responsibilities, we have certain rights: to be independent and free to choose where we want to go and what we want to do, to have a voice in how the community functions (through voting, participation, or both, in community politics), to have access to community amenities (ranging from utilities to transportation to shopping malls), and to be protected from infringements on our rights by others.

Most of us take these rights and responsibilities for granted, but for adults with disabilities that may not be the case. Because of their limitations, adults with disabilities may only be expected to fulfill their responsibilities to the best of their ability. And because of structural and attitudinal barriers, adults with disabilities often are not guaranteed their full rights as citizens. The upshot is that adults with disabilities may live *in* a community, but may not necessarily be a *part* of that community. That is why it is important to plan for this aspect of life for your son or daughter.

There are three major issues to consider in planning for your son's or daughter's future as a citizen in the community. First, it is important to know your son's or daughter's legal rights and how to assure that those rights will be respected. Second is the question of how best to nourish your son's or daughter's freedom to make decisions about his or her day-to-day life. Third, you should consider what aspects of life in the community your son or daughter might most enjoy as a participant—that is, what religious, leisure, and cultural activities he or she might want to pursue.

WHAT LEGAL RIGHTS DOES MY
SON OR DAUGHTER HAVE AS AN ADULT?

Most parents of young people with disabilities are familiar with their son's and daughter's rights under the Education for All Handicapped Children Act, also known as PL (for Public Law) 94-142. You may be aware that your son or daughter has a right to a free and appropriate public education that is individually designed to meet his or her needs. You may also know that you as a parent have a great deal of power over decisions about what will be taught, where your son or daughter will be taught (in special classes or in the mainstream, for example), and what special services he or she will receive. When there are disagreements between families and the school, there are clearly specified *due processes* to resolve the dispute. As a parent, you have rights to notification, to have your rights explained to you, to see you son's or daughter's confidential records, and to demand that any material you find objectionable in that record be removed.

The rights of adults who have left school are not as clear. Most adult community programs offering vocational, residential, or leisure services are under no obligation to accept everyone. For example, they may exclude adults with behavior problems, or may restrict their clientele to persons with one particular type of disability. Some vocational rehabilitation programs may restrict services to clients considered to have potential for employment according to certain narrow criteria. Parent rights (unless parents are legally named guardians, as was discussed in Chapters 6–8) are not as clear, either. Many agencies try to involve parents in planning individualized programs, but the parent (or the adult) may not have the same right to demand services that are offered under the Education of the Handicapped Act.

Despite these ambiguities, adults with disabilities do have some protections. The Rehabilitation Act of 1973, which prohibits discrimination on the basis of disability, requires that a person must not be excluded on the basis of some arbitrary judgment and allows for an administrative hearing on claims of discrimination. Every state has a protection and advocacy agency to defend the rights of persons with developmental disabilities. Most states also have regulations that protect the rights of adults with disabilities. Also, most states have adult protective services that require that suspected abuse incidents be reported and investigated. These are general protections built in as a condition of accepting certain federal funds for a program. For example, programs funded under Medicaid have requirements for individualized active treatment plans, least restrictive treatment, and so on. These protections may vary from program to program depending on the funding source. Agencies may be required to specify careful procedures, with rights of appeal, for termination of services. Many agencies have formal human rights committees that review treatment plans to make certain that they do not place the person in any danger, that appropriate consent has been obtained, and that the treatment or training is designed to achieve its goals in the least restrictive way. Suppose, for example, that a person has a habit of injuring himself by chewing on his hands. The human rights committee may rule that the staff cannot drug or tie down the person to stop him from injuring himself, but must use less drastic means (perhaps heavy cotton mittens) while they also develop a behavior modification program to stop the behavior.

Also, many agencies have policies to involve families in decisions about the adult's program. It may also be agency policy to include the adult himself or herself in the decision-making. Families may be on the boards of directors of some community agencies. Families may be welcome to visit the program at any time, and the staff may make special efforts to involve families in the day-to-day program to the extent they can or want to be involved. Also, most agencies have strict policies about the confidentiality of records that allow only those people who really need to know the information in a person's file to see it, and that specify that information may be released only upon the explicit consent of the person, his or her family, or both.

Some communities have citizen advocacy programs. These are programs in which a volunteer is paired with an adult with a disability in a sort of "big brother" or "big sister" role. The citizen advocate may help the person with such matters as negotiating with a landlord for repairs or doing business with a bank, or may make certain that a service agency is meeting the person's needs. Beyond that (and perhaps even more important), the citizen advocate serves in the role of a friend, including the person in family activities or hobbies, going shopping or to ball games, or doing any other things of interest to them both.

Finally, there is a growing number of self-advocacy groups. In these groups, adults with disabilities can come together to learn about their rights and responsibilities and how to advocate change. We know of one self-advocacy group, for example, that successfully negotiated for bigger lockers and a better snack bar in their sheltered workshop. Some self-advocacy groups have taken an active interest in politics, have learned about voting, and even invited candidates to come to meetings to explain their positions.

It is extremely important for your son or daughter to be assured of these civil and social rights as a firm foundation for a successful life in the community. "Things That Are Important in My Life in the Community," the checklist at the end of this chapter, contains some specific points relevant to the rights an agency is willing to assure. You may want to consider which of these are important to you. You may want to use the items in this section of the checklist that you and your son or daughter consider most important as a guide when you ask questions of the management and staff of any prospective vocational, residential, leisure, or other program being considered. For instance, you may ask to see the agency's written policies about confidentiality and about the procedures followed when a client is being considered for termination from a program. For example, if the capacity (and willingness) to work with persons who have behavior problems is important to you, you need to ask for specific examples of behaviors an agency is willing to tolerate. After all, "behavior problems" covers a wide range of possible behaviors, from passive resistance to violent attacks on others. When some agencies say they can manage behavior problems, they really mean milder ones.

If it is important to you and your son or daughter that your family be involved in a program, you should ask to see any written policies concerning family involvement. How often may you visit? What procedures are followed if you or your son or daughter disagree with a proposed individualized program goal? Are there family members on the board? Is there a human rights review committee? Is there a self-advocacy group? Is there a citizen advocacy program? You may wish to talk with other parents who have a son or daughter in the program. All of these are issues you may wish to consider as you and your son or daughter search for options in the community.

HOW MAY MY SON'S OR DAUGHTER'S
RIGHTS TO PERSONAL AUTONOMY BE ASSURED?

Beyond legal rights, there are rights people in our society possess by virtue of their humanity. These are rights that cannot be cataloged in laws, primarily because the list is endless. They are the rights that are observed when someone calls you "sir" or "ma'am" at the store, or when people say "excuse me" when they bump into you. Most of your neighbors don't pick your flowers from your yard unless you offer them. Likewise, coworkers don't take paper or pencils from your desk or tools from your workbench without asking. In most families, family members don't open mail addressed to another person, or enter a bedroom when the door is closed without knocking first. Someone asks your opinion about how much ice cream you want in your dish ("Say when!"), or allows you to serve yourself. When you are shopping, a friend may give an opinion about a dress or shirt you take from the rack, but ultimately the choice is up to you.

All of these are rights, but we don't usually call them that. We may refer to them as "giving people space," "being polite," "showing respect," or "allowing dignity." Taken together, they are the rights we have to be autonomous human beings, with bodies people cannot touch at will, space people cannot invade, personal possessions people cannot take from us, private thoughts people may not know unless we choose to share them, and choices we may make without interference.

Unfortunately, and sometimes despite others' best intentions, adults with disabilities do not always receive their full share of their rights to autonomy. Especially in the case of persons with severe disabilities, it is easy to cross the line from caretaking to disrespect. Lillian Weber encountered this problem one day. An old school chum she hadn't seen in years was visiting when David called her to his bedroom; he needed his diaper changed. This was a routine chore for Lillian, and she was about to ask her friend to come to David's room with her so they could keep on talking. But suddenly she checked herself—would *she* like to have a stranger watching while she attended to her own toileting needs? Lillian realized that it was such an easy thing to forget that David had his right to privacy, too. "And," she said to Henry later on that evening, "I'm his own mother! If it were someone else, it might be even easier for them to forget he's a person, too!"

The loss of some of these basic autonomy rights is also frequently experienced by people with milder disabilities. All of us have from time to time eaten at a restaurant with friends who use wheelchairs. Very often we are asked by the waiter or waitress, "And what would *he* like today?" Inevitably, the waitress gets an embarrassed look on her face when we respond, "I don't know, why don't you ask him?" Adults with developmental disabilities are often treated the same way, ignored by sales clerks or summarily presented with a selection of clothes or food. In some adult service agencies (fewer, we hope, as times goes by), staff convenience may take precedence over a person's autonomy. Thus, for example, there may be rules requiring that doors be left open, or that everyone have an enforced bedtime. Choices about menus and recreation may be made by staff rather than residents.

Part C of the checklist that appears at the end of this chapter is titled, "About How I Am Treated." This part of the checklist gives you and your son or daughter an opportunity to decide how important some of these autonomy issues are to you. As in Part A, you may want to use those items you consider most important as a guide to asking questions about prospective adult services. In some of these cases, however, it may be a bit more difficult to determine just how an agency treats the people it serves. For example, it is difficult to imagine an administrator telling you, "No, we don't respect our clients' opinions." You may need to observe staff interacting with adults in the program, if possible for an hour or so at different times of the day.

Barbara Hughes used some of these principles to choose a tennis instructor for

Brian. She had two applicants for the job, and she invited each one to spend an hour or two with her and Brian at the club. She watched as they interacted with Brian, noting how comfortable they seemed, and how much they fell in with Brian's mood rather than try to direct him. One young man kept trying to interest Brian in a variety of activities. The other simply sat back and talked to Brian, then followed him as Brian wandered over to a lounge chair. They sat together, talking and laughing like two boys. Barbara hired the second young man.

IN WHAT MANNER WOULD MY SON OR DAUGHTER LIKE TO PARTICIPATE IN THE COMMUNITY?

Once you've considered the issues of legal and basic autonomy rights, you'll have a foundation on which to base consideration of *what* your son or daughter wants to do as a participant in the community. Professionals are most often concerned with vocational issues, that is, where a person will work and what he or she will do. They may also be concerned with residential issues, that is, where a person will live and with whom. These are important issues, but there are other aspects of life besides where one works and sleeps. After all, most people only work to be able to enjoy life during the other 18 hours of the day. These hours include one's religious activities, leisure interests, and hobbies. Often, the responsibility for helping a young person with a disability cultivate this part of his or her life falls on the family—for example, Barbara Hughes hired a tennis instructor rather than the school physical education teacher. Brian's sister Abby was the one who taught him to play the guitar, not the school's music therapist. Likewise, Odessa Harris is the one who takes her daughter to church and who talks to her about the Bible, not Jolene's special education teacher.

Religion, like politics, is a touchy subject and is usually left undiscussed. Yet, it is a crucial part of life for many families. Adults with disabilities have spiritual needs as much as any other person, and can gain many benefits from participation in a religious organization.

An increasing number of religious organizations are trying to accommodate the needs of persons with disabilities. As more and more parents take their children with disabilities to religious services, the other members of the congregation or synagogue become exposed to persons with disabilities. As Odessa Harris told her Aunt Jewell, Jolene has "educated the church." She said, "When Jolene was little, she fit right in with all the other kids. Now they're finding out that Jolene can learn her catechism and be part of the worship like anybody else." Odessa is working with her minister to help Jolene prepare for her baptism in the church.

Almost all the major denominations have materials related to disabilities available through their national offices. These include materials for clergy to help them in counseling, other materials and ideas for sermons and discussions, and curricula for special instructional or Sunday school classes. If you are interested in providing these materials to your own religious organization, the addresses of these groups are listed in the resource section at the back of this book.

Leisure, by definition, is something we do by choice for relaxation, rather then for money as part of our job. We generally discover our leisure interests by sampling a variety of activities and learning which ones "push our buttons," so to speak. Parents of boys and girls of preschool and elementary school age talk of exposing their children to a variety of experiences, such as museum classes, music lessons, little league, and scouting. As we grow older, the process of sampling leisure interests depends less on parents, and more on our widening circle of friends. For young people with disabilities, however, parents and other family members may continue to engineer leisure experiences. For example, Barbara Hughes hired a tennis instructor for Brian, but now it is clear his heart really isn't in the game. But since she firmly believes Brian ought to have some sort of activity that helps keep him physically fit, she is thinking of switching to swimming lessons. In the meantime, Brian himself is spending an increasing amount of time with his music, playing the guitar, listening to records and tapes, watching Abby dance. It occurred to Abby that maybe her mom's concern about Brian's physical fitness and his own interest in music could be brought together by teaching him to dance. She taught him a few modern dance steps, and Brian was positively ecstatic. Now Barbara has launched a search for a music therapist who can teach Brian to dance.

One additional leisure issue that families confront is illustrated by the exchange between Barbara and Lowell at the beginning of this chapter. That is the question of whether the person with a disability should participate in activities designed specifically for people with disabilities, or should be part of the mainstream, participating with people who do not have disabilities. On the plus side of special programs, as Barbara pointed out, is the fact that without special programs the person may be excluded from any activity at all. Programs such as Special Olympics, or the coffeehouse being organized by Barbara's Association for Retarded Citizens chapter, provide opportunities that people with disabilities may not otherwise have. On the minus side, special programs may not always be available when a person with a disability wants to use them. Also, large groups of people with disabilities congregating together may intensify community stereotypes and may result in a little, mobile island of segregated activity in the midst of the larger community.

The bottom line in the issue of special versus "regular" leisure programs is the larger issue of protection versus risk-taking. Barbara and Lowell's perennial disagreement about this is echoed everywhere as families and service agencies alike grapple with the question. At what point does "freedom of choice" become exclusion, or worse, danger for the person with the disability? On the other hand, at what point does "protection" become oppression and unnecessary restriction? This can only be answered by individuals with disabilities and their families.

Part D of the checklist at the end of this chapter lists a few leisure and life-style activities your son or daughter may want to consider. Since the variety of leisure activities is endless, we have only been able to list possibilities in major groups (e.g., sports, arts). It will be up to you and your son or daughter to consider specific possible interests within these larger categories. But whatever you do, remember that leisure should be fun, not work. Trying out a variety of activities with your son or daughter should be approached as an adventure. After all, that's what life is all about.

SECTION 2: THINGS THAT ARE IMPORTANT IN MY LIFE IN THE COMMUNITY

	Absolutely yes			Don't care			Absolutely no

A. About My Legal Rights and Programs

1. I may attend my own IEP, IPP, IHP, or other meetings.

+3	+2	+1	0	−1	−2	−3

		Absolutely yes			Don't care			Absolutely no
2.	I may refuse to have certain goals or objectives included in my IEP, IPP, IHP or other programs if I feel that they are not right for me.	+3	+2	+1	0	−1	−2	−3
3.	My own programs and goals are fully explained to me.	+3	+2	+1	0	−1	−2	−3
4.	I have a say about the times I work on my programs and goals.	+3	+2	+1	0	−1	−2	−3
5.	I may see the records on my progress in my programs.	+3	+2	+1	0	−1	−2	−3
6.	I have a say over who can see my records.	+3	+2	+1	0	−1	−2	−3
7.	Only people who really need to know may see my records or files.	+3	+2	+1	0	−1	−2	−3
8.	Someone explains my rights to me about my own records or files.	+3	+2	+1	0	−1	−2	−3
9.	I may vote.	+3	+2	+1	0	−1	−2	−3
10.	I may work or campaign for a candidate of my choice.	+3	+2	+1	0	−1	−2	−3
11.	I may choose my own lawyer.	+3	+2	+1	0	−1	−2	−3
12.	I may join a self-advocacy group.	+3	+2	+1	0	−1	−2	−3
13.	I may join other support groups.	+3	+2	+1	0	−1	−2	−3
14.	I may go to classes or get advice about being my own advocate.	+3	+2	+1	0	−1	−2	−3
15.	I may go to classes or get advice about my voting rights and responsibilities.	+3	+2	+1	0	−1	−2	−3
16.	I may get advice about my duty to register for Selective Service.	+3	+2	+1	0	−1	−2	−3
17.	I may go to classes or get advice to help me understand laws about crimes, contracts, personal injuries, federal and state assistance, etc.	+3	+2	+1	0	−1	−2	−3
18.	I may go to classes or get advice about how to pay my income taxes.	+3	+2	+1	0	−1	−2	−3
19.	Someone acts as my advocate regarding my human rights.	+3	+2	+1	0	−1	−2	−3
20.	My family and friends may visit me at any time.	+3	+2	+1	0	−1	−2	−3
21.	My family and friends feel comfortable about making suggestions to the staff.	+3	+2	+1	0	−1	−2	−3
22.	My family and friends are told about my programs and goals.	+3	+2	+1	0	−1	−2	−3
23.	My family and friends have a say about the kinds of programs I may participate in.	+3	+2	+1	0	−1	−2	−3
24.	My family and friends are told about the good things I do as well as the problems I may have.	+3	+2	+1	0	−1	−2	−3
25.	The rights of my family to see my records are explained.	+3	+2	+1	0	−1	−2	−3
26.	There is a family support group available.	+3	+2	+1	0	−1	−2	−3
27.	The needs of my family are considered to be as important as my needs.	+3	+2	+1	0	−1	−2	−3
28.	The state or federal government pays for respite care for my family.	+3	+2	+1	0	−1	−2	−3
29.	_____	+3	+2	+1	0	−1	−2	−3
30.	_____	+3	+2	+1	0	−1	−2	−3
31.	_____	+3	+2	+1	0	−1	−2	−3

	Absolutely yes			Don't care		Absolutely no	

B. About My Health Needs and Rights

1. I may decide who will give me advice about my health needs. +3 +2 +1 0 −1 −2 −3
2. I may decide not to follow a diet that other people think I should. +3 +2 +1 0 −1 −2 −3
3. I may decide not to do exercises that other people think I should. +3 +2 +1 0 −1 −2 −3
4. I may decide who my doctor, dentist, and other specialist will be. +3 +2 +1 0 −1 −2 −3
5. I may schedule my own appointments with a doctor or dentist. +3 +2 +1 0 −1 −2 −3
6. I can decide not to see a doctor or dentist. +3 +2 +1 0 −1 −2 −3
7. I have a say over who can see my medical records. +3 +2 +1 0 −1 −2 −3
8. I am responsible for my own medications given by a doctor (e.g., pills for pain or seizures, pills to help me act calm). +3 +2 +1 0 −1 −2 −3
9. I may decline to take any medications. +3 +2 +1 0 −1 −2 −3
10. I may buy my own medicines at drug stores or supermarkets (e.g., aspirin; cough syrup; creams for insect bites, sunburn, rashes). +3 +2 +1 0 −1 −2 −3
11. I may decide to have operations (like having my tonsils taken out, having tumors removed, or other operations if some part of my body has a problem) without advice from other people. +3 +2 +1 0 −1 −2 −3
12. I may decide not to have an operation that a doctor or someone else, for example my parents, thinks I should have. +3 +2 +1 0 −1 −2 −3
13. I may decide other things that a doctor may do for me (like fix a broken leg, or put a bandage on a bad cut). +3 +2 +1 0 −1 −2 −3
14. I may decide not to let a doctor do anything to me. +3 +2 +1 0 −1 −2 −3
15. I may decide to let a dentist pull a tooth. +3 +2 +1 0 −1 −2 −3
16. I may decide not to let a dentist do anything to me. +3 +2 +1 0 −1 −2 −3
17. _____ +3 +2 +1 0 −1 −2 −3
18. _____ +3 +2 +1 0 −1 −2 −3
19. _____ +3 +2 +1 0 −1 −2 −3

C. About How I Am Treated

1. I may talk and show both my good (positive) and bad (negative) feelings. +3 +2 +1 0 −1 −2 −3
2. People respect my opinions. +3 +2 +1 0 −1 −2 −3
3. I may make a deal about (negotiate) whether I will carry out what people tell me to do. +3 +2 +1 0 −1 −2 −3
4. People take my feelings (such as loneliness, anger, sadness, happiness) seriously. +3 +2 +1 0 −1 −2 −3
5. Somebody helps me to understand my emotions or feelings. +3 +2 +1 0 −1 −2 −3
6. I may take moderate risks or chances. +3 +2 +1 0 −1 −2 −3
7. I can have as much responsibility as I can handle. +3 +2 +1 0 −1 −2 −3

		Absolutely yes			Don't care			Absolutely no
8.	I may decide how much I want to depend on other people.	+3	+2	+1	0	−1	−2	−3
9.	I have control over my life.	+3	+2	+1	0	−1	−2	−3
10.	Nobody checks on my incoming and outgoing mail or phone calls.	+3	+2	+1	0	−1	−2	−3
11.	No one may use the things I own without my permission.	+3	+2	+1	0	−1	−2	−3
12.	Nobody can take away my personal things as a punishment.	+3	+2	+1	0	−1	−2	−3
13.	I may choose what clothes I wear each day.	+3	+2	+1	0	−1	−2	−3
14.	I may buy clothing, food, and other things I want without someone else's okay.	+3	+2	+1	0	−1	−2	−3
15.	I may pick out the kinds of clothes I will buy.	+3	+2	+1	0	−1	−2	−3
16.	I may spend small amounts of money however I want to.	+3	+2	+1	0	−1	−2	−3
17.	I may handle my savings account or checking account by myself.	+3	+2	+1	0	−1	−2	−3
18.	Somebody else takes care of all my money.	+3	+2	+1	0	−1	−2	−3
19.	I may spend large amounts of money however I want to.	+3	+2	+1	0	−1	−2	−3
20.	_____	+3	+2	+1	0	−1	−2	−3
21.	_____	+3	+2	+1	0	−1	−2	−3
22.	_____	+3	+2	+1	0	−1	−2	−3

D. About My Free Time

		Absolutely yes			Don't care			Absolutely no
1.	I may practice my own religion, or no religion at all.	+3	+2	+1	0	−1	−2	−3
2.	I may do things that other people think are childlike.	+3	+2	+1	0	−1	−2	−3
3.	I may spend my free time doing quiet things like watching TV, playing cards, doing puzzles, reading, or listening to music.	+3	+2	+1	0	−1	−2	−3
4.	I may spend my free time doing nothing.	+3	+2	+1	0	−1	−2	−3
5.	I may go anyplace in my community that is open to the public.	+3	+2	+1	0	−1	−2	−3
6.	I may go anyplace in my community where I have been invited.	+3	+2	+1	0	−1	−2	−3
7.	The community where I live is easy to get around in. (Curb cuts, handicap parking, wheelchair ramps, etc., are present.)	+3	+2	+1	0	−1	−2	−3
8.	I may take part in any recreation in my community.	+3	+2	+1	0	−1	−2	−3
9.	I have chances to do fun things with people who do not have disabilities.	+3	+2	+1	0	−1	−2	−3
10.	I have chances to do fun things with people who have disabilities.	+3	+2	+1	0	−1	−2	−3
11.	I may schedule my own activities and fun things for weekends and evenings.	+3	+2	+1	0	−1	−2	−3
12.	I may smoke cigarettes, cigars, or pipes.	+3	+2	+1	0	−1	−2	−3
13.	I may drink alcoholic beverages if I am of legal age.	+3	+2	+1	0	−1	−2	−3
14.	I may go to taverns, bars, and night clubs.	+3	+2	+1	0	−1	−2	−3

		Absolutely yes			Don't care			Absolutely no
15.	I may gamble if it is legal.	+3	+2	+1	0	−1	−2	−3
16.	I may go shopping anywhere in my community.	+3	+2	+1	0	−1	−2	−3
17.	I may take part in or go watch sports events of any kind.	+3	+2	+1	0	−1	−2	−3
18.	I may go to any art event (like movies, arts and crafts, museums, concerts).	+3	+2	+1	0	−1	−2	−3
19.	I may go to classes to learn hobbies (like gardening, wood carving, collecting things).	+3	+2	+1	0	−1	−2	−3
20.	I may eat out anywhere in my community, if I can afford it.	+3	+2	+1	0	−1	−2	−3
21.	_____	+3	+2	+1	0	−1	−2	−3
22.	_____	+3	+2	+1	0	−1	−2	−3
23.	_____	+3	+2	+1	0	−1	−2	−3

19 WHAT ARE MY SON'S OR DAUGHTER'S INTERPERSONAL PREFERENCES?

The air was tense around the Rodriguez family dinner table. Luis ate slowly and thoughtfully, as if every bite were a weighty responsibility. Eloisa kept fluttering to and from the kitchen, remembering this or that dish, going back to check the stove. Maria sat quietly eating, her eyes intent on her plate and her shoulders hunched.

Luis cleared his throat before he spoke. "How was work today, Maria?"

"Fine." Maria didn't look up.

"Mama says you came in late last night."

No answer.

"Who were you with? Where did you go?"

"Sophia." Maria looked up at her father. "I was with Sophia and we went to a movie." Her voice was icy. "Is that all right with you?"

"You were at a movie until 2 A.M.?" Luis put down his fork and returned her stare.

"Where I go and when I come back is none of your business!," she hissed.

Luis's face turned purple. He slammed his fist on the table, making the dishes clink. "You don't talk to your father that way, young lady!" Sullenly, Maria looked down at her plate.

Eloisa nervously covered her mouth with her napkin. "Maria," she said gently, "your father is only looking out for your welfare."

Luis leaned forward. "That was Ramon Guerra's car you were getting out of, wasn't it?"

Maria glared at her father. "So what if it was? He's my friend, too! I can do what I want with my friends!"

Geraldo's told me about that Ramon!" Luis was shouting now. "He's no good! He's a dopehead and he's been mixed up with the law. All he wants from you is . . ."

"Luis!" Eloisa put her hand on her husband's arm and shook her head.

But it was too late. Maria's face reddened and, throwing her napkin on the table, she jumped up. "I don't have to take this from you! He's my boyfriend and he loves me! He said so! If I can't live my life the way I want to in this house, I'll just . . ." she faltered, caught short by her mother's gasp. "I'm sorry," she mumbled. She looked down and twisted her skirt in her fingers.

But Luis pressed on. "I don't want you seeing him, Maria!"

Maria lifted her chin defiantly and squared her shoulders. She turned deliberately away from her father and spoke quietly to her mother. "Thank you for the dinner, mama, I'm going out now. Don't wait up for me." She turned and swept from the room.

The sound of the front door slamming echoed back from the living room. Eloisa sobbed quietly and rattled dishes as she began to stack the dirty plates, still half full of food. Luis leaned his elbows on the table and buried his head in his hands. What a heartache! Where had he gone wrong? And why could Maria never understand that he only had her welfare at heart?

*   *   *

The scene was very different in the Levine household. Ruth came home from work to find Anna flushed with happiness and humming a little tune as she carefully unloaded the dishwasher.

"Hello, dear," Ruth said, brushing her daughter's cheek with a kiss. "How was school today?"

"Just fine, mother." Anna smiled happily. "There's a new girl in my homeroom. Her name's Sarah. We ate lunch together, and guess what? She said she'd call me sometime and we'd go to a movie or something!"

Ruth hugged her daughter. "That's so nice, dear." Anna had so few friends, and almost none of the youngsters in the regular classes ever paid attention to her. Ruth found herself humming along with Anna as the two of them began preparing dinner.

But as the days went by and Sarah didn't call, that happy feeling was slowly replaced by gloom. Ruth watched Anna spring to the phone every time it rang and answer it with a hopeful "Hello?," only to turn it over to Ruth or Ben with a despondent "Oh, it's for you."

A week later, Arnold and Saundra invited the Levines to a backyard barbecue at their new home. As Ruth packed a cake in its carrier she noticed that Anna had quietly settled herself in the big easy chair next to the phone. Ben, standing by the door with car keys in hand, asked, "Are you ready, Princess?"

"I'm not going," Anna said, "Sarah might call, you know."

Ben and Ruth looked at each other. Ben shrugged. "Suit yourself."

When the Levines returned, Anna was still in the chair, surrounded by soda cans and a half-eaten bag of potato chips. "Sarah didn't call," Anna told her mother. "Do you think I gave her the wrong number?"

Ruth bit her lip and turned away quickly so that Anna wouldn't see the pity on her face. "I don't know, dear. But I hope the next time you'll come with us. You always have a nice time at Arnold's house."

Ruth sighed. How could this Sarah be so thoughtless? But no, she checked herself, how could she know how her careless words would affect Anna? Every day people tell each other they'll call sometime, and everybody understands it is just a polite social convention. Except Anna. How could Ruth help Anna understand? More to the point, how could she help Anna make some friends?

*   *   *

The problems Anna and Maria are experiencing are not uncommon. Especially during adolescence, almost all of us face a certain amount of stormy weather in our interpersonal relationships. You probably remember disagreements with your parents about your friends, or waiting in vain by the telephone for someone to call. Why, then, should interpersonal relationships require special attention as you plan for the future?

It is, we believe, precisely because interpersonal relationships are so vitally important that they cannot be left to chance.

Very few people go through daily life without any contact with others. We are all surrounded by family, friends, neighbors, coworkers, and strangers on the sidewalk. With all these people we establish relationships. Some are tenuous and fleeting, like the moment of contact with the small boy who smiled shyly at you yesterday while you were in the grocery check-out line. Others are deep and enduring, like the relationships between parents and children and between husbands and wives. Between these two types are all degrees of relationships along a wide range of long- to short-term, intimate to impersonal, positive to negative. We call the web of relationships people spin with others their *social support network*.

Psychologists believe that a high-quality social support network is vital to mental health. From our support network we receive all those tangible and practical things that help us get through the day, like help with a difficult task at work, babysitting, or directions to a destination in an unfamiliar part of town. But even more important, we receive those intangible things, like a pat on the back, respect and admiration, a sympathetic ear when things go wrong, a feeling of belonging to a group. Isolated people— or those whose support network for some reason doesn't provide those intangible benefits—are more prone to a host of social ills such as alcoholism, abuse, depression, and suicide.

It should not be surprising that a strong social network is just as vital to adults with disabilities as it is to anyone else. People who get to know someone with mental retardation usually learn very quickly that the desire and ability to form friendships has no relationship to one's intelligence. In fact, parents have often told us that their sons and daughters have taught them a thing or two about unconditional love and acceptance. Think of Steve Stuart's strong attachment to his family, and his desire to interact with others and be useful to them. Jolene Harris thinks of friends and relationships before she thinks of jobs. And David Weber feels and acts more alert whenever his mother is able to arrange for a companion to visit him.

Another important part of an adult's life is his or her social-sexual relationships. For the vast majority of us, sexual identity is very much a part of our social relationships. From early childhood we learn how to behave as little girls or little boys in a myriad of ways, ranging from playing with particular toys to imitating men and women in their mannerisms and roles. Even though our society is changing and sex roles may not be as rigid as they once were, it is still true that our orientation to daily life as men or as women is very much a part of who we think we are and how we respond to others.

A very important part of adult social-sexual relationships is the intimacy and affection we experience with a partner. It is through social-sexual relationships that most of us learn to share our most intimate selves, to express and receive affection, to communicate in an atmosphere of trust—in short, to love and be loved.

The point is that there is a great deal more to sexual relationships than the physiology and mechanics of sex. Social-sexual relationships fulfill basic physical needs, to be sure. But they also fulfill the equally human needs to have affection and intimacy and to establish a sense of who we are in a social context.

As much as anyone else, adults with disabilities experience all these physical, emotional, and identity needs. That statement seems so obvious that we may wonder why it needs to be said. Yet the topic of sexuality and disability was for many years shrouded in myth, fear, and prejudice. In the early decades of this century, adults with mental retardation were thought to be naturally promiscuous and "morally degenerate." Alternatively, some believed that people with disabilities had no sexual feelings at all. The belief in the hereditary nature of disabilities led to widespread sterilization, and the segregation of adult men and women in isolated institutions. Many of these beliefs have lingered on into the present, with the general public seeing people with disabilities as either "sexless" or "oversexed." As of 1981, 38 states still had laws prohibiting or restricting the marriage of people with mental retardation.

Research and experience now tell us that, except for individuals with the most profound impairments, adolescents and adults with disabilities have social-sexual interests and needs that are very similar to everyone else's. Most people with delays or impairments in their thinking processes have nothing at all wrong with their bodies—including their hormones and their reproductive systems. Young people with mental retardation are influenced by the same messages about sexuality and relationships that everyone receives from TV shows and advertisements. Those messages are that people have boyfriends or girlfriends, they date, they hold hands and kiss, and they go to bed with each other. It is no more "right" to exclude people with disabilities from opportunities to have those experiences than it is to exclude them from jobs or a homelike living environment.

In our society, marriage is considered the most satisfactory social-sexual relationship. We now know that many people with disabilities are perfectly capable of having a successful marriage. In fact, the divorce rate among couples with disabilities seems to be no better or worse than that for the population in general. Adults with mental retardation often think of marriage as a badge of "normality." They speak of being able to help one another, of companionship, and of feeling "just as good as anybody else." Though they may need continued support from family and professionals, there is no reason to suppose that marriage is not a realistic goal for many adults with disabilities.

At one time, the inevitable outcome of marriage was children. That is no longer necessarily so. For adults with disabilities, this means that the question of whether or not to marry can be separate from the question of whether or not to have children. Contrary to prevailing beliefs in the earlier part of this century, we now know that most causes of mental retardation are not hereditary, and that children born to parents with mental retardation usually have normal intelligence. Many parents and professionals, however, do express concerns about the ability of parents with disabilities to care for children properly. When it is a struggle to care for oneself, it may certainly be even more of a struggle to be responsible for children. There are training programs designed to teach parenting skills to adults with disabilities, and in some parts of the country services are available to provide support to families in which the parents have disabilities. Professionals who work with these adults say that their ability to be good parents depends less on IQ than it does on their willingness to put their own needs aside in favor of meeting their children's needs. Our point is that, while it may be difficult for adults with disabilities to raise children, the decision to have them should not be ruled out automatically.

WHAT IS IMPORTANT IN MY SON'S OR DAUGHTER'S INTERPERSONAL RELATIONSHIPS?

The ability of an adult with a disability to form social relationships is complicated by the attitudes and prejudices of society. It seems likely that the more people an adult with a disability is able to meet, the more likely he or she is to form meaningful social relationships. Yet it also seems likely that the more people an individual meets, the more likely it is that he or she will face rejection, rudeness, or other forms of public stigmatization.

Families react to stigmatization differently. Some find the stares or rude comments of strangers very unpleasant, and withdraw from situations in which such things are likely to occur. Other families may ignore any discomfort and continue to take their child with a disability wherever he or she wants to go. When that child is an adult, the same principle applies. How much does your son or daughter value opportunities to have friendships with people who do not have disabilities? How much does he or she want to avoid rejection and unpleasantness? Every opportunity can be a risk; every avoidance of risk can be a missed opportunity. Most people try to balance protection with opportunity, but how much of each is "right" varies from person to person.

As we think about opportunities for adults with disabilities to form social relationships, this effort to find a balance between risk and opportunity may be behind every decision. If it is important to your son or daughter to have friends who do not have disabilities, that may have a bearing on the choice of an employment program. Also, residential programs, even those that may seem alike in many other respects, may vary in the number of integration opportunities they make possible for residents.

Another important aspect of forming personal relationships is the degree to which an adult with a disability is free to choose the people with whom he or she may associate, and when those associations occur. All of us make these choices on a daily basis; it is how we balance our need for privacy with our need for social relationships. Some programs for adults with disabilities are more structured than others, in that they require group participation with other residents or employees. Others allow for residents or employees to make many of their own decisions about participation. Some adults with disabilities are more comfortable with structured programs that provide guidance in the development of their social relationships. Others want to have as much freedom of choice as possible in the matter of their social relationships. Still others are concerned about freedom to choose to participate (or choose not to participate) in social activities that have a religious connotation, for example, Christmas parties.

Still another factor in considering what's important in social relationships is the degree to which your son or daughter may participate in social situations, and the degree to which he or she may be able to learn appropriate skills to enhance social relationships. Jolene Harris, for example, has a tendency to walk up to strangers and give them a hug. Odessa knows this behavior can be considered offensive by even the friendliest people. Steve Stuart's occasional hand-flapping when he gets nervous makes people think he's "weird," and makes them want to avoid him. Anna Levine's shyness, and her inability to take the initiative in reaching out to friends, may be part of the reason she is sitting home by the phone. Some of these traits and behaviors can be changed by teaching social skills to the affected individuals. Others may be personality characteristics or deficits related to severe handicap, that may not be so easily changed. It may be relatively easy to teach Jolene not to hug strangers, and a little more difficult to modify Steve's hand-flapping behaivor. But helping Anna get over her shyness may be extremely difficult, and teaching Steve to engage in meaningful conversations may be beyond our current teaching ability. It's important to consider what your son or daughter may learn to do, and what he or she may not learn, as choices are made concerning social relationships.

An uncomfortable topic for most parents, social-sexual relationships may be even more difficult to discuss for the parents of young adults with disabilities. Parents of youths with mild to moderate disabilities, especially daughters, often express fears that their child may be exploited sexually. This, indeed, is the fear that Luis Rodriguez has for his daughter. For him, the issue is how to balance his daughter's right to associate with whomever she chooses with the need to protect her from someone he knows is not good for her. In a society in which about half the general population experiences divorce, the risks of being hurt emotionally by venturing into a social-sexual relationship are pretty high. Whether those risks are higher for an adult with a disability is a matter of conjecture. However, many families, like the Rodriguezes, feel a greater need to protect their sons and daughters from exploitation and rejection. This need to protect, balanced against the need to provide opportunities for a fulfilling relationship, may be a factor in considering what's important to your family.

Other parents are concerned that their sons or daughters may manifest inappropriate sexual behaviors in public. The Hughes family was faced with this problem one day when the teacher called to say that Brian was masturbating in class. Barbara and Lowell Hughes believe that masturbation is a normal and natural part of sexuality, but they know Brian will face all kinds of censure and rejection if he masturbates in public. For the Hughes family, the problem is how to help Brian understand he must not touch his genitals in public without making him think he is forbidden to masturbate, even in private.

In the area of social-sexual relationships, two of the most important issues are how to teach appropriate behavior, and how to balance risk and opportunity. The most important guides, perhaps, are your family's beliefs and values. Beliefs about what a person should and should not do in the area of social-sexual relationships are very closely tied to religious and other social and cultural values, and therefore are very individual things.

The type and severity of your child's disability is also a very relevant concern. For someone with a profound disability, social-sexual options are limited just as every other area of life is restricted. For an adult with a mild disability, the issues of sexuality, marriage, and parenthood need to be thought out especially carefully. For those in between (individuals with moderate to severe disabilities), however, there is a broad gray area—it is difficult to say, without knowing an individual, just how capable he or she may be of having social-sexual relationships, or even of marrying and raising children. Another factor to consider might be the degree of support you as a family are willing to give your son or daughter. Some families are heavily committed to helping a couple with a disability make a successful life, with the parents on both sides working together to make a sturdy support network. Other families, for one reason or another, cannot be as intensively involved.

There is a checklist at the end of this chapter titled, "Things That Are Important in My Relationships with Other People." It is designed to help you and your son or daughter think through his or her preferences concerning interpersonal relationships. As with the checklist on life in the community presented in Chapter 17, we hope you will use this checklist in a way that is most comfortable for you.

*   *   *

Ben and Ruth Levine sat down with Anna and asked her how she felt about each one of the items in the checklist. It was clear that Anna wanted to have friends who do not have disabilities, that she wanted people to take her feelings seriously, and that she wanted somebody to help her understand her feelings. But when Ruth read her the questions on dating and sexuality, Anna blushed and wouldn't answer. Ruth decided not to push her. But a few days later, while the two were cleaning up the kitchen after dinner, Anna asked hesitantly, "Mom . . . do they really have a class where I can go and learn about . . . uh, sex?"

"Yes, dear," Ruth told her. "And it's about more than just sex. You can learn about going out with boys, what to say and how to talk to them. Would you like that?"

"Oh, but I can't talk to boys! They make me feel all nervous and I can't even say one word!"

"That's just it, honey," Ruth said. "You can practice talking in these classes and then maybe you won't feel so shy when you know what to say."

"Well . . . " Anna chewed her lower lip. Ruth thought about how pretty she looked . . . if only she had a little more confidence.

"Do you want me to see if you can go to one of those classes?" Ruth asked.

Anna flushed and looked down at the towel in her hand. "Yes," she whispered. "Thank you, Mother."

*   *   *

Barbara and Lowell Hughes used the checklist a little differently—they took the Shoes Test. As they looked at each item, they tried to keep in mind what Brian would want. Of course, Barbara and Lowell were not in total agreement about some of the items. Barbara thought Brian would prefer to be in a situation in which lots of group activities were scheduled for him (see Section 3, Part C, Number 4), while Lowell thought Brian would rather schedule his own activities (Section 3, Part C, Number 7).

"I know him better than you do," Barbara said. "He just wouldn't be able to set up fun things by himself."

"You just want to baby him," Lowell told her. "He could learn how to do things like that by himself. Anyway, who wants to go around in a herd of people with disabilities?"

"Brian would, that's who. He likes being with a large group of people."

"Okay, okay," Lowell said, giving in. "But listen, why wouldn't he like both options? If he learned how to set up fun things by himself, he could choose more freely."

"Yeah," Barbara said. "That's probably the most sensible response." Together, they circled +3 for "Lots of group activities or fun times are scheduled each month," and a +2 for "I may schedule my own activities and fun things for weekends and evenings." They made a note to ask Brian's teacher if there were any materials they could use to teach him more about how to call friends and decide about fun things they could do together. Barbara decided to make a conscious effort to help Brian set up activities on weekends or evenings with friends.

SECTION 3: THINGS THAT ARE IMPORTANT IN MY RELATIONSHIPS WITH OTHER PEOPLE

	Absolutely yes			Don't care			Absolutely no

A. About My Family and Friends

1. I may choose my friends.　　+3　+2　+1　0　−1　−2　−3
2. I may visit friends and family at any time it is okay with them.　　+3　+2　+1　0　−1　−2　−3

		Absolutely yes			Don't care			Absolutely no
3.	I have chances to meet and make friends with people who do not have disabilities.	+3	+2	+1	0	−1	−2	−3
4.	I have chances to meet and make friends with people who have disabilities.	+3	+2	+1	0	−1	−2	−3
5.	I have chances to meet and make friends with people outside my home and other homes like mine.	+3	+2	+1	0	−1	−2	−3
6.	My family and friends may, within reason, visit me at my house at any time.	+3	+2	+1	0	−1	−2	−3
7.	I may refuse to visit or be visited by friends and family at my home.	+3	+2	+1	0	−1	−2	−3
8.	My family and friends may take part in special events with me (like birthdays).	+3	+2	+1	0	−1	−2	−3
9.	I may decide how much I want to depend on other people.	+3	+2	+1	0	−1	−2	−3
10.	I may choose who will help me with my personal care.	+3	+2	+1	0	−1	−2	−3
11.	I may choose who will help me with my mail and telephone calls.	+3	+2	+1	0	−1	−2	−3
12.	People respect my opinions.	+3	+2	+1	0	−1	−2	−3
13.	I may make a deal about (negotiate) whether I will carry out what people tell me to do.	+3	+2	+1	0	−1	−2	−3
14.	People take my feelings (such as loneliness, anger, sadness, happiness) seriously.	+3	+2	+1	0	−1	−2	−3
15.	Somebody helps me understand my feelings.	+3	+2	+1	0	−1	−2	−3
16.	_____	+3	+2	+1	0	−1	−2	−3
17.	_____	+3	+2	+1	0	−1	−2	−3
18.	_____	+3	+2	+1	0	−1	−2	−3

B. About My Sexual Needs

		Absolutely yes			Don't care			Absolutely no
1.	I may go to classes or get advice about sexuality.	+3	+2	+1	0	−1	−2	−3
2.	I may go to classes or get advice about how to be a good parent.	+3	+2	+1	0	−1	−2	−3
3.	I may go to classes or get advice about diseases I can get from having sex.	+3	+2	+1	0	−1	−2	−3
4.	I may go to classes or get advice about homosexuality or lesbianism.	+3	+2	+1	0	−1	−2	−3
5.	I may go to classes or get advice about masturbation.	+3	+2	+1	0	−1	−2	−3
6.	I may go to classes or get advice about how to protect myself if somebody wants to be sexual with me and I don't want to.	+3	+2	+1	0	−1	−2	−3
7.	I may go to classes or get advice about birth control.	+3	+2	+1	0	−1	−2	−3
8.	I may make my own choice about birth control.	+3	+2	+1	0	−1	−2	−3
9.	I may decide whether or not I want to get married.	+3	+2	+1	0	−1	−2	−3
10.	I may decide whether or not to have my own children.	+3	+2	+1	0	−1	−2	−3
11.	I have a private place where I may masturbate.	+3	+2	+1	0	−1	−2	−3

		Absolutely yes			Don't care			Absolutely no

12.	I may choose to look at "adult" books, magazines, and movies.	+3	+2	+1	0	−1	−2	−3
13.	I may go on dates.	+3	+2	+1	0	−1	−2	−3
14.	I may have sex with another person of the opposite sex if we both want to.	+3	+2	+1	0	−1	−2	−3
15.	I may have sex with another person of my own sex if we both want to.	+3	+2	+1	0	−1	−2	−3
16.	I may choose not to be sexual.	+3	+2	+1	0	−1	−2	−3
17.	No one will pressure me to go on dates.	+3	+2	+1	0	−1	−2	−3
18.	No one will pressure me to do sexual things with other people.	+3	+2	+1	0	−1	−2	−3
19.	People respect my decisions about sexual things.	+3	+2	+1	0	−1	−2	−3
20.	_____	+3	+2	+1	0	−1	−2	−3
21.	_____	+3	+2	+1	0	−1	−2	−3
22.	_____	+3	+2	+1	0	−1	−2	−3

C. About Other People and Things in My Life

1.	I may ask for and get help (such as counseling) from persons other than my family or paid staff.	+3	+2	+1	0	−1	−2	−3
2.	I may decline to take part in any special religious holidays or celebrations that the other people are doing together.	+3	+2	+1	0	−1	−2	−3
3.	I may choose not to take part in group recreational and fun times.	+3	+2	+1	0	−1	−2	−3
4.	Lots of group activities are scheduled each month.	+3	+2	+1	0	−1	−2	−3
5.	I have a say over who can see my records or files.	+3	+2	+1	0	−1	−2	−3
6.	I have a say about the times I work on my programs and goals.	+3	+2	+1	0	−1	−2	−3
7.	I may schedule my own activities and fun things for weekends and evenings.	+3	+2	+1	0	−1	−2	−3
8.	I may do things that other people think are childish if I want to.	+3	+2	+1	0	−1	−2	−3
9.	I may send and get mail (letters, cards, gifts) at any time.	+3	+2	+1	0	−1	−2	−3
10.	I may take moderate risks or chances.	+3	+2	+1	0	−1	−2	−3
11.	I may stay out as late as I want to.	+3	+2	+1	0	−1	−2	−3
12.	I may go anywhere I want if I am of legal age.	+3	+2	+1	0	−1	−2	−3
13.	_____	+3	+2	+1	0	−1	−2	−3
14.	_____	+3	+2	+1	0	−1	−2	−3
15.	_____	+3	+2	+1	0	−1	−2	−3

20 WHY LOOK FOR RESIDENTIAL OPTIONS?

Where a person chooses to live is influenced by a number of factors that will be different for different people. One person may choose an apartment complex because yard and building maintenance is provided, while another will be motivated to buy a house because he or she finds the idea of a garden and yard work very appealing. For families with younger children, school district boundaries may be a consideration. Others may be more interested in proximity to shopping malls or their place of employment.

Finances are a major consideration, but within the range of what is affordable a number of options exist. Each of us has explored options and found places to live that best suited our individual needs and preferences. Perhaps some of us are not completely happy; our houses, apartments or other dwellings may be lacking in some ways, but undoubtedly most of our individual necessities have been secured.

Residential options can provide the same opportunities to meet the individual needs and preference of your son or daughter. Searching for the ideal residential placement can, however, be confusing. A large part of this confusion is attributable to the many terms used to describe available programs. For example, *group home, community residence,* and *ICF/MR* are all terms used to describe the same type of program. This chapter and the 6 following chapters (21–26) will help you reduce the confusion caused by the different labels placed on residential options.

When you select a residence, other factors may add to the initial confusion. Depending on the capabilities of the residents, two group homes located adjacent to one another can offer vastly different residence programs. Consider this example:

Located in a residential neighborhood are two identical structures on adjacent lots. Both provide homes for six people with mental retardation. Both houses have bedrooms, a spacious kitchen, a large dining room, a living and recreation roon, laundry facilities, and a big back yard. However, the similarity abruptly ends with the physical structure and surroundings.

In one house, six men and women with mild mental retardation live almost independently of the sponsoring agency. They cook their own meals, maintain the house, and tend an extensive vegetable garden in the back yard. These people take a pulic bus to jobs in the community and plan their own leisure activities. Staff hired by the sponsoring agency provide minimal supervision. The main function of the staff is to help the residents find apartments for two or three to share in an even more independent life-style.

The other house presents a vastly different picture. The six men and women living there have moderate to severe mental retardation and considerably fewer skills. Staff closely supervise many aspects of daily living, especially hygiene and meal preparation. A large van is parked in front of this house; it is used to transport residents to and from sheltered employment settings as well as agency-organized recreational activities. Both homes may be considered "group homes", but they share few traits beyond the number of residents and their family-style living activities.

When attempting to sort out and properly describe living options, it is necessary to construct some framework. Prior to constructing the framework, a review of some broad issues which will influence the form that the framework takes will be useful. The discussion of the issues that follows in Chapters 21–26 will provide a base of knowledge to help you evaluate residential options.

21 | HOW CAN I FIND RESIDENTIAL OPTIONS?

In this chapter we describe different methods of locating and evaluating residential options. You may choose to use some of these methods, while other families may find different methods more suited to their needs. As we have stressed before, there are no right or wrong ways to plan for your family's needs. If the end result produces a plan that satisfies family members, then you have used the process best suited to you. The methods we describe are your menu, so choose according to your taste.

Pick up your telephone book and turn to the Yellow Pages. Now, look for residential options. How many listings do you find under "Community Living Arrangements," "Group Homes," "ICF/MR," "Residential Options," or "Supervised Apartments"? The typical answer would be "none." Yet, you will see that the common telephone book can be a valuable resource as you begin your search.

Knowing where to look will enable you to find contacts who can answer your questions. If is also helpful to use the first contact to get to another, which will lead to still others. When you begin your search for residential options, your goal is to identify as many as possible. At this stage, you simply want to know what is available so that you can begin evaluating the different options to determine how well they meet the needs of your son or daughter.

WHAT ARE SOME LOCAL RESOURCES?

Every state has numerous public agencies responsible for meeting the various needs of people with disabilities and their families as well as the general health needs of others living in the state. The names of the agencies vary from state to state, within the District of Columbia, and throughout the U.S. territories. In the resource section at the back of this book you will find a list of public agencies in each of the various U.S. jurisdictions (Appendix 2). This list can serve as your first contact in locating residential programs in your community.

Another source of information might be the Association for Retarded Citizens (ARC), a national organization of parents, family members, and professionals. The organization seeks to influence policies relating to youth and adults with mental retardation and to provide support to families. The state and local chapters of the ARC have information about programs. Some state and local ARCs even manage residential and vocational settings that provide direct services.

Local chapters of the ARC are usually listed in your local telephone directory. They can usually provide information on residential options in the vicinity. Local chapters can offer further information on a variety of services, such as parent and sibling support groups, respite care, and recreational programs.

Many colleges and universities operate programs for people with disabilities and their families. A number of universities operate federally supported University Affiliated Programs (UAPs). The UAPs provide information and services. Research relating to disability issues, training, and education techniques is the emphasis at most UAPs. You can obtain more information on UAPs and other university services by contacting the American Association of UAPs, at the address in the resource section at the back of this book (Appendix 2).

Personnel in your local school district (in some states referred to as education agencies) can be a valuable source of information on residential options. If your son or daughter attends school, discussing future residential programs with his or her teacher can help guide you. Some school districts have special transition specialists who can help you locate and evaluate residential programs.

WHAT ARE SOME SOURCES OUTSIDE MY STATE?

A list of public agencies responsible for services for people with disabilities may be found in the resource section at the end of this book (Appendix 2). These agencies may be helpful in providing information about residential programs outside your state. Your local ARC might also be able to put you in contact with similar groups in other states.

Some residential programs are run by private agencies. While state agencies are usually aware of the private programs in their states, there are national organizations that can provide details on non–state-supported options. In the resource section some organizations are listed that you may wish to contact concerning residential options.

The National Information Center for Handicapped Children and Youth (NICHCY) is a federally sponsored clearinghouse. The program is authorized by Congress under the Education of the Handicapped Act (PL 94-142 as amended by PL 98-199). NICHCY provides a range of services to family members and professionals, including: information on education issues; referrals to other local, state, and national services agencies; support groups; technical assistance through workshops and consultations; and information packets. The information packets answer commonly asked questions concerning the needs of people with disabilities. NICHCY also provides up-to-date publications dealing with educational, vocational, transitional, and other issues. Material from NICHCY is available in large print, Braille, or on tape. Most of the services and information available from NICHCY are free. The address and phone number of NICHCY are provided in Appendix 2. This excellent national clearinghouse can become a valuable ally as you plan for your family's future.

WHAT ABOUT OTHER PARENTS AND FRIENDS?

If you know other people who are parents or relatives of someone with a disability, they may also be able to provide information that will help you in your search for residential options. These people may be able to do far more than simply inform you of one or more specific residential possiblities in your community. Meeting with other people who have been or are involved in planning for the future needs for their relatives can also be an important source of support. These people can help you understand that you and your family are not alone; other people, much like yourself, are facing the same situation. You can gain strength from sharing your experiences.

Some people have successfully searched for residential programs that meet their unique family needs. They can point out the roadblocks and pitfalls they encountered so that you might be able to avoid similar situations in your search. We all can (and should) learn from our mistakes—this holds true for the experiences of others, not just our own.

You and other parents and other family members may choose to work as a team in locating and evaluating residential options. You may decide to divide the tasks involved in the search. Perhaps you could contact half the agencies providing residential programs while another parent contacts the other half. The more parents and family members become involved, the less work there will be for all. Meanwhile, the information you collect will cover the widest range possible.

You may decide to continue using a group approach when you evaluate residential options. Remember, two heads are better than one. You may help someone else by noticing some aspect of a group home that the other person has missed. Other people will return such favors through their own insights.

The team approach does not work for everyone—some people prefer to work alone. If that is the most comfortable approach for you, it is also the best approach. Yet you may decide that working with other parents would best fit your style and serve your needs.

HOW DO I OBTAIN INFORMATION ON RESIDENTIAL OPTIONS?

Whether you telephone agencies and programs or write letters, you will find it helpful to maintain some type of master list of the programs you contact. It is easy to forget the names of programs, especially if there are many of them. A master list will make follow-up contacts much easier.

It may also be helpful to note the date you initially requested information, the kind of information requested, and the date you received the information. Noting the name of the person you spoke to or corresponded with may make later contacts easier. Dealing with the same person each time can eliminate confusion concerning the specifics of the information you requested, and can be the first step in establishing a working relationship with contact persons in different agencies.

As you begin receiving information from different programs, you may find it useful to develop a system for organizing the materials. Many people store the information in folders and rely on the master list to note the date it was received and the nature of the material (e.g., entry criteria, information on cost, and waiting list descriptions). The way you organize your search is less important than devising a system that will ensure that you get the information that helps you best evaluate your options.

WHAT SPECIFIC INFORMATION WILL I NEED?

Most programs offering residential placements provide brochures that should provide you with enough information to begin your evaluation. However, leave nothing to chance. You may want to specify the range of information you will need.

The following list includes the information you will need to begin evaluating residential options:

> What types of residential programs are provided (e.g., group homes, supervised apartments)?
>
> What types of disabling conditions (e.g., mental retardation, autism) make a person eligible for services?
>
> What degree of disability do the residents have (e.g., severe, moderate)?
>
> What are the specific admission criteria?
>
> What is the cost?
>
> Is there a waiting list?
>
> What are the procedures for initiating a placement?
>
> What levels of supervision are provided?

The list is not extensive because you should be primarily interested in finding as many options as possible at this point. If you do not receive the information you have requested from a program, a follow-up letter or phone call is in order. You may want to request additional information from responding programs as well. A follow-up request may result in the discovery of an ideal program for your son or daughter; it may be worth the extra effort.

As you contact agencies that operate residential programs, you will find that the quality of service varies widely. Yet, it is advisable to ask to be placed on mailing lists— even the mailing lists of programs you might consider inadequate. Programs change, new services are added, personnel change, and other aspects of the overall program evolve. Being on various agency mailing lists allows you to keep abreast of changes.

Some residential options have ownership or management characteristics that make it more difficult to contact them. Residences owned by the people with disabilities who live in them while offering to rent to other people are one example. Because they are private homes, these options seldom advertise their existence, unlike more traditional residential programs. The families or philanthropic organizations that make available living arrangements for people with disabilities often operate without advertising for residents.

As more people explore the possibility of private ownership of residences, this option is bound to become available to greater numbers of people. Whether such residences choose to advertise their services remains to be seen. Word of mouth from people who have relatives or friends living in such arrangements may lead you to them. You may ask to visit or talk with people in such programs. In Chapters 22–26, we discuss established private residential programs exclusively.

22 WHAT SHOULD I KNOW ABOUT RESIDENTIAL SERVICES?

Three broad issues will be discussed in this chapter: 1) *owner-ship*, 2) *size*, and 3) *licensure*. To varying degrees these three issues affect all residential options available to people with disabilities.

OWNERSHIP

The issue of who owns the residence your son or daughter may choose to live in may be important to you. Different types of ownership arrangements are possible and each results in different types of residences. We discuss three broad issues in this section on ownership: 1) *consumer and family ownership*, 2) *public ownership*, and 3) *private ownership*.

Consumer and Family Ownership

Lowell Hughes ambled up the front walk toward his house with a spring in his gait and a smile tugging at the corners of his mouth. He threw open the front door and called his wife, Barbara, whom he heard rummaging through the antique drop front desk in the study, "Hey Babs, I'm home!"

Barbara met him in the foyer, where he was hanging his tweed jacket in the closet. "My, aren't we in a good mood," she said laughing. "You're smiling like the cat that ate the canary."

Doing a bad W. C. Fields impression, Lowell answered, "No, my little chickadee, there's no canary, but we've caught the system by the tail. Brian is going to buy his own house."

"And I," said Barbara, "am going to London to be crowned queen."

"Well, Your Royal Highness," Lowell continued, as he bowed deeply from the waist, "I shall prepare you a small predinner cordial and explain it all. Brian really is going to buy a house!"

Barbara suddenly thought, "He's serious." But how could it be? Brian had severe problems. In fact, in the process of doing some preliminary searching into possible residental programs, Barbara and Lowell had been told that Brian's multiple needs might be hard to serve in some community settings. Buy his own house? He needs so much attention; who would take care of Brian in this house? Who would take care of the house, the maintenance, upkeep, repairs . . . No, Lowell could not possibly have thought the situation through.

"Lowell," Barbara said, as she joined him the family room, "what in the world are you thinking? Have you forgotten all it takes to own and run a home?"

Lowell asked his wife to sit down so that he could outline the situation for her. As he explained, Barbara began to understand that it was not only possible, it was actually in Brian's best interests to own his own home.

Because of Brian's severe disabilities, lack of personal resources, and low income, he represented the lower end of the low-income category within the human services system, and qualified for almost every low-interest housing program available from the state of Indiana and the federal government. Lowell, with the help of financial planners at his bank, tax accountants, and knowledgeable lawyers, had worked out a plan to qualify Brian for a low-interest loan from the U.S. Department of Housing and Urban Development (HUD) Direct Loans for Housing for the Elderly or Handicapped program. By serving as cosigners, which would satisfy the down payment requirements, Lowell and Barbara would guarantee the loan for their son.

Brian would purchase a three-bedroom house and "rent" two of the bedrooms to other people with disabilities while also living in the house himself. Brian qualified for a low-interest loan from the local municipal housing authority. Brian's parents financially assisted the venture through the development of a shared equity arrangement. Under this time-limited co-ownership arrangement, Brian would gain an increased share of the house as rental and mortgage payments were paid. Support services (i.e., staff, financial assistance, transportation, living skills programming) needed by the people living in the home would be provided by existing adult service agencies through arrangements made as part of the overall plan. Any necessary overnight staff would sleep in finished rooms in the basement of the house. Through careful legal planning, Brian would not face the loss of existing benefits due to his ownership of the home or the "income" he would receive from the other two tenants.

Brian would have his own home and the adult service agency providing residential programs in Brian's community would have two openings for other people with disabilities needing residential services. These openings would not strain existing options, but rather add to them. The Hughes family would not have the burden of running the home, but would have the assurance that Brian would have a residence and the services he needed.

The arrangements made by the Hughes family are not described in detail because each situation is unique. There are a number of creative financial arrangements that can be made to provide for individual ownership of real property.

Types of Ownership Arrangements Possible through Creative Financing

Through creative financing arrangements, the availability of quality, community-based residences for people with disabilities can be greatly expanded. Five categories of real estate ownership that can be facilitated by creative financing are:

1. **Agency ownership**   By *agency*, we mean a private or public nonprofit organization that wishes to acquire or build residences for people with disabilities.
2. **Social investing**   *Social investing* includes procedures that can be used by foundations and other philanthropic organizations to use capital for the social values gained from investments while maximizing financial resources. The foundations may hold title to the properties, or an arrangement may be

made that allows existing adult service agencies eventually to purchase these properties from the foundations.

3. **Private investor**   *Private investors* are individuals, corporations, partnerships, or other legal entities that may rent or lease residences for the purpose of producing income. In the process of gaining income for the investor, people with disabilities reap many benefits.

4. **Consumer ownership**   The term, *consumer*, is used here to note ownership by both the individual with a disability and families or guardians who act on behalf of that individual.

5. **Housing cooperative ventures**   *Cooperatives* represent joint corporation ownership of residences. Housing cooperatives offer people with disabilities and those without disabilities living at these cooperatives the opportunity to participate jointly in the ownership and management of their homes, to control their living environments, and to reap the mutual benefits of associating with each other.

Important Aspects of Creative Financing   Creative financial arrangements require careful, detailed planning. It is imperative to understand the following points fully if you are considering such arrangements for yourself or your son or daughter with a disability:

1. Creative financing is an absolutely legal but complicated procedure. You must involve professionals who have thorough knowledge of all complexities involved. Financial planners, tax accountants, bank officials, lawyers, and insurance underwriters must be active participants in such ventures. The Tax Reform Act of 1986 significantly changed many aspects of real estate ownership, and people involved in creative financing must understand the implications of the new tax regulations.

2. Consumer ownership and cooperative housing ventures should not be viewed as alternatives to existing systems, but as additions to these systems. Some experts have repeatedly warned against families trying to create parallel service systems for their sons and daughters with disabilities. Ideally, creative management procedures should aim at providing for the physical residential needs of people while maintaining reliance upon existing services such as vocational rehabilitation, medical programs, recreational programs, and case management. The position of these experts presupposes that existing adult service agencies are providing services that meet an individual's needs and preferences. This may not always be the case. In such situations, family members may want to take responsibility for supervising the residence, as well as become actively involved in the provision of other services such as recreation and leisure activities. This can be very time-consuming. Families are advised to undertake such endeavors only after they have fully investigated everything that may be required of them.

3. Creative management procedures will not be possible for all people with disabilities and their families, but they represent a new and exciting alternative. Cooperation among legal, financial, and adult service professionals can create quality adult options for many.

In summary, Lowell and Barbara Hughes were able to create an opportunity for their son and add to the existing system. They are not alone in having accomplished this, but they were nonetheless able to do so only through extensive, careful planning. You may want to consider an arrangement similar to that used by the Hughes family. Contacting the right individuals and agencies is the first step.

The information presented in the description of the Hughes family and that presented in the remainder of this chapter was made possible by the kind permission of Robert J. Laux, president of Creative Management Associates of Portsmouth, New Hampshire. Additional information is provided in the resource section at the end of this book (Appendix 2). Private arrangements may be made to secure Laux's services or those of similar firms in your area. Laux or his associates can provide help in locating such firms.

Public Ownership

As recently as the early 1980s, most people with mental retardation and other developmental disabilities who were living outside family homes resided in large, publicly owned institutions. Although the deinstitutionalization movement has resulted in the closing of many of these large facilities, or at least a reduction in their size, publicly owned institutions still account for a significant percentage of residential alternatives for people with disabilities. Although large numbers of people continue to live in these facilities, for some time now this group has represented a minority of the total population with mental retardation and other developmental disabilities.

As we note throughout this chapter, public residential facilities differ from state to state as well as within states. Public facilities, however, continue to share several features: 1) They tend to have large populations. In 1982 at least half of all people living in public facilities lived in ones with populations of 64 or more residents. 2) They are generally isolated. Many public facilities continue to be located in rural settings far removed from access to community opportunities, and most older public facilities, wherever located, continue to be characterized by a style that emphasizes self-containment and large buildings in a campus-like setting set apart from the community. 3) Public institutions usually depend on self-contained services. Medical, transportation, and recreational services are often provided within the facility. This latter characteristic is often dictated by certification standards and is discussed later in this chapter.

Large public institutions have come under increasing criticism. If the trend toward depopulating them continues, these facilities will eventually be replaced by smaller facilities located where residents can use services available to the community at large. A key to this trend lies in state funding patterns. Still, as recently as 1984, the 50 states spent 1.5 times as many dollars on their publicly owned facilities as they did on community-based options. If the states would provide more funding for community alternatives, then families would have a greater range of options from which to choose. More money needs to be directed to community-based options as an alternative to institutions.

Private Ownership

There are two forms of private ownership of residential options: *nonprofit* and *profit*. It is not possible to say that one facility is better than another solely on the basis of that factor. Often, both types of facilities will operate under the same licensure requirements, and thus be virtually identical. Determinations can be made only after one considers the total program and its full range of services.

The most prevalent form of private ownership continues to be the nonprofit model. Nonprofit facilities operate under state charters and are usually directly controlled by a board of directors composed of representatives from the community, the private business sector and, in some cases, the public sector. The latter is especially true if the state in which the facility is located provides significant funding for residential programs in its communities. Some nonprofit facilities include consumers (the people who live in these facilities and use the organization's services) and their families on the governing boards.

Group homes are commonly run as nonprofit organizations, as are large intermediate care facilities for people with mental retardation and developmental disabilities (ICFs/MR). These residential models are discussed more fully in Chapter 23.

Profit facilities for people with developmental disabilities have become common, especially in the nursing home sector. Corporations run for profit have gradually expanded into other service areas, such as group homes, but they still represent the minority. As different options continue to be created, both nonprofit and profit models can be expected to offer an increasing array of services.

In evaluating residential options, you should be aware that you have the right to know the status of ownership. Feel free to ask questions about this factor. It is important to feel that you have at least a working understanding of the financial structure of the facility in which your son or daughter may choose to live.

WHAT ABOUT SIZE?

The number of people who reside within a facility is important for two reasons. First, population size directly affects the licensure standard under which a facility may operate. Licensure is discussed in greater detail in the next section of this chapter. Here, it is sufficient to say that regulations under Title XIX of the (Social Security) Medicaid programs for facilities with 15 or fewer residents are less medically oriented than those for facilities with 16 or more residents. The second reason is that size may affect the quality of relationships and habilitation. Numerous studies have documented that the smaller the population of a facility, the better the quality of care and the progress made by the people living in that facility will be. Among the areas in which gains have been noted in smaller facilities are communication skills, self-help capability, social ability, physical development, home care skills, financial management skills, independent travel, and behavior management. These gains have been noted in people with varying degrees of disabilities and have been recorded over periods ranging from 1 to 4 years.

Others assert that current information is incomplete and inconclusive, and that other factors are more important than size in determining both quality of care and rate of development. These factors include: quality of training received by facility staff, the quality of facility training programs for residents, and the amount of direct interaction a person has with others in the facility.

Some studies suggest that smaller settings are most beneficial to people with severe to mild mental retardation, while individuals with profound retardation achieve few significant gains in such settings. Some studies further suggest that the novelty of a new setting for people transferred from a large institution to a smaller community placement may be the primary cause of positive change. A final argument stresses that the medical and nutritional needs of some people with severe and multiple handicaps can best be met in larger settings that provide a concentration of medical personnel and equipment.

The issue of size will be resolved only after further studies provide families and professionals with more information. Proponents of smaller settings insist that to date the burden of proof has rested with smaller settings. That is, smaller settings have been expected to prove that they are providing better habilitation. These proponents insist that the larger settings be required to demonstrate their advantages over smaller, community-based programs.

Determining which type of setting is best for your son or daughter will require a careful assessment of individual needs. The kinds of medical services available in a given setting will vary greatly. You may want to discuss your son's or daughter's medical needs with your personal physician. Perhaps your physician would be willing to help you evaluate an option. A good rule of thumb is to seek competent medical advice whenever confronted with doubt concerning health or safety issues.

Aside from cases involving medical necessities, the process of determining the ideal size of a residence should be guided in large part by your son's or daughter's personal needs and preferences. In Chapter 24, we introduce some strategies you may find helpful in determining these personal needs and preferences. The ideas we offer are intended to allow maximum input from your son or daughter. He or she will, after all, be the one who will live in the residence, and should have a say in the final decision.

LICENSURE

There are three general categories of licensure for residential programs: *state and local, federal,* and *private*. These are discussed individually in the following section.

State and Local Licensure

State and local agencies have licensure regulations which differ according to the type of residential services provided by a program. Likewise, regulations will vary from state to state. Certification at this level will cover two broad areas—*health and safety*, and *programmatic issues*.

Residential programs are required to meet minimal health and safety guidelines. These guidelines cover such matters as fire codes, provisions for dealing with natural disasters such as storms, sanitation standards pertaining to food preparation, physical upkeep of the home or facility, and health practices for the residents. The agencies responsible for enforcing health and safety regulations vary from state to state, and in some cases may be county or city agencies.

When evaluating residential options, keep in mind that their regulations are open to public scrutiny. You or other members of your family may ask to review these regulations and discuss the program's compliance with them.

Licensure regulations that cover programmatic issues also differ from state to state. The agency responsible for investigation and documentation will carry a different title depending on which state you live in. In general, the agency will be the one charged by your state with providing social services funding, such as a department of social rehabilitation services or a department of human resources.

These state agencies set standards for programs concerning issues such as the quality of training for program staff, staff-to-client ratios, the quality of individual habilitation plans, access to confidential records, documentation procedures for training programs, and fiscal accountability.

   Like health and safety codes, programmatic regulations are open to public scrutiny. You may inquire as to the extent of such regulations and determine the degree of compliance with the regulations by a prospective residential program. In almost all cases, programs will need to meet regulations at the state and local level (e.g., fire codes) to be able to continue offering services. Regular re-evaluations (usually annual) of a program's compliance is the rule.

Federal Licensure

Programs that receive funding under Title XIX of the (Social Security) Medicaid program must follow specific federal guidelines. These guidelines place heavy emphasis on medical issues and procedures because the purpose of Title XIX is to provide for the medical needs of people living in these facilities. These facilities are called *intermediate care facilities for the mentally retarded* (ICFs/MR).

   Guidelines for such facilities are based on size of client population. The regulations that apply to facilities that house 15 or fewer clients are different from the regulations that affect facilities serving 16 or more residents. The guidelines for larger facilities are more stringent. Because most persons living in ICFs/MR have ongoing medical needs, the bulk of the federal regulations are medically oriented.

   ICF/MR programs with 15 beds or fewer operate under less rigid standards than those imposed on larger (16 beds or more) ICFs/MR. For example, there might not be a 24-hour nursing staff. Instead, nurses might be on call. Some professional services such as psychiatry or other medical specialties may be contracted for rather than available from staff, and training requirements for paraprofessional or direct care staff may be less rigid. The medical needs of the clients in these facilities may not be as great as those of clients in the larger facilities.

   Most ICFs/MR are of the larger (16 beds or more) type, although smaller facilities are increasing in number. The increase is due, in part, to the fact that more states are receiving waivers that are enabling them to use Title XIX funds in facilities that place less emphasis on the availability of ongoing, in-house medical care. The people residing in these small ICFs/MR have fewer medical needs; consequently, emphasis is placed on programming and habilitation plans.

   In evaluating residential options for your son or daughter with a disability, you may encounter facilities that are certified as ICF/MR programs. Again, you may freely inquire about the specific regulations that apply to such facilities. Knowing the extent of such regulations and an agency's compliance with them may help you evaluate residential options more effectively.

Private Accreditation

Private accreditation is granted by agencies that have no affiliation with either governmental regulatory agencies or the individual service agencies charged with maintaining residential programs. The best known, most respected, and most widely-employed private accreditation agencies for residential facilities are the Accreditation Council for Facilities for the Developmentally Disabled (ACDD) and the Commission on Accreditation of Rehabilitation Facilities (CARF).

   Both these agencies have detailed standards that have been developed by their respective governing boards, whose membership is drawn from professional and consumer associations in the field of developmental disabilities. For example, CARF is supported by the American Hospital Association, the American Occupational Therapy Association, Goodwill Industries of America, Inc., the National Association of Jewish Vocational Services, the National Easter Seal Society, and the United Cerebral Palsy Association, among other organizations. Each of these sponsoring members appoints one person to the governing board. In addition, the CARF board of trustees appoints at-large members who have professional expertise in different areas.

The residential programs pay the accreditation agencies a fee to survey their various activities. The accreditation agencies send teams of professionals who employ the highest standards of objectivity and integrity in their on-site evaluations. Deficits are noted and thoroughly explained to the program administrators. The program is given a specific deadline by which it must correct any deficits, or else risk denial or loss of accreditation.

Once a facility is accredited, frequent follow-up reviews are conducted (some annually, others every 2–3 years). These reviews are designed to ensure continuous delivery of quality human services. As a rule, accreditation through a private agency indicates a genuine commitment to high standards.

If the residential option you are investigating has private accreditation, you will probably find out early in your conversations with program staff. Because of the rigor of the standards involved, the staff will undoubtedly be proud that their program has met the criteria. You might ask for copies of the private accreditation regulations to understand the full range of the certification process and to appreciate the efforts an agency has expended to meet them.

If an agency does not have private accreditation, this does not mean it could not meet such regulations. Many facilities opt not to seek private accreditation. One reason may be the expense involved. Such fees sometimes dissuade completely reliable agencies from participating.

23 WHAT ARE SOME RESIDENTIAL MODELS?

Now that you are armed with a general understanding of how size, licensure regulations, and types of ownership affect residential options, it is time to review some of the options themselves. As we stated earlier, a framework for grouping and differentiating between options is necessary to the search for an appropriate residence. The framework we present in this chapter is based on a continuum. The models described have progressively more elaborate organizations, policies, and certification standards.

We do not endorse one model over another. Nor do we attempt to evaluate the benefits of one model as compared to those of another model. You and your family have unique needs that will be met in unique ways. We simply describe the options so that you will be better prepared to evaluate them. The six models we describe are:

1. Independent living
2. Natural and adoptive homes
3. Intentional communities
4. Adult care and board-and-care homes
5. The group home continuum
6. Intermediate care facilities for the mentally retarded (ICFs/MR)

As you begin to evaluate residential options in your community, you will discover that, even within categories, considerable differences can exist. The purpose of the framework we use is only to provide you with broad categories to consider.

INDEPENDENT LIVING

Independent living involves people residing in their own apartments, trailers, and houses, caring for their own daily needs, and requiring very limited assistance. The assistance can take the form of periodic visits from adult agency personnel to ensure that all is running smoothly. Staff may assist in areas that require higher skills, such as problem-solving and money management. As its name indicates, minimal supervision is the key characteristic of independent living.

A recent trend in independent living involves helping people with disabilities locate in proximity to one another, for example, in apartments within walking distance. Such arrangements allow people to give both material and emotional support to each other while maintaining independent life-styles. A key element in ensuring success is that, in addition to easy access to social support, there must be access to transportation, shops and businesses, recreation facilities, and other aspects of community life.

Another trend related to independent living is that growing numbers of people with disabilities are choosing to marry. Marriage can provide a great deal of social support and can enable a couple to live more independently by enabling them to pool their strengths, skills, and resources. Some individuals are also choosing to raise families. Additional outside support for these people may be indicated, and appropriate planning must be part of the total package.

The skills needed for independent living may rule out this option for some people with severe disabilities. However, considering independent living may provide families with a greater insight into the full range of residential options.

NATURAL AND ADOPTIVE HOMES

Both natural and adoptive homes are common residential options for many adults with disabilities. In fact, there is some evidence that the popularity of these living arrangements has grown in recent years.

Four factors appear to be responsible for the trend toward family-style living arrangements. First, the passage in 1974 of The Education for All Handicapped Children Act (PL 94-142) made educational services available to all school-age children and adolescents regardless of disability. In the past, some families placed their children in residential facilities of one type or another to obtain educational services. However, education in one's home community is now a reality for the great majority of students with disabilities.

The availability of full-day public school programs has benefited the family unit in other ways. With the student in school, family members have been freed from direct care responsibilitites for long periods during the day. Frequently, both parents choose to work outside the home while their children are in school, a choice which can mean a greater family income. This greater availability of time and money has combined to enable more families to keep school-aged members with disabilities at home. Often, when the person with a disability reaches adulthood, these families continue the same living arrangements.

The second factor in the trend toward natural and adoptive homes is a gradual change in community attitudes towards people with disabilities. Physicians and other health professionals are less likely today to encourage institutionalization of youngsters with disabilities. Other segments of the community have also become more supportive, which has led to a greater availability of services and programs to help maintain people in the community.

An increasing number of professional services, such as medical care, counseling, and therapies, are now available locally. Likewise; the expansion of programs such as organized respite care, which provides temporary supervision and direct care for members with disabilities so that other family members can have a break from their responsibilities, has enabled more people to work and therefore augment family income.

The third factor relates to an individual's preferences and choices, and those of his or her family, regarding where he or she will live. The family may believe that "taking care of our own" is important. The person with a disability may choose to provide companionship for aging family members as well as help with household chores and finances. Once adulthood is reached, disability insurance benefits can augment the family income. For some families, this money may constitute a vital resource to help meet the entire family's needs. As we have repeatedly stressed, every family has unique needs and preferences and any decision in this area will reflect unique family characteristics.

The last factor is indicative of a less pleasant situation. Families may be keeping their members at home because acceptable alternatives simply do not exist. But if a family is offered no alternatives to their own home, then that home is not a real choice.

INTENTIONAL COMMUNITIES

In the late 1960s, news from France, Belgium, and other European countries reached North America about a revolutionary new concept concerning people with disabilities. People both with and without disabilities were choosing to live together in small communities designed so they could support one another. This residential option has been collectively called the *intentional community*. Two types exist in the United States— L'Arche (described below) and Camp Hill. Located in New York, Pennsylvania, and Wisconsin, Camp Hill communities generally have about 100 residents, both with and without disabilities, living as families in homes on common ground.

One of the founders of the intentional community movement was Jean Vanier, who in 1964 invited two men, Raphael and Phillipe, to live with him in a suburb of Paris. Both men had lived for many years in a large institution for people with mental disabilities. Vanier's goal was to start a movement to provide a residential alternative for people with disabilities. The alternative is a home within a community that strives for the integration and happiness of those living within the home. Vanier called the movement *L'Arche* (The Ark).

The L'Arche model grew as new homes were established in France and other European countries. The first L'Arche community in North America was founded in 1969 in Richmond Hill, a small town near Toronto. Today, L'Arche is an international federation of more than 50 communities in Belgium, Canada, Denmark, France, Great Britain, Haiti, Honduras, India, the Ivory Coast, Norway, and the United States. There are more than 20 permanent L'Arche communities in North America, each one operating 1–7 district homes.

The size of the communities varies, but most are small, consisting of single family units located within established residential neighborhoods. Some rural L'Arche communities stress agricultural activities. The most distinctive characteristic of the model is the personal conviction of its proponents that people with disabilities can and do add uniquely to the lives of others. There is an emphasis on personal relationships that are mutually beneficial. Residence in a L'Arche model home is viewed as permanent; bonds are formed that cannot be easily severed.

Another noteworthy characteristic of L'Arche communities is the lack of emphasis on salaried staff. In homes that do have salaried personnel, the staff are called assistants, while the people with disabilities are never referred to as "clients," "patients," or "residents." While the movement maintains and stresses its Christian roots, it is not affiliated with any single religion or faith.

Funding sources for the homes vary. Many receive government subsidies such as the Social Security benefits of the residents. The International Council of the Federation of L'Arche provides varying degrees of support. Private payments and funds raised through different activities, as well as contributions from a diversity of sources, complete the funding picture. Information that will enable you to contact individual programs for details is provided in the resource section at the back of this book (see Appendix 2).

ADULT FOSTER CARE AND BOARD-AND-CARE HOMES

Adult Foster Care

Adult foster care homes differ from natural homes in two ways. First, the residents of these homes consist of families and other people (usually not relatives) whom the families have invited to live with them. Second, these homes receive government reimbursement. This means that, unlike natural homes, foster care homes must follow special regulations. Unlike foster care for youngsters, adult foster care is intended to be more or less permanent.

One of the positive features of adult foster care is the family-like environment it provides. Often, families accepting adults into foster care tend to have well-established community ties. This may enhance the integration of the person with a disability into the community mainstream. Foster families usually have fewer members than group homes or other facilities. The number of adults that may be placed in a home varies according to state regulations, but the current range is 2–6 people per home.

The people who choose to open their homes to adult foster placements usually are not "in it for the money." Some foster care families cite religious convictions as the basis for their actions, and others are just interested in helping others.

One couple who have served as foster parents for many years made the following observations when asked why they were working with young adults with disabilities: "We are only doing what we believe God wants us to do. We do not attend an organized church on a regular basis, but we are Christians and lead our lives accordingly. Our own children, Brent, age 9, and Holly, who is now 12, have gained so much from our family experiences. They have learned the meaning of compassion and charity, and they have learned that their abilities are gifts to be shared with others. Does that sound hokey? Well, it's the truth."

Foster care homes for adults are not required to provide training in skill areas where the adults may be lacking. Although some foster care providers are adept at teaching independent living skills and providing systematic training to the people living with them, this is not required by most state regulations. For this reason, foster care placement may not be appropriate for adults for whom extensive training is a priority.

Foster care homes have other potential negative aspects. Although adult foster care is intended to be a long-term arrangement, few guarantees actually exist. Families may choose to cease providing foster care, or changes in their own families may require them to stop. Adults with disabilities living in these arrangements may have formed strong emotional bonds with their foster families. The need to move to another home can be very upsetting. If you or others are concerned about the permanence of a residential option, you are not alone. Many parents share this concern and it is an issue that you can investigate when exploring residential options.

Another potentially troublesome aspect of foster home placement is inherent in the model itself. It is the parents and other family members who will determine how good a foster home will be. Close supervision by state agencies cannot guarantee that every foster care home will be a desirable placement. While the majority of foster homes undoubtedly strive for quality and offer a viable residential option, the same care that is exercised in considering other placements should apply to this option.

It is possible that some families may feel threatened by the concept of adult foster care. Some families may be seeking a placement outside the home because their physical or psychological ability to continue to live with and care for the member with a disability has been exhausted. The members of the foster family may present themselves as people who can do what the natural parents and other family members can no longer manage. This, of course, will not be the case for all families, but the possibility exists. As we show throughout this chapter, individual families will make decisions based on their own unique needs.

Boarding Homes

Boarding homes will vary appreciably as to the type of residents living in them and the training and supervision provided. In some boarding facilities, sleeping rooms and meals are provided, while in others meal preparation may be the residents' own responsibility. Some training in daily living skills may be provided, but such training is usually not required by licensing agencies.

The level of supervision at boarding homes will vary, but will generally be determined by the needs of relatively independent adults. Some smaller, family-operated boarding homes more closely resemble foster care homes. Often, these boarding facilities will have a varied clientele with a variety of disabilities.

Boarding homes will vary as to licensing requirements, but safety, health, and fire codes must be observed. The boarding home option is important in that it can provide independent settings for some people while freeing rooms in more structured facilities for those who require closer supervision and training.

GROUP HOMES

With the recent expansion of living arrangements for people with disabilities, the group home continuum has expanded to include many forms. The use of different names to describe these living arrangements (for example, *group home, community residence,* and *community care home* all can describe similar options) has caused confusion among families planning for future residential options.

Before discussing the individual options within the group home continuum, we must discuss general characteristics that apply to all the options. First, although some descriptions of group homes include large facilities (from 16 to more than 300 residents within the group home continuum), that is not the case here. Throughout, when we discuss group homes, we mean only those facilities serving fewer than 16 people.

The second characteristic of most group homes is that they are more or less family-like; that is, the actual physical structure of the house or apartment and the activities of the people living in it are similar to the structure and activities of other homes in the community. The house, although sometimes larger than an average family home, generally looks like others in the neighborhood. Inside is found the usual array of rooms.

For the most part, the tasks of everyday living are performed by the people who reside in the home to the extent of their abilities. Residents frequently prepare meals, perform maintenance chores such as cleaning, mowing lawns, and washing dishes, and take care of their personal needs according to their individual capabilities.

The third important characteristic of group homes is that emphasis is placed on formal habilitation and training programs. Through individual plans, training objectives stressing independent living skills are developed and usually implemented. The group home continuum model stresses continued growth in the competence and capabilities of the residents. People begin within an environment designed to meet their levels of needs in both structure and supervision. The expectation is that they will "graduate" to a more independent situation that meets their individual needs and preferences. For some people, this may mean complete independence outside adult service programs.

What follows is a brief review of the two broad options within the continuum. The breakdown of the options is based on the amount of structure, supervision, and assistance provided at each level. Within each option, expect programs to differ among themselves in the manner in which they strive to meet the unique needs of the people living and learning within the residences. The two broad options are *supervised group living* and *semi-independent living arrangements*.

Supervised Group Living

The term, *group home*, has taken on a generic meaning much in the same manner that aspirin today means a general headache remedy while originally it was a specific drug produced by only one company. In general, a group home refers to a family-style home designed to house up to 15 people and usually located in a residential neighborhood. The number of residents will vary, although current attitudes stress smaller homes serving fewer residents. Experts in the field and many advocacy groups point out that the more a group home mirrors the size of other residences in the neighborhood, the greater are the chances for full assimilation. So, number of residents is an issue, with lower numbers (e.g., five or six people) being preferable. It would be wrong, however, to attempt to set a specific number for an "ideal" supervised group living arrangement. Individual preferences and needs should dictate the ideal. For one person, a residential setting for four or five people may be appropriate. For another person such an arrangment may be too large. Some people prefer or need residential programs on even smaller scales.

The home may be a renovated structure or one that is specifically built to serve adults with disabilities. The home may likewise be an apartment or other such structure that meets individual needs. In some communities, the high cost of renovating older homes to meet fire and safety codes has resulted in more new structures being built as group homes. Nationally, the majority of these homes continue to be older dwellings in established neighborhoods.

The group home may be staffed in different ways. The home may have live-in house managers augmented by relief staff. Some house managers are married couples with children of their own. In this arrangement, a part of the house actually may be set aside for the house manager and his or her family. The managers are responsible for seeing to the needs of the house and the residents and implementing training programs. The relief staff provide the resident managers time off from their duties on a regular weekly schedule.

Another common staffing arrangement involves rotating shifts. In some settings, staff work at the home for 8-hour shifts and are replaced by other shifts, thereby covering the hours staff are needed when residents are at home. Still other settings employ a rotation model in which staff work several days on and several days off, replaced by other staff to cover the need for supervision and training of residents.

Ideally, the supervision needs of the various residents will influence the staffing patterns within group homes. In exemplary programs, the number of staff who are present will depend upon the time of day. Additional staff may be present to assist residents during meal preparations or to help implement specific residents' programs. Some group homes even employ special trainers to augment the supervisory staff.

Semi-Independent Living

We use the term *semi-independent living* to describe a range of residential options that share some characteristics, while differing in other aspects. The physical structure of such arrangements is as varied as the imagination allows. Groups of apartments offered at subsidized rents may be clustered within established apartment buildings or complexes. Buildings designed specifically for use as semi-independent settings may be constructed. Houses may be converted for this use, as may mobile homes or condominiums. Residents may have one or more roommates or may live alone within an apartment complex.

The key characteristic is that staff do not live or stay for a specific shift in the semi-independent setting occupied by people with disabilities. Staff may live in apartments within a semi-independent living complex and be available to assist with supervision and training at specific times of the day (for example, at mealtime). In other situations, staff can be on call to handle certain duties or emergencies.

Ideally, levels of supervision are designed to meet individual needs. For the most part, residents have the ability to perform many everyday tasks independently, but require some assistance in limited areas. Many semi-independent living facilities are designed for people with mild disabilities, while some are appropriate for those with more severe disabilities. The emphasis in these settings is on continued growth in independent living skills. The goal is to "graduate" to independent living.

INTERMEDIATE CARE FACILITIES
FOR THE MENTALLY RETARDED (ICFs/MR)

Within the ICF/MR category are several types of residential programs that share the distinguishing characteristic that they are funded by Title XIX of the Social Security Medicaid program. These programs are designed to meet the medical needs of people and as a result a strict medical orientation is the norm. As we noted earlier, these programs must meet the stringent requirements of the funding source.

To make our review of the options within this broad category easier, we group them according to shared characteristics. Our groupings are 1) *small ICF/MR*, 2) *nursing home*, 3) *large ICF/MR*.

Small ICFs/MR

Small ICFs/MR serve 15 or fewer people and must meet the somewhat relaxed standards that were discussed in Chapter 22, which deals with licensure. These federal standards, although more stringent than state and local standards for typical group homes, are more relaxed than those required for large ICFs/MR. The standards may be appropriate for clients with chronic health needs who do not require stringent medical care. Also, as more states obtain waivers to use Medicaid funds in less typically medical settings, such facilities are serving people with milder disabilities.

Some small ICFs/MR resemble group homes, and their required habilitation plans may address nonmedical goals. An issue nationwide is the cost of providing residential options. The *reimbursement rate* (i.e., the monetary rate per person per day that is paid from government programs such as Medicaid) for small ICFs usually exceeds that for non-ICF–certified group homes. The continued growth of small ICFs/MR will remain closely tied to the overall economic conditions affecting residential providers.

Nursing Homes

The main emphasis in nursing homes is on the provision of medical care to the residents. Accreditation standards will differ depending on the medical needs of the people living in these facilities. The two most common designations are *intermediate care* and *skilled care*.

Intermediate care homes are staffed to care for individuals with mentally or physically disabling conditions (or both) that require medical treatment under the supervision of doctors and other licensed medical personnel. The facilities are staffed to provide at least 8 hours a day and 5 days a week of care by licensed nurses and other required staff. Residents are generally of advanced years.

Skilled care homes serve people whose medical condition requires 24-hour nursing care and treatment on a daily basis that must be provided by licensed medical/ nursing personnel. The skilled nursing care includes observation, care and counseling, the administration of medications and treatments, and other nursing functions that require substantial specialized judgment and skill.

Except for those people with disabilities who are elderly or have chronic health problems, these facilities are not appropriate placements. The number of placements in such facilities continues to decrease.

Large ICFs/MR

In the late 1960s, the population of state-owned and state-operated institutions stood at approximately 200,000 people with developmental disabilities. By the late 1980s, the deinstitutionalization movement had reduced this number to a population of less than half that number. This is, however, only part of the whole picture because another aspect of large institutions, the growth of private facilities, has not been reported as accurately as the decline of public facilities.

There have always been private facilities which were indistinguishable from the numerous state institutions. In fact, these private facilities have grown in number as the state facilities have been gradually depopulated. Many of the large private facilities are now licensed ICFs/MR, and new facilities continue the growth pattern. Today, more than half of all people with developmental disabilities who are not living at home are housed in facilities serving in excess of 60 people.

The gamut of large ICFs/MR includes a combination of publicly owned institutions as well as privately owned and operated facilities. Some of the private facilities are nursing homes which have been adapted to meet Title XIX regulations. Newer facilities have been built specifically to meet the regulations, so that they may serve people with disabilities. Chronic medical needs are often an issue for some people with disabilities and many large ICFs/MR are staffed to address these needs specifically. Some experts in the field, however, question the extent of the medical needs of many people living in these facilities. These experts argue that many of these people could live in smaller residences where the programming is not medically oriented. They further argue that the smaller settings would be far less costly to maintain and would still meet resident needs.

Many of these facilities have educational programs associated with them for school-aged residents, although it is not uncommon for many residents to attend community schools. Training programs are usually offered in most such facilities and target various social, domestic, and academic skills. Chronic medical needs are often an issue for some residents and many facilities have adequate medical staff to handle them.

The resident populations of large ICF/MR-certified facilities range from 16 to more than 400. The states are gradually getting out of the business of running these facilities and pressure is on the larger private facilities to depopulate also. The trend is to close or "streamline" these facilities in favor of community-based options.

24 NOW THAT I HAVE THE INFORMATION, HOW DO I EVALUATE THE OPTIONS?

Locating an appropriate residential placement for their son or daughter remains an important concern for many parents. This chapter was designed to provide a framework to use when identifying types of options, and to help you begin your own planning. As we have shown, the different models vary substantially at times. Ideally, your son's or daughter's preferences and needs should guide program evaluation. However, matching preferences to programs may result in the determination that an ideal program does not exist.

In this chapter, procedures are identified to help you with the evaluation process. These procedures will enable you to rate programs by identifying those aspects that are most important to your son or daughter. At the same time, shortcomings can be clearly identified. Ultimately the choice is yours to make in the manner that best suits your family's decision-making style, preferences, and needs.

As you make contacts with programs providing residential services, you will find yourself accumulating a lot of information. You will undoubtedly scan through the information as you receive it and form preliminary impressions of available programs. However, comparisons will be difficult until you have compiled information on a number of programs. If asked, "How well does a particular agency meet your family's needs?", you should be able to respond, "Compared to what?"

The manner in which you evaluate residential programs will reflect your decision-making style. This first section of Chapter 24 suggests some tactics you may find useful. Consider it a buffet line; feel free to adopt what you find to your liking and disregard those aspects that would not serve your needs. Modify approaches as you see fit, mix and match—there are no set rules in this buffet, if you wish to mix the French and blue cheese dressings, then by all means proceed.

Initial Review

Early in their search for an ideal residential program for their son, Lowell and Barbara Hughes had an experience you might find instructive. A private agency in the Midwest that they had contacted mailed them a brochure. In part, the program was described as follows:

> Small, homelike cottages provided for the unique needs of the hard-to-handle adolescent and young adult. We have a fully trained staff of professionals who provide around-the-clock care and training. Come see our beautiful campus—40 rolling, wooded acres providing space to play, learn, and grow.

Barbara commented that the program sounded perfect, and that she wanted to visit the facility. Lowell, skeptical, feared that the description was too perfect to be true. The agency was 300 miles from the Hughes' home, but they decided that a first-hand look would be in order. Sadly, their visit proved that the description was indeed not true. The "small, homelike cottages" were two-story dormitories housing 90 people each. The "fully trained staff of professionals" consisted of direct care workers augmented by consultants who spent little time working directly with the residents. The "40 rolling, wooded acres" were in fact flat farmland with less than a dozen newly-planted saplings. Only 5 acres were available to the agency. The remaining 35 acres were leased to a nearby farmer who grew corn and strictly enforced the "No Trespassing" signs posted on the barbed wire fence enclosing his leased land.

After the visit, Lowell commented, "The brochure for that program must have been put together by fiction writers!" The point is simple—sometimes the information you receive may be misleading. Agencies will attempt to present the best possible picture of their programs and facilities, something that is not always done in a responsible manner.

Visiting residential options will expose most deceptive descriptions, but you may find it impossible to visit every option you have located. Time may be a factor as well as cost. Lost wages resulting from time off from work and the cost of traveling can be prohibitive. The different personal schedules of family members involved in the planning process may prevent some from visiting certain residential programs. You can imagine the problems this might cause: you visit a program and consider it fantastic; how can you convey your enthusiasm adequately to others in your family who could not visit?

After reviewing the information you have gathered up to this point, it may be obvious that certain programs are completely inappropriate. Consider the two following situations involving the Stuart and Harris families.

HOW DO I DETERMINE MY SON'S OR DAUGHTER'S PREFERENCES?

The checklist presented at the end of this chapter (titled, "Things That Are Important about the Place Where I Live") is designed to help you determine the range and the intensity of your son's or daughter's preferences concerning a place to live. You will notice a few particularly important aspects of the checklist as you read through it. First, there are many items which should not be surprising given the importance of residential arrangements in our lives. The environment of the particular home your son or daughter will live in will largely determine his or her quality of life.

The second thing you will notice in reviewing the checklist is that there may be some items that may not be important to your son or daughter becase he or she may be unable to understand the complexities these items entail. Yet these items represent issues of vital importance to you. The checklist has been specifically designed to allow you to determine your own preferences and those of other family members in regard to residential options, as well as the preferences of your son or daughter.

As an example, look at two items from Part C of the checklist:

2) Someone in the house or the people who run the house act as an advocate of my human rights.

17) The house has an active human rights committee with representatives from the community.

Your son or daughter may be unprepared to understand the concept of a human rights committee and what such a committee may add to a residential program. Likewise, the concept of an advocate may be foreign to your son or daughter, who knows only that there has always been someone around to stand up for his or her rights. That someone may have been another family member, but someone was always there when needed. You may feel strongly that a group of people from outside an adult service agency can provide the needed review process to prevent abuses of human rights. A human rights committee may represent a must for you in this case. Furthermore, by figuratively stepping into your son's or daughter's shoes you might determine that Item 2 of Part C is very important as well, and that your son or daughter would want this situation to continue.

The last thing you will notice about the checklist is that there are blank spaces to allow you to fill in those items that are uniquely important to you or your son or daughter. As one mother put it after completing the checklist with her 20-year-old son who has moderate mental retardation, "Why, this list doesn't mention being able to have a bike. That's very important to Tom; he gets around town that way, so you can see it's very important because the house can't be on a busy highway or in a part of town where he'd have to contend with a lot of traffic." We are all different; the blank spaces will allow you to spell out those differences.

In the following pages, you'll see how two of the families used the checklist to help them plan. You will begin to see how the checklist was used in the early stages of planning and through the rest of the process, leading to different decisions for different families.

*   *   *

Rose, Jack, Sally, and Theresa Stuart sat around the kitchen table reviewing the information that had arrived in that day's mail. Rose had requested information on residential programs from several agencies, and the response had been good. These review sessions brought the family together in a common cause—the best for Steve. Sally thought of her role in this process and felt tremendous pride. Her parents respected her opinions and treated her as . . . well, as an adult. She had much to add to the planning and her parents listened when she spoke and openly discussed their own feelings, doubts, and desires in regard to Steve's future.

Sally loved Steve and the rest of her family deeply. The knowledge that she was helping those she loved made her tremble slightly. Her mother noticed and asked, "Are you all right, dear? Not coming down with anything, I hope." Sally beamed. Shaking her head "No," she replied, "I'm just fine; what kind of program sent info today? Let's check out this Ridge Valley Community Homes."

Everyone started reading the materials sent that day from an agency called Ridge Valley Community Homes, and commented on aspects of the program that caught their interest. "Kind of far away," said Jack. Jack had indicated earlier on the checklist that Steve would want to continue regular contact with his family. Note how the Stuarts responded to the following items from Part C of "Things That Are Important about the Place Where I Live":

23) My family and friends can visit me any time.
      +3   +2   +1   0   −1   −2   −3

28) My family and friends can become involved in boards and committees that supervise the running of the house.
      +3   +2   +1   0   −1   −2   −3

29) My family and friends may take part in special events with me (birthdays, celebrations, etc.).

(+3) +2 +1 0 −1 −2 −3

The Ridge Valley program, being some distance from the Stuart's home, might make it difficult to meet the preferences expressed in the above items.

"The pictures of the different houses look nice, real clean," added Theresa. The preferences noted on the items below from Part B seemed to have been satisfied by the flattering pictures of the homes:

19) The house is in a neighborhood that is like my family's.

+3 (+2) +1 0 −1 −2 −3

20) The house has a yard.

(+3) +2 +1 0 −1 −2 −3

22) The house is in a safe neighborhood.

(+3) +2 +1 0 −1 −2 −3

"Hey, they have speech therapists!" Rose exclaimed. "And PTs," added Theresa. Note the importance placed on this aspect in the checklist (from Part C):

10) Other (ancillary) services (such as physical and occupational therapy, respite care, personal care attendants) are reasonably available.

(+3) +2 +1 0 −1 −2 −3

Steve's continued need for habilitation to improve his walking required that physical therapy be available.

"It's not right for Steve." Sally's insistent voice penetrated the rising chatter. "Look at this," Sally said, passing the part of the brochure she had been reading across the table to her mother. "The part at the bottom of the second page," Sally indicated.

Rose read aloud: "Ridge Valley provides for the total needs of the elderly who are mentally retarded. Although we accept people who are younger, most of your residents are over 50 years old . . . "

The Stuart family had talked at length about Steve's likes, dislikes, and needs. He liked older people and interacted well with them, yet he clearly preferred the company of those closer to his age. They had decided in many items that this was important to Steve (from Part B):

1) I have a say in who my housemates will be.

+3 (+2) +1 0 −1 −2 −3

Steve's decision for Item 4 would be to have housemates nearer his own age:

4) The people who live with me are as capable as I am.

+3 (+2) +1 0 −1 −2 −3

To Steve, capability meant similar likes and dislikes, such as music, television programs, and leisure activities. People considerably older than him might not be compatible with the young man.

Finally, there was an item they had added to Part B.

27) Other residents in my house are near me in age.

(+3) +2 +1 0 −1 −2 −3

The Ridge Valley program had many positive features and would meet the needs of another family, but it was obviously inappropriate for Steve. The decision was easy—file the information away and wait for tomorrow's mail.

* * *

Odessa Harris pushed open the back door with the sound of the phone ringing in her ears. She hurriedly placed the sack of groceries on the small dinette table, started toward the phone, and suddenly stopped, remembering the remaining groceries in the trunk of her car. "They'll keep," she thought.

Picking up the phone, she heard her brother's voice: "Where've you been? Haven't you learned that phones aren't any good unless you answer them?"

"Okay, Owen, what does this sound like, a recording?," she said, chuckling at her brother's impatience.

"I just got back from Atlanta, and I have some news," Owen said. "I looked at a place, real nice place, where Jolene might want to live."

Odessa thought about how helpful Owen had always been. His concern for her and Jolene had been the source of her strength on more than one occasion. Owen had always been close to his niece, and more and more, he took on the role of the father she had never known.

Owen excitedly described the boarding home he had visited in Atlanta. He had heard about the program from a friend and he tried to get Odessa to go to Atlanta to see the place for herself, but she had always refused, saying it was too far from West Point. So, he made up an excuse—he had to go to Atlanta on business. The only business he had was a long visit to the boarding home and a Braves double-header. At least half the trip was successful. The residential program was top notch—the Braves dropped both games.

Odessa finally interrupted Owen's nonstop description, saying, "We've been through this all before. Atlanta is too far away. Now just let it rest!" As soon as she said it, she wished the bite in her voice hadn't been there. "Owen, thank you, really. But I want her close to me, and we decided that Jolene wants that also."

One item Jolene added to the checklist clearly summed up her preferences regarding the distance issue (Part B, "About Where and with Whom I Will Live"):

27)   I must be able to attend services at my church every weekend.
     (+3)   +2   +1   0   −1   −2   −3

Jolene's involvement with the First Baptist Church was very important. She was in the youth choir, took part in helping run early morning child care on Sundays, and never missed a Sunday service. She was very fond of the Reverend Davis and his wife. She often spent Saturday evenings with them helping in any way she could to prepare for Sunday's activities. There might be other Baptist churches in Atlanta, but Jolene's heart and soul belonged with her church family in West Point.

"Look, I know you've probably gathered a ton of things that describe the place you visited," Odessa said. "Bring it over, and I'll look at it. But for now, Atlanta will have to wait." She paused. "How was the rest of your business trip? Did the Braves win?" Owen chuckled. They said their good-byes and hung up.

Going to the car to retrieve the rest of the groceries, Odessa was just in time to see her neighbor's dog fleeing her open trunk. She knew what had happened—he had jumped his fence again. She found the remains of a package lying on the ground. The hint of a smile curled one corner of her mouth as she thought, "Best bird dog in the county—can sniff out a package of breakfast sausage a mile away."

* * *

Like the Harris and Stuart families, you may determine that there are aspects of certain residential programs that make them totally inappropriate for your family. You should save information on such programs so that you can re-evaluate them later. Remember, programs change over time so you may want to recontact apparently inappropriate programs at some later point.

At this stage, however, your goal is to identify programs that you and others can visit that appear to meet the preferences of all involved. You may want to use a broad rating scheme at this stage. For example, you could separate the programs after your initial evaluation into the following three categories:

Appear to meet your son's or daughter's preferences and needs—*Must visit.*
May be appropriate for our son's or daughter's preferences and needs—*May visit later.*
Appears to be inappropriate—*No visit, but keep in touch.*

SECTION 4: THINGS THAT ARE IMPORTANT ABOUT THE PLACE WHERE I LIVE

	Absolutely yes			Don't care			Absolutely no
A. About the Things I May Do in My House							
1. I may have my own TV, stereo, and radio in my bedroom.	+3	+2	+1	0	−1	−2	−3
2. I may have my own furniture in my room.	+3	+2	+1	0	−1	−2	−3
3. I may put posters and pictures on my bedroom walls.	+3	+2	+1	0	−1	−2	−3
4. I may have my own bedroom.	+3	+2	+1	0	−1	−2	−3
5. I may have any other personal things that I want.	+3	+2	+1	0	−1	−2	−3
6. I have a say in how the rest of my house will be decorated.	+3	+2	+1	0	−1	−2	−3
7. I may have a larger pet (such as a cat or dog).	+3	+2	+1	0	−1	−2	−3
8. I may have smaller pets (such as birds, fish, or gerbils).	+3	+2	+1	0	−1	−2	−3
9. The staff that work in my house respect my opinions.	+3	+2	+1	0	−1	−2	−3
10. There is a place and time in my house where I can be by myself if I want to.	+3	+2	+1	0	−1	−2	−3
11. I may choose who takes care of my personal needs.	+3	+2	+1	0	−1	−2	−3
12. Someone of my sex takes care of my personal needs.	+3	+2	+1	0	−1	−2	−3
13. I may continue to use my family physician, dentist, and other specialists.	+3	+2	+1	0	−1	−2	−3
14. I have chances to meet and make friends with people outside my home and other homes like mine.	+3	+2	+1	0	−1	−2	−3
15. I may use the telephone whenever I want to.	+3	+2	+1	0	−1	−2	−3
16. Nobody checks on my incoming and outgoing mail or phone calls.	+3	+2	+1	0	−1	−2	−3
17. I may decline to take part in any special religious or holiday celebrations that other people in my house are doing together.	+3	+2	+1	0	−1	−2	−3
18. I may pay my rent and utilities without someone else's okay.	+3	+2	+1	0	−1	−2	−3

		Absolutely yes		Don't care			Absolutely no	
19.	I may request special meals and diets.	+3	+2	+1	0	−1	−2	−3
20.	I may spend long periods of time away from the house with my family or friends (for vacations, trips, or special occasions).	+3	+2	+1	0	−1	−2	−3
21.	Punishments, if used, do not humiliate or embarrass me.	+3	+2	+1	0	−1	−2	−3
22.	The chores the staff ask me to do around the house are important or useful.	+3	+2	+1	0	−1	−2	−3
23.	I have a say about what chores or duties I do around the house.	+3	+2	+1	0	−1	−2	−3
24.	I may refuse to do any chores or duties around the house.	+3	+2	+1	0	−1	−2	−3
25.	My family and friends can become involved in boards and committees that supervise the running of the house.	+3	+2	+1	0	−1	−2	−3
26.	_____	+3	+2	+1	0	−1	−2	−3
27.	_____	+3	+2	+1	0	−1	−2	−3
28.	_____	+3	+2	+1	0	−1	−2	−3

B. About Where and With Whom I Will Live

		Absolutely yes		Don't care			Absolutely no	
1.	I have a say in who my housemates will be.	+3	+2	+1	0	−1	−2	−3
2.	I have a say in who my roommates will be.	+3	+2	+1	0	−1	−2	−3
3.	Fewer than six people live in my house.	+3	+2	+1	0	−1	−2	−3
4.	The people who live with me are as capable as I am.	+3	+2	+1	0	−1	−2	−3
5.	Those living in the house are of different sexes.	+3	+2	+1	0	−1	−2	−3
6.	People in my house appear to care for one another.	+3	+2	+1	0	−1	−2	−3
7.	I may live in a house where nobody smokes.	+3	+2	+1	0	−1	−2	−3
8.	I do not have to follow the same schedule that everyone else has.	+3	+2	+1	0	−1	−2	−3
9.	I may stay in the house for several years without having to move.	+3	+2	+1	0	−1	−2	−3
10.	I may choose whether to move from one house to another.	+3	+2	+1	0	−1	−2	−3
11.	When I learn certain skills, I may move to another house where housemates are more independent.	+3	+2	+1	0	−1	−2	−3
12.	I may move back to my old house if the new place does not work out for me.	+3	+2	+1	0	−1	−2	−3
13.	If I get married, my spouse and I can still live in the house.	+3	+2	+1	0	−1	−2	−3
14.	If I have a nonmarital intimate relationship, my partner and I can still live in the same house.	+3	+2	+1	0	−1	−2	−3
15.	I may live by myself.	+3	+2	+1	0	−1	−2	−3
16.	The house is close to school and work.	+3	+2	+1	0	−1	−2	−3
17.	The house is close to public transportation.	+3	+2	+1	0	−1	−2	−3
18.	The house is close to shopping and recreational sites.	+3	+2	+1	0	−1	−2	−3
19.	The house is in a neighborhood that is like my family's.	+3	+2	+1	0	−1	−2	−3

		Absolutely yes			Don't care			Absolutely no
20.	The house has a yard.	+3	+2	+1	0	−1	−2	−3
21.	The house has space for a garden.	+3	+2	+1	0	−1	−2	−3
22.	The house is in a safe neighborhood.	+3	+2	+1	0	−1	−2	−3
23.	My house has a work program that is part of the overall program.	+3	+2	+1	0	−1	−2	−3
24.	The staff at my house provides transportation to and from my job.	+3	+2	+1	0	−1	−2	−3
25.	Most of my neighbors do not have a disability.	+3	+2	+1	0	−1	−2	−3
26.	Most of my neighbors are friendly and helpful.	+3	+2	+1	0	−1	−2	−3
27.	_____	+3	+2	+1	0	−1	−2	−3
28.	_____	+3	+2	+1	0	−1	−2	−3
29.	_____	+3	+2	+1	0	−1	−2	−3

C. About Staff and the Way My House is Run

		Absolutely yes			Don't care			Absolutely no
1.	There is somebody in the house who knows how to give emergency first aid.	+3	+2	+1	0	−1	−2	−3
2.	Someone in the house or the people who run the house act as an advocate of my human rights.	+3	+2	+1	0	−1	−2	−3
3.	Someone in the house knows how to teach independent living skills.	+3	+2	+1	0	−1	−2	−3
4.	Someone in the house knows how to handle behavior problems.	+3	+2	+1	0	−1	−2	−3
5.	Staff are well-paid.	+3	+2	+1	0	−1	−2	−3
6.	Staff take part in regular training to learn how to do their jobs better.	+3	+2	+1	0	−1	−2	−3
7.	Staff members are employed over a long period of time; there is low staff turnover.	+3	+2	+1	0	−1	−2	−3
8.	There are three or fewer staff changes within each week.	+3	+2	+1	0	−1	−2	−3
9.	The house hires people of both sexes as staff.	+3	+2	+1	0	−1	−2	−3
10.	Other (ancillary) services (such as physical and occupational therapy, respite care, personal care attendants) are reasonably available.	+3	+2	+1	0	−1	−2	−3
11.	Staff meet all licensing requirements.	+3	+2	+1	0	−1	−2	−3
12.	Staff or family members will not enter my bedroom or the bathroom when I close the door without knocking first and asking me if they can come in.	+3	+2	+1	0	−1	−2	−3
13.	If I am in the bedroom or bathroom and do not answer repeated knocks, someone will come in and check to see if I'm all right.	+3	+2	+1	0	−1	−2	−3
14.	The house is owned by a nonprofit organization.	+3	+2	+1	0	−1	−2	−3
15.	Smoking is not allowed in the house.	+3	+2	+1	0	−1	−2	−3
16.	The house is not closed during major holidays or during staff vacation times.	+3	+2	+1	0	−1	−2	−3

	Absolutely yes			Don't care			Absolutely no
17. The house has an active human rights committee with representatives from the community.	+3	+2	+1	0	−1	−2	−3
18. My house is certified by an independent accreditation agency (such as ACMR-DD or CARF).	+3	+2	+1	0	−1	−2	−3
19. The state or federal government pays for my living expenses.	+3	+2	+1	0	−1	−2	−3
20. I have to pay less than $100 per month for my living expenses.	+3	+2	+1	0	−1	−2	−3
21. The state or federal government pays for my personal care attendant.	+3	+2	+1	0	−1	−2	−3
22. The total cost of living in the house is explained clearly and does not change from month to month.	+3	+2	+1	0	−1	−2	−3
23. My family and friends can visit me any time.	+3	+2	+1	0	−1	−2	−3
24. My family and friends feel comfortable about making suggestions to the staff who work in my house.	+3	+2	+1	0	−1	−2	−3
25. My family and friends are told about my programs and goals.	+3	+2	+1	0	−1	−2	−3
26. My family and friends have a say in the kinds of programs and goals I may have.	+3	+2	+1	0	−1	−2	−3
27. My family and friends are told about the good things I do as well as about the problems I may have.	+3	+2	+1	0	−1	−2	−3
28. My family and friends can become involved in boards and committees that supervise the running of the house.	+3	+2	+1	0	−1	−2	−3
29. My family and friends may take part in special events with me (birthdays, celebrations, etc.).	+3	+2	+1	0	−1	−2	−3
30. The rights of my family to see my records and files are explained.	+3	+2	+1	0	−1	−2	−3
31. _____	+3	+2	+1	0	−1	−2	−3
32. _____	+3	+2	+1	0	−1	−2	−3
33. _____	+3	+2	+1	0	−1	−2	−3

25 WHAT SHOULD I DO WHEN I VISIT A PROGRAM?

After you've completed your preliminary evaluation of potential programs at home, you'll be ready to move forward. Remember Lowell Hughes's remark about the brochure that was done by "fiction writers." You will want to visit residential programs to get a firsthand look. Properly preparing for a visit may be one of the most important things you do at this point. A number of questions may come to mind, such as when to visit, who should visit, and what to ask on a visit. In this chapter we cover these and other important questions.

WHAT ABOUT THE PRIVACY ISSUE?

Because you will be visiting residences that are people's homes, you will be a guest and carry the responsibilities of a guest. It is quite possible that you will be considered an uninvited guest by the people living in the various residences. Sensitivity to this issue will go a long way toward making your visits comfortable for you and others.

The agency operating the residential programs you visit will provide the necessary staff to answer your questions and guide you and others who accompany you through the different residences. A good rule of thumb is to take your lead from the staff person guiding you. Closed doors in a house should be respected and visitors should ask permission before opening and looking. Never open bedroom doors without knocking. Once in a person's bedroom, be mindful of personal spaces such as closets and dresser drawers. In short, show the same respect for the privacy of your hosts that you would expect of guests in your own home.

HOW DO I ARRANGE A VISIT?

All agencies that operate residential programs understand and respect families' need to inspect their facilities. A phone call to an agency expressing your desire to visit should put you in contact with the staff member responsible for making the arrangements. You should let this person know who will be visiting and the kinds of information you are looking for—for example, in-depth data on costs. In this way, the agency can prepare to have the appropriate personnel available when you visit.

Who Should Visit?

The decision on who will make the visit will depend on your individual needs, the characteristics of your family, and your personal decision-making style. Certain people definitely should be included on such visits. Your son or daughter is one. His or her participation in this process gives him or her control over an important decision. Again, it cannot be said too often—your son or daughter will have to live in the residence that is eventually selected.

Your son's or daughter's reactions to the physical environment of a residence and the people living and working there may provide some indications of how happy he or she would be if that particular option were chosen. Allowing other residents to meet potential housemates gives them meaningful input into the conduct of their lives as well. Staff working in a residential program will be greatly aided by your son's or daughter's presence when determining if the program meets his or her individual needs and preferences.

You should consider other family members and friends who have been or may want to be involved in your planning, especially if this makes you feel more at ease. Having other people with you provides the chance to hear other views on a program. Another person may see something you missed or may ask an important question that you forgot.

When Should I Visit?

Houses are toured, but homes are for living. You should arrange a visit during times that will allow you to get a feel for a typical day in the residence. Touring a house when all the people who normally live there have gone to their job sites will help you learn about the physical layout and furnishings, but little more. To get a feeling for daily life in the residence, be sure to ask the following questions:

> How do the people living there get along with one another?
> How do residents and staff interact?
> What's the atmosphere of the house? Chaotic? Noisy? Laid back?
> What are some of the routines and normal activities?

Insist that your visit be scheduled at a time when residents and staff are there. If other agency staff need to answer specific questions and are not available during the busiest living times in the residence, you can make special arrangements. For example, if you need to speak with the staff physician and the person responsible for determining program costs, you could meet them during the agency's afternoon work hours and visit residences in the early evening.

Some families find it useful to visit a residence more than once, and at different times of day. An evening visit followed by a weekend visit may offer a clearer picture of a residential program. Multiple visits can confirm or correct first impressions. For example, when Lillian Weber returned from a visit to a group home with glowing reports, her husband Henry made a good point: "I remember my days in the Marine Corps," he said. "When strangers come inspecting, you do things differently."

WHAT SHOULD I DO ON A VISIT?

The purpose of visiting a program is to evaluate how well it meets the preferences and needs of your son or daughter and other family members. Having a clear idea of what is important to you and others will help you make the most of your visit. Completing the checklist of important things about a place to live, which appeared at the end of Chapter 24, can help you identify aspects of residential programs that require your attention.

For example, Steve Stuart has occasional problems controlling his behavior. He does not become violent with other people, but does destroy property. He has on past occasions broken windows by throwing shoes, books, and other objects through them. His parents understand that his behavior might easily lead to Steve's expulsion from a residential program. For them, an item they added to the checklist ("Someone in the house knows how to handle behavior problems") is crucial. Rose and Jack Stuart have identified a list of concerns relating to that specific item. Beyond knowing that someone in the house has training in behavior management, they have further concerns:

> What specific training does that person have?
> What specific procedures would be used with Steve?
> Would a behavior management program be a part of his individualized program?
> Would all residence staff be able to follow and carry out the management procedures?
> Under which criteria would Steve be asked to leave a program because of his behavior?
> Who is financially responsible if Steve damages property?

Jack and Rose decided to go through the checklist, noting things that were absolute necessities. Then, they developed a list of questions for each important item. You may find this helpful, or you may have a different style. Whatever your approach, it is important to emphasize that there are a few questions you may not ask during your visit. Questions that would violate another person's privacy should be avoided. For example, asking questions about another resident's specific medical diagnosis or arrangements to pay for program services is inappropriate. Yet, general questions can provide the needed information. These include:

> Are there people who live here who have behavior problems?
> What are some of the problems?
> How are the problems handled?
> What are the costs per month for your services?
> What types of payment arrangements have other people made?

You should be able to ask questions freely of the residential staff during your visit. You may wish to know how long they have worked there, what professional training they have, what their specific duties are, and perhaps their personal philosophies on their work with people who have disabilities. Questions such as the following can give you an insight into some unseen qualities:

> Why have you chosen to work with people with disabilities?
> What do you see as the most pressing needs of people with disabilities?
> What is the best aspect of the program here? What is the worst aspect?
> If you could change one part of the program here, what would you change?

Speaking with other people who live in a residence can also provide valuable information. How happy are the people who live there? What changes would they suggest, if any? How are they treated by staff and housemates? What life-style preferences do they share with your son or daughter? How do they differ from your son or daughter? Are the residents comfortable around your son or daughter?

Some residential programs maintain lists of people who are willing to talk with family members and potential housemates about the residence. These people are usually relatives or friends of the residents. Volunteering to be contacted does not necessarily mean that someone will have biased, pro-agency views—the "everything is beautiful" syndrome. It is to the agency's advantage to maintain lists of people who will present an honest assessment. Ask if there are such people you may contact. If there are, call them and feel free to ask about their experiences and share any concerns you may have.

WHAT SHOULD I DO AFTER MY VISIT?

All right, you, your son or daughter, and two friends have just spent a weekday afternoon and evening visiting a residential program. What now? Many people find it helpful to take time soon after a visit to compare reactions and insights. Let's look at the Rodriguez family and how they evaluated their experiences after looking at some apartments that a local adult agency operates . . .

Luis, Eloisa, Maria, and her brother, Geraldo, drove to their favorite restaurant directly from the apartment complex they had just visited. After the waiter took their orders, Eloisa said to her husband, *"Digame, ¿que te parecen, los apartamentos?"*

Geraldo interrupted, with a sigh, *"Por favor, en inglés."*

How quickly he has become an American, Eloisa thought. He speaks Spanish so infrequently that he no longer knows the language well. He would someday regret his loss, but for now there were more important matters.

Luis answered his wife, "I don't know, something about the apartments just didn't seem right. Maria, what did you think?"

"Too small," said Geraldo.

"Since when have you become Maria's voice?," Luis said, chiding his son. Turning again to his daughter, he said, "Maria, did you like the apartments?"

"No, papa. I don't want to move in with people I don't know. I want to live with my friend Carmen."

"Too many rules, too much 'do this, do that.' Maria doesn't need all those rules," added Eloisa.

"No one there could speak Spanish," Luis noted.

"This is America, Papa. Here we speak English," Geraldo interjected.

"You speak English, *hijo,* but your sister wants to speak Spanish, too," Eloisa said, in a tone that made it perfectly clear that the apartment program they had just visited had serious shortcomings.

"I'll call tomorrow and ask if Maria could choose a roommate, perhaps her friend Carmen. Oh, and I'll see if Maria could have more freedom. You know, fewer rules," Eloisa said, summarizing as the food arrived. They spent the rest of the evening discussing what they saw during their visit and realized Maria would probably not be happy with the apartment program unless a lot of changes could be made.

Debriefing as the Rodriguez family did can help you identify strong points and weaknesses in a program. You may also remember questions you forgot to ask that you want to follow up on with another visit or telephone call. Debriefing can also enable you to rate a program. How you choose to rate a program will again be based on your needs. For example, you may simply rate a program as good, fair, or poor. Some families choose to go back through the checklist and note how a program meets the preferences of their son or daughter.

Whatever your feelings after visiting a program, you should consider visits to other programs that offer similar services. Being able to make a comparison between at least two programs can help put residential issues in perspective. Programs differ and you may discover aspects of one program that can be incorporated into another program that will greatly improve it.

One mother, upon completing an extensive tour of a group home, was asked by the person guiding her what she thought of the program. This mother's reply may express your feelings: "How do I like it? As compared to what?"

26 | I'M READY TO DECIDE— WHAT'S THE BEST WAY?

If you and others involved in the planning believe you have found a residential option that meets all or most of your requirements, you should meet with the residential coordinator, admissions director, or staff person responsible, to determine the agency's requirements. You may often encounter waiting lists, so it is important to begin admissions procedures as soon as possible so that your son or daughter may get a placement at the appropriate time. Other matters will also need attention, such as arranging for payment plans, physical examinations, and agency evaluations, and filling out permission forms.

Involving your son or daughter in completing the preparations for moving can make the transition easier. Stress often accompanies major change and should be expected. Maybe discussing your fears or those of other family members can help you deal with them. Parent and family support groups have helped many people deal with transitions. Your son or daughter may need this kind of help as well.

What if, after evaluating different options, you conclude that there may be no suitable placement for your son or daughter? You may be discouraged at this point, but at least you'll have a better understanding of the situation.

You may decide to continue looking for other options. You may decide to postpone planning in this area and concentrate on other areas such as employment or legal planning. It may be possible that you and others are willing to take a placement that is less than completely satisfactory until something better comes along. Or, you may work to change a placement so that it meets more of your preferences and needs. Suggestions for working within an established system and suggestions for working completely outside a given system are discussed in Chapters 36–37.

27 | WHY SHOULD I LOOK AT EMPLOYMENT OPTIONS?

Odessa Harris sat down on her front porch swing. It was a warm Sunday afternoon in spring. She watched as her daughter, Jolene, went into the house to change from her Sunday dress. They had just returned from church; Jolene looked so grown up in that new dress. Just 17, she was already taller than her mother. Odessa began to think about a conversation she'd had with her brother Owen a few weeks earlier. Owen had sparked one of his sister's old fears. "What would become of Jolene if something should happen to you?," he'd asked Odessa. Jolene had Down syndrome and a heart condition.

Odessa knew that if anything happened to her, the rest of the family would make sure that Jolene was cared for. But she also knew that Jolene wanted a life of her own. She wouldn't be happy just being "cared for." Besides, Odessa didn't want Jolene to become a burden to anybody.

Maybe Owen was right. Maybe it was time to look at some training programs and talk to Jolene seriously about working and making a life for herself. Odessa called to Jolene to come and sit beside her on the swing.

"I've been noticing how tall you are and how grown up you're looking," she told her daughter. "You know, honey, you're practically grown, and pretty, too. It's almost time for you to start your own life."

"Almost, mama," Jolene agreed.

"Well now, what would you think if I gave your Uncle Owen a call about some of those training schools he was telling us about, the ones that help you find work?"

"That would be okay, mama, long as I could still go to church and sing in the choir. And I want a job that pays me money to go shopping. I want my own money, mama, so I can buy what I want. Other girls go shopping with their own money and they go by themselves. I want to do that."

Odessa called her brother later that day. Owen had not forgotten his conversation with her. He had, in fact, done some more investigating. He recommended that Odessa start with vocational rehabilitation and vocational counseling because Jolene didn't know what she wanted to do or whether she wanted to work. No one really knew if Jolene would be able to work.

Owen offered to make Jolene an appointment with a counselor at the regional office of the state vocational rehabilitation agency.

* * *

Think a moment about the following situation and how you might respond to it. You are in a crowded diner and have taken a seat at the counter. As you wait for your order to arrive you initiate a conversation with the pleasant stranger sitting next to you. You quickly exhaust the introductory topics: the weather, the fact that the restaurant is crowded, and the hope that tomorrow's weather will be different.

The stranger then asks, "What do you do?" If you are like most people, you will respond by saying what you do for a living. So the answer might be, "I'm a teller at the First National Bank," or "I work at a machine shop." Work is prized in our culture.

Work provides a number of things. First, it is the source of the money we need to support ourselves and our families. Beyond the essentials such as food, clothing, and shelter, however, our wages help us to enrich our lives with all those things that constitute a life-style. We may invest some of our income with an eye toward future needs or goals such as our retirement. We spend our so-called extra money for entertainment, vacations, or to purchase furniture, appliances, and other things that enhance the quality of life.

Holding a job makes many of us good credit risks, so we can borrow money to acquire other possessions such as cars and houses that again are part of a certain life-style. At this point you might be thinking, "Wait, money isn't everything." You're right, work provides much more than just money.

Employment provides a sense of being a productive member of society. Our different jobs contribute needed services and goods to our communities. We help fill the needs of others while our own needs are met by others' labors. Employment fulfills the need people have to know they are taking care of themselves, and that they are not dependent on society; it enhances our self-respect. We hold our own, pay our taxes, and have a right to expect our government to provide certain services and protections.

Employment provides many of us with an avenue for socialization. Often, coworkers become friends with whom we share the personal aspects of our lives. The very process of getting to our workplaces and doing our jobs offers a variety of opportunities to interact with other people. You may take a bus to get to your office, or perhaps your job involves working with the public. We eat lunch in a cafeteria or a restaurant and take coffee breaks with our coworkers. Employment brings us all into contact with others.

Our careers provide us with an identification. We are plumbers, teachers, carpenters, scientists, farmers, nurses, and salespersons. We belong to unions and professional organizations. We identify with the companies for which we work. We identify with our coworkers. Through this identification process, we come to realize we are part of a team or a larger group and our concept of ourselves is enhanced.

For most of us, employment provides security. We know the money that we'll need for next week will come from our work. We may have a pension plan that will be there when we retire. There may be a hospitalization policy with our jobs that relieves some of the worry over possible illnesses and accidents.

If we add together all the things that a job provides, the sum could best be described as independence. Through our work we are able to make choices concerning where we live, what we do for recreation, the people we will have as friends, and how we feel about ourselves. Employment is an avenue for growth and fulfillment, and it is equally important for people with disabilities.

The last 10 years or so have been a period of rapid, positive change in the area of employment for people with disabilities. Families and professionals have recognized the importance of work and many options have been created. The situation has improved, but it is evident that further gains are needed when U.S. Department of Labor figures are considered. These figures show that in 1983, 50%–80% of all people with disabilities were unemployed or underemployed. This is a significant loss for both the people involved and society.

28 | WHAT ARE SOME ALTERNATIVES TO EMPLOYMENT?

We believe that people with disabilities have the same employment rights as the general population, including the right not to work or to work in an unpaid, volunteer position.

A careful review of your son's or daughter's finances is crucial to determining if enough income from nonwork sources will be available to cover daily living expenses should you, your son or daughter, or others in your family consider not working.

A second and equally important consideration involves choosing the exact form that the alternative will entail. Total inactivity can hardly be viewed as an acceptable alternative to employment. In the following sections of this chapter, we discuss three alternatives to paid employment that may meet your son's or daughter's individual needs: *day activity programs, volunteer work*, and *retirement*.

DAY ACTIVITY PROGRAMS

Day activity programs can comprise either structured programs or informal activities. Either way, for the individual who chooses not to work, the amount of free time is greatly increased. Day programs combining adult educational activities (for example, self-care, reading, and social skills) with recreational activities can meet the diverse needs of people who choose not to work.

Leisure time options are discussed in Chapter 18. Read (or re-read) that chapter carefully if you are considering nonwork options.

VOLUNTEER WORK

For some people, volunteer work may be an alternative to employment. Volunteer work provides many of the benefits derived from salaried work: being a productive member of society, getting opportunities to socialize, and interacting with other people who work and volunteer in the same setting. The person who chooses to volunteer learns the importance of adhering to a schedule, interacting with coworkers, accepting responsibility, and other job-related skills. For some people, volunteer work serves as a type of training that enables them to become more employable. Also, a volunteer position can sometimes evolve into a paid position.

Volunteer work has benefits, not found in salaried employment, that can enhance a person's overall quality of life. The volunteer is often found in situations that involve providing for other people's needs. Volunteers are often found working in hospitals and other health care facilities such as nursing homes, or visiting people confined to their homes. The volunteer's duties often center on meeting some other person's need for companionship, assistance with everyday tasks such as preparing meals, or generally ensuring that another person is neither alone nor made to feel unimportant.

Some volunteer positions include working for service agencies such as Boy Scouts, Girl Scouts, Big Brothers/Big Sisters, United Way, neighborhood improvement organizations, church groups, and youth recreation programs such as Little League baseball. Other people choose to become involved in the political process by working for candidates for public office. The volunteer often provides a valuable service that an organization could not otherwise provide because of the lack of finances. The volunteer donates time and talent and the reward is knowing that others benefit. Your son or daughter can be in a position to help others who, in a real sense, are less capable in some areas.

Close friendships often form between volunteers and the people with whom they work. Volunteers may receive help in areas in which they lack skills. For example, a volunteer may help an elderly person prepare one meal each week and, during the visit, get help with balancing his or her checking account. Volunteering can provide situations which benefit everyone involved.

RETIREMENT

Concerning retirement, a true story comes to mind concerning a friend of ours who has moderate mental retardation. Millie was experiencing problems in her group home and the staff had asked for help. The staff reported that she was resistive and even aggressive each morning, and refused to cooperate with others as she prepared to go to her sheltered workshop. At the workshop, her production rate had fallen and her work habits had deteriorated. Everyone was concerned because Millie had always been a gentle person and a very hard worker.

Sitting down and talking with Millie made the cause of her "problems" become clear. Millie said, "I'm tired, I've worked hard all of my life. I'm 62 years old; I want to retire." Millie wanted what many others in our society take for granted, the right to retire. Her situation has a happy ending. She did retire and now enjoys other interests. She remains active, yet on some days, as she puts it, "I do nothing, I am happy."

Millie was 62 years old when she retired, but what about people who are younger and would still like to be able to do what Millie did? Many people without disabilities retire early, while others choose to work part-time. The same possibilities should exist for people with disabilities.

Certainly a person's individual preferences should be considered and alternatives to employment should be explored and planned. Provisions for a person's financial security and health care needs must be made. This is one reason the in-depth information on financial planning provided in this book is important to you.

In summary, a key element in nontraditional alternatives to employment is *individuality*. Employment needs will vary from person to person. Choosing not to work represents an individual decision made by people with disabilities and their families.

This alternative, like all options involving employment and other life-style components, will be right for some but not for others.

In the next two chapters we describe two broad vocational/work models: *sheltered employment* and *integrated employment*.

29 | WHAT IS SHELTERED EMPLOYMENT?

$\qquad$ In the *sheltered employment* model, workers are placed in settings where the work force is composed entirely of people with disabilities. Supervision is provided by persons without disabilities who are employed by the agency that received the work contract or is operating the sheltered sites. The person with the disability is an employee of the adult service agency. In many cases, he or she is called a *client* rather than an employee.

$\qquad$ The sheltered employment options described in this chapter are:

1. Prevocational activity center
2. Sheltered workshop
3. Work station/enclave

Specific issues related to sheltered employment that are discussed in this chapter include organization and funding, and problems and shortcomings.

PREVOCATIONAL ACTIVITY CENTERS

The goal of the *prevocational activity center* is to provide an educational program that emphasizes the teaching of vocational skills to people who are not yet ready to enter the job market. In the past, many people with severe and multiple disabilities were perceived as unemployable and were involved in day activity centers that varied greatly in organization and emphasis on vocational skills training. For many, transition to paid employment never occurred.

$\qquad$ Today, many knowledgeable people claim that all individuals, regardless of their level of disability, are employable. Great strides have been made in training techniques which have resulted in the successful placement of people with the severest disabilities in wage-earning positions. Often, this option represents the bottom tier of sheltered workshop employment, an entry-level position. Some of the work performed may be part of a paid contract and at times workers receive some wages. These wages are invariably very low. The majority of the employees' time is spent practicing work tasks such as sorting, collating, matching, and minor assembly that presumably will be needed in other areas of sheltered workshop employment.

$\qquad$ The repetitive nature of the tasks makes them unsuitable for many people, and the sense of accomplishment derived from producing real finished products is too often absent. In one such setting, for example, there were two crews. The morning crew, using an assembly line technique, produced bicycle brakes. The afternoon crew then disassembled these brakes so the morning crew could again assemble them so the afternoon crew could . . . Unfortunately, such a system is more common than one might expect.

The activity center option may, however, provide an opportunity to evaluate a person's vocational strengths and weaknesses before placement at a work site, and thus may represent a genuine step toward employment. Such centers may also provide intensive training to enable clients to enter the job market more quickly. As a long-term option, however, the prevocational activity center may not meet the needs of the majority of people with disabilities.

SHELTERED WORKSHOPS

The term, *sheltered workshop*, has taken on a generic definition that covers a variety of work settings for people with disabilities. Ideally, a sheltered work setting provides employment opportunities along with training to enable clients eventually to move into community jobs. The sheltered workshop's goal should be to enhance the employability of people with disabilities in community settings. However, certain aspects of sheltered workshops have combined to prevent the transition of people with disabilities into community employment.

Organization and Funding

The average sheltered workshop employs people with disabilities in the role of production workers, and staff who do not have disabilities are responsible for supervision and training. If the workshop is licensed by the U.S. Department of Labor, the production workers must be paid at least 50% of the federal minimum wage. Workshops that are not licensed may pay a wage considerably below the minimum hourly rate. Most workshops today are nonlicensed, and depend on contracts from community businesses and industries to provide work for their clients.

The nature of the contracts completed by workshops varies greatly. They do, however, share some general characteristics. Contracts tend to emphasize the packaging, assembly, and shipping of products, rather than actual manufacturing. For example, a contract may require the shipment of complete first aid kits. The components of the kits (e.g., adhesive bandages, sunburn lotion, antiseptic) would be provided to the workshop along with the containers and packing materials. Workers would collate the components into completed kits and prepare them for shipping.

Contracts also tend to be tied to piece-rate production quotas. A contract might require that a certain number of finished first aid kits be shipped each week. The workshop would probably be paid according to a formula of so much money for each completed kit. The workers in turn would probably be paid according to their rate of production, rather than receive an hourly wage. These contracts allow the job to be broken into smaller tasks that can be performed by many people in assembly-line fashion. Ideally, this provides employment opportunities for people with the severest mental and physical disabilities.

Several shortcomings of the sheltered workshop model have been identified.

Some agencies that operate the workshops have attempted to change their approaches to overcome these problems, while others have been unwilling or unable to change.

Problems and Shortcomings

Employment practices in many job settings limit opportunities for clients to interact with people who do not have disabilities. This is a two-way street in that the community is also deprived of seeing people with disabilities as capable and productive individuals. Many workers who do not have disabilities have little knowledge of what occurs in the sheltered workshop setting.

Some settings have addressed these problems by attempting to hire some workers who do not have a disability. Others have located their sheltered workshops near other businesses and industries. Despite such moves, many people continue to be concerned about the isolation of individuals with disabilities in many sheltered settings.

The nature of the funding for sheltered settings continues to be a major issue. Low wages remain the norm in these settings. One recent study reported that the average workshop employee earned 81¢ per hour. Contracts are often difficult to find and may be short-term or sporadic. Many workshops are subject to long periods when no work is available. During these "down times," clients sometimes "practice" assembly and disassembly tasks, but too often down time is filled only with idle time when nothing happens. Meanwhile, overhead expenses (e.g., utilities, staff salaries, administrative costs) tend to remain constant, which increases the financial pressure on sheltered settings. Layoffs sometimes result, which cause severe disruptions and setbacks in people's lives.

Some sheltered workshops are seeking to obtain contracts that last longer and offer greater income potential. However, the skills required to meet some contracts preclude industries from awarding them to facilities serving people with more severe disabilities. Some contracts may require initial investments for machinery that many sheltered workshops cannot afford. The limited contracts that are consequently available force sheltered workshops to compete with each other. This keeps income potentials generally low.

The limited training capacities of workshops represents a Catch-22 situation— unskilled work forces cause workshops to seek contracts that require few skilled workers; the workers continue to have few skills because the opportunity does not exist to upgrade personal skills. Although most workshops would opt to pursue contracts that would allow them to provide better training opportunities, the need to provide work to large numbers of clients forces them to compete for contracts requiring repetitive, low-paying operations. Scant attention can be given to matching the preferences of clients to jobs in these situations.

Despite their general problems, we must stress that sheltered workshops vary greatly. Within your community you may find a sheltered setting that meets both your family's requirements and the preferences of your son or daughter.

Some people have identified aspects of sheltered work settings that have been positive for themselves and others employed within such settings. For some, the lack of emphasis on speed associated with some contract work has enabled them to be employed. Although their income from such work may be very low, socialization with peers and others while at work may be as important to them as wages. Others have observed that some people with disabilities do best at highly structured, repetitive tasks.

WORK STATIONS (ENCLAVES)

Work stations, also known as *enclaves*, are a bridge between the traditional sheltered work setting and the employment of people with disabilities in community businesses and industries. In this option, a group of individuals work in a community-based business or industry under the supervision of a trained employee of the adult service agency responsible for people with disabilities. The group would ideally work alongside other workers without disabilities, with ample opportunity for interaction.

Often, the work station model involves a business contracting for specific tasks to be done by groups of people with disabilities. These contracts may be for varying lengths of time. This is not an ideal situation in that it tends to separate workers with disabilities into the category of temporary help. Also, the model tends to deny these workers benefits such as vacation and sick leave which are enjoyed by regular employees. This is because enclave workers remain on the payrolls of the sheltered workshops or adult service agencies. Generally, they are not considered full-fledged employees of the business or industry.

Many advocates in the field of employment for people with disabilities urge that work stations in industry be structured to minimize differences between the regular employees and those with disabilities. The employees would not only work in proximity, but would be responsible for similar tasks. Pay scales would not vary on the basis of disability, and as many job-related benefits as possible would be available to the workers with disabilities. Further, work station/enclave special crews would be employed with the understanding that the arrangement would be long-term. The special crew could gradually be assimilated into the total work force. The goal would be full employment by the business or industry rather than continued supervision by the adult service agency.

The work station model exposes workers with disabilities to real job situations and offers opportunities to develop skills that may be useful in gaining other employment. This model also demonstrates the capabilities of workers with disabilities to the community at large. The work station remains an interesting option, combining aspects of sheltered employment and community-based employment.

30 WHAT IS INTEGRATED EMPLOYMENT?

In the *integrated employment* model, people are employed in a setting where the work force consists mostly of people without disabilities. Workers with disabilities may receive varying degrees of support from outside service agencies, but they are still employees of the businesses in which they work. They are not employed by adult service agencies.

We introduce the integrated employment model by first discussing the role of the job coach in vocational education for people with a disability. This is followed by a review of two broad options:

1. Supported employment
2. Competitive employment

WHAT IS A JOB COACH?

Before we discuss the two integrated employment models, we will describe a recent development in vocational training for people with disabilities, the *job coach*. The person filling this role is often crucial to the success of people in supported and competitive employment.

The job coach may be employed by traditional rehabilitation facilities such as nonprofit placement agencies (i.e., adult service agencies that operate placement services), state vocational rehabilitation departments, or special education agencies. They might also be employed privately by people with disabilites or their families. The job coach performs multiple tasks designed to meet the individual needs of people so as to prepare them for employment in the community.

Another role assumed by some job coaches is that of liaison between the person with a disability, the employer, the family, and the adult service agencies. In some agencies, the job coach functions as a case manager who ensures that a person's vocational needs fit into an overall plan including residential, recreational, and social-interpersonal components.

In most agencies that employ job coaches, the person with a disability is hired immediately for a real job in a community business or industry. The coach then begins an on-the-job training program with the person to teach the skills that will be needed for retention of the position. The two of them work side by side. The requirements of the job are broken into component steps, and the person with a disability is taught one step at a time.

In the beginning the coach may do many of the person's job tasks, to ensure that the immediate requirements of the employer are met. As the person's skills increase, the job coach gradually fades out of the picture. Ideally, the person receiving job coaching eventually reaches the stage where only minimal contact with the coach is needed. If he or she slips in performance, the job coach immediately re-enters to correct the situation.

In addition to on-the-job training and follow-up, the job coach may be involved in other vocationally related training. The coach may teach independent use of public transportation so the person can get to and from work. The coach may also be involved in social-interpersonal skills training aimed at encouraging appropriate interaction with coworkers. Money management, the use of checking and savings accounts, and learning workplace policies may be other areas in which the job coach functions.

Ongoing counseling of family members may be needed to address concerns related to the employment of the member with a disability. Continual contacts with employers and other workers, both nondisabled and disabled, may be crucial to the success of the client in a workplace. The job coach can be a key element in securing community employment for most people with disabilities, regardless of the level of severity.

SUPPORTED EMPLOYMENT

The *supported employment* model involves working for pay in community settings with support in the form of training and assistance. The use of job coaches is the most common form of support in such situations. Supported employment opportunities are found in every area of business and industry. Successful programs have been reported in the manufacturing, food service, janitorial, clerical, yard maintenance, sales, and child care fields. Further success is limited only by the imaginations of families, employees, and professionals.

Some interesting variations on the job coach model have been developed in recent years in the area of supported employment. Several businesses have established training courses designed specifically to prepare people with disabilities for employment. In some cases, prospective employees have been paid to attend these training courses. In cases where private businesses have taken the lead in providing specialized training, the beneficiaries mostly have been people with physical disabilities or mild mental retardation.

Another variation on the job coach model was implemented by an adult service agency is a rural community in western Kansas. The agency placed two individuals in a local manufacturing business which specialized in custom wood products. Two current employees were recruited to serve as on-the-job trainers. With the agreement of the employers, the employees who provided the training received extra hourly pay provided by the adult service agency. This averaged $1–$2 extra per hour per person. Such an arrangement has many positive aspects. In addition to receiving job training, the people with disabilities receive help in learning to deal with the day-to-day politics involved in employment. An understanding of the likes, dislikes, and pet peeves of supervisors and coworkers can come only from someone familiar with others on the job. The employee who acts as a job coach can be very helpful in integrating the new employee into the social aspects of the job. Further, the employee job coach can be an effective advocate for the person with a disability as well as a friend outside the workplace.

For most people with disabilities, supported employment can serve as a transition stage leading to full competitive employment and greater personal freedom in other areas of life. Because supported employment can be adapted to meet individual needs, it offers a potentially limitless range of options.

COMPETITIVE EMPLOYMENT

Competitive employment means obtaining a job for pay in the general work force by virtue of being the person most qualified for the position. In a sense, the supported employment model just reviewed is competitive employment. In supported employment, the person works in an integrated community setting and earns a wage comparable to that of fellow employees. However, reserve the term *competitive employment* for those situations in which a person holds a job without outside support such as that provided by a job coach.

Many people with severe disabilities would be unable to hold some jobs without varying degrees of support. This is not the case for people with less severe disabilities, and this is why the competitive employment model may be appropriate for your son or daughter. Many people with disabilities can successfully obtain competitive jobs and work alongside people without a disability.

Perhaps someone with a disability would need some assistance in completing the application form and other work-related documents such as the W-4 or health insurance forms. Others might need help in developing job interviewing skills, while others might only need assistance getting to and from work. Some might also require guidance in managing their income.

Competitive employment will not be appropriate for all people with disabilities, but more and more of such individuals are working in community jobs, earning competitive wages, and leading lives that differ little from those of their neighbors who do not have disabilities. In the following chapter, we review the processes you may choose to follow in planning for the vocational needs of the member of your family with a disability.

31 HOW DO I LOCATE AND EVALUATE JOB OPPORTUNITIES?

The preceding chapter was intended to provide an overview of the diverse vocational models that exist in various parts of the United States. The same models and variations may exist in your community. As is the case in planning for residential placements, the needs and preferences of your son or daughter should guide you as you evaluate employment options.

In the following pages, a procedure similar to the one for evaluating residential options is described to help you find, review, and choose employment options. The procedure will help you match the preferences and needs of your son or daughter to an appropriate type of employment. Some positive and negative aspects of different work options will become clearer as you proceed.

In some ways, planning for a person's employment future requires some of the same steps involved in exploring residential options (such as determining personal preferences, visiting potential settings, and determining the pros and cons of various options). But there are some important differences. Most people with disabilities have access to a formal, government-sponsored system to assist them in obtaining employment—the *Vocational Rehabilitation* (VR) system. There are also formal systems sponsored by adult service agencies serving people with disabilities that provide job opportunities. Finally, there is the informal system—finding a job by oneself, with the assistance of a friend or a relative, or through other means. These three systems, 1) Vocational Rehabilitation, 2) adult services for people with disabilities, and 3) informal approaches to finding employment, are discussed in detail in the following pages.

HOW DO I DETERMINE MY SON'S OR DAUGHTER'S VOCATIONAL PREFERENCES AND CHOICES?

Enjoying one's work involves more than simply choosing a type of job to do. Two machine shops may have openings for a skilled press operator at comparable salaries. Yet Shop A has rigid rules regarding vacations, the press operator's duties are repetitive, and, while the work area is clean, the building has few windows. Shop B involves employees in the scheduling of work hours and vacations, the operator's duties are varied, and the clean work area is well-ventilated and lighted by ample windows and skylights. The shops are quite different.

Perhaps you picked your present job only after evaluating the different aspects of similar job openings. Like yourself, your son or daughter has individual choices and preferences concerning employment options. In selecting the right option you may choose to seek the help of the vocational rehabilitation agency in your state or you may work with adult service agencies that provide vocational programs. You may even decide to forego formal systems and use your own resources to locate an appropriate job.

Regardless of the method you use, it is important to consider the choices and preferences of your son or daughter as well as other relevant work issues. To help you do this, a preference checklist ("Things That Are Important about My Job") is provided at the end of this chapter.

HOW DO I USE THE PREFERENCE CHECKLIST TO HELP DETERMINE EMPLOYMENT OPTIONS FOR MY SON OR DAUGHTER?

The portion of the checklist provided at the end of this chapter will help you identify the preferences your son or daughter has pertaining to employment options. The checklist covers two broad areas: 1) type of work and nature of employment option, and 2) finances and other employment-related issues. Like the checklist presented in Chapter 24 pertaining to residential options, it is not exhaustive. It lists issues that have been identified as important concerns by other families planning for the employment future of members with disabilities. Some of the issues identified in the checklist may be of little importance to your son or daughter or other members of your family, while others may matter a great deal.

In addition, you may identify employment-related issues that are not included in the checklist. Blank spaces are provided so that you may add and rate these additional concerns. For example, one father completed the checklist for his son who has moderate mental retardation. He noted early that his son Jesse would want to work in a setting where he could wear a sportcoat and tie. "I wear a tie and coat to my job," explained the father, "I guess Jesse simply wants to be like me." With the help of his family and a job coach, Jesse got a job in a large college library where he may, if he wishes, wear a tie and sportcoat. Jesse's preferences guided his job selection.

You will notice that some of the checklist items concern issues that, because of their complex nature, may be difficult for your son or daughter to comprehend. Because they do not quite understand them, your son or daughter may not consider these items important, yet you may recognize them as such. The checklist allows you to determine your own preferences and those of other family members as well.

For an example, consider the following items from Part C of the checklist:

7) I can control how much I earn so I don't lose my Social Security Disability Insurance (SSDI) benefits.
8) I can control how much I earn so I don't lose my Supplemental Security Income (SSI) benefits.
9) I will get help in planning to use SSI benefits for special job-related expenses.
13) My job will provide me with special insurance (disability/worker's compensation) in case I get hurt.

Your son or daughter may not fully understand the intricacies of the SSI and SSDI programs. He or she may also fail to recognize the importance of insurance for medical needs. At the same time, you may realize that without the proper assistance, your son or daughter might find a job that results in the loss of important benefits. The job setting may meet your son's or daughter's preferences in many ways, but the risks might exceed the benefits. In this case, you may determine that Items 7, 8, 9, and 13 are crucial, so any employment option must provide protection for your son or daughter in these matters.

There are other checklist items that you may feel do not pertain to your son or daughter because a proper response requires the understanding of other concepts. For example, consider Items 23 and 24 from Part B:

    23)   I may, within reason, schedule my own work hours.
    24)   I may, within reason, schedule my own vacation times.

Let's say that you initially decide that neither item is important to your son or daughter because he or she does not understand the concept of time. But if you use the Shoes Test you may arrive at a different conclusion. Your son or daughter may not be able to tell time, but preferred times may be discernible. If your son or daughter prefers to sleep late but is active through early evening hours, then an employment option calling for afternoon work hours would be preferable to one requiring earlier hours. In this case, your son or daughter does, in fact, have a preference for a job that allows input into the setting of his or her schedule. Simply put, the preference is "Yes, let me schedule my hours for the afternoon."

Consider Part B, Item 24. Your son or daughter may not understand the concept of months, but consider the following scenario: If your family has traditionally taken a group vacation during mid-July at that beautiful spot on the shores of Lake Superior, the situation changes. Use the Shoes Test again. Given the family vacation that your son or daughter thoroughly enjoys, what would be the preference—a work setting where all workers get their vacations during a one month shutdown in August, or a job placement in which workers may schedule vacation time throughout the summer?

*   *   *

"If today was a harbinger of the summer to come," thought Odessa Harris, "then two things are foregone conclusions. The dogs will spend the summer lying under the oak trees, and I'll spend it paying huge electric bills for air-conditioning." The day was stifling—98 degrees and rising, with humidity as thick as a wet wool blanket.

Jolene came running out the front door past her mother, who was swinging gently on the old porch swing. Jolene stopped in the middle of the front yard under the full heat of the sun and, raising her arms skyward, blurted out, "Oh, what a great day!"

Her skin longing for a breeze, Odessa smiled. Jolene was an outdoor child. Be it spring, summer, winter, or fall, she would rather be outside than anywhere else. Although the summer might turn out to be a scorcher, it would be an exciting one for Jolene. Two possible summer jobs were available and Odessa wanted to help her daughter decide today which one to accept.

Reverend Davis wanted Jolene to help with the day care program that the church operated. Jolene would work from 8 A.M. to 11:30 A.M., 5 days a week. The job involved helping supervise morning snacks and organizing nature activities for about 15 children ages 4–8. Jolene would help with trail hikes, nature studies, and outdoor games. And the pay seemed fair, $3.50 per hour. Reverend Davis was a wonderful man, thought Odessa. He was always doing things to set up opportunities for Jolene to learn and grow.

Odessa's aunt, Jewell Weeks, was also a caring person. She had convinced a friend of hers who owned and operated Andy's Steakhouse that he needed extra summer help and that Jolene was the person he should hire. This job would require Jolene to help with general kitchen chores and do some busing in the dining roon. Jolene would work 4 P.M. to 7 P.M. Tuesdays through Saturdays. Andy was offering a staggering $4.50 per hour, plus a free meal each night. "Humph," Odessa thought aloud, "with his prices, heaven knows he can afford such wages." However, Andy Martel, the owner, was one of the nicest men in town, always doing good things for other people.

"Jolene, honey, come on up here and sit beside me," Odessa called to her daughter. "Let's talk about the things you want to do this summer."

"I want to work to get money," Jolene said matter-of-factly, as she climbed the front steps to sit down in the swing. "I want to work for Reverend Davis," she added.

"What about Mr. Martel's restaurant? He wants you to work there, too, remember?" Odessa said, prompting a discussion.

"Oh, mama, what should I do?" Jolene asked.

"What you want to do," her mother said, smiling.

"Tell me, mama," Jolene begged.

"No, my little girl," answered her mother. "I'll help you decide, but in the end, you will do what you want. That's the way it should be."

*   *   *

Let's see how Jolene and her mother might use the checklist to help them with a decision. Because Odessa insisted that her daughter play a major role in the decision, what Jolene wants to do will largely determine which summer job she takes.

The responses to Items 2, 3, 4, and 5 (Part A) have been made obvious by Jolene's statements:

2) I may choose not to work.
    +3   +2   +1   0   −1   −2   (−3)
3) I may choose a nonwork activity program, like day recreation.
    +3   +2   +1   0   −1   −2   (−3)
4) I may work in a sheltered workshop.
    +3   +2   +1   0   (−1)   −2   −3
7) I may get a job in the community.
    (+3)   +2   +1   0   −1   −1   −3

Now consider these items from Part B:

23) I may, within reason, schedule my own work hours.
     +3   (+2)   +1   0   −1   −2   −3
25) My work schedule will allow me to take part in social events and fun things at my house.
     (+3)   +2   +1   0   −1   −2   −3

The hours at both jobs are established, so that no latitude is left for Jolene in this area, yet the hours at the restaurant would mean that she would miss the frequent early evening get-togethers when her relatives come to visit. Her Uncle Owen and her grandparents often came on weekday evenings to sit on the big front porch. Jolene so enjoys these times that the thought of missing them made her lean strongly toward scheduling her own hours by choosing the morning job at the day care center.

Now, consider Item 21, Part B:

21) My job has few changes in duties from day to day.
     +3   +2   +1   0   −1   −2   (−3)

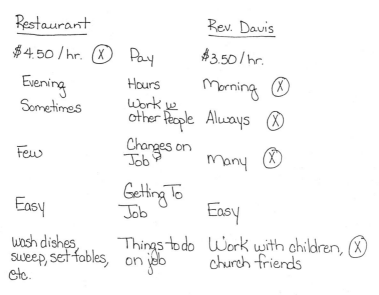

Figure 31.1. Odessa made a list to help Jolene decide which job she liked best. Jolene made an *X* next to the features she preferred.

Jolene answered as she did because she likes variety, although she does very well with more routine tasks. The day care job clearly would offer greater variety, and Jolene could spend time outdoors.

After some additional discussion, Odessa and Jolene were ready to make a decision. "Okay, let's do this," suggested Odessa. "We'll list the important things about each job. Then Jolene, you'll have to decide."

On a piece of paper, Odessa laid out the situation, asking questions and helping her daughter make the choice that would be best for her (Figure 31.1).

Odessa put an *X* after each item on the list that Jolene chose to help her make a decision. Jolene could count the *X*'s and see for herself which job she preferred.

Jolene chose to work at the day care center. The pay was less, but she felt that the work was more rewarding. She had a most enjoyable summer. She learned that she could do things that her younger charges could not do. Her self-esteem grew in that summer of maturity. The 17-year-old neighbor boy, Kyle, took the job at Andy's Steakhouse.

SECTION 5: THINGS THAT ARE IMPORTANT ABOUT MY JOB

	Absolutely yes			Don't care			Absolutely no
A. About the Kind of Job I Will Have							
1. I may choose the kind of work I want to do.	+3	+2	+1	0	−1	−2	−3
2. I may choose not to work.	+3	+2	+1	·0	−1	−2	−3
3. I may choose a nonwork activity program, like day recreation.	+3	+2	+1	0	−1	−2	−3
4. I may work in a sheltered workshop.	+3	+2	+1	0	−1	−2	−3
5. I may get the help of a job coach on my job.	+3	+2	+1	0	−1	−2	−3
6. I may choose my own job coach.	+3	+2	+1	0	−1	−2	−3

		Absolutely yes			Don't care			Absolutely no
7.	I may get a job in the community.	+3	+2	+1	0	−1	−2	−3
8.	I may go to a vocational training school instead of an actual job.	+3	+2	+1	0	−1	−2	−3
9.	I may work in a place where nobody smokes.	+3	+2	+1	0	−1	−2	−3
10.	I may quit my job.	+3	+2	+1	0	−1	−2	−3
11.	_____	+3	+2	+1	0	−1	−2	−3
12.	_____	+3	+2	+1	0	−1	−2	−3
13.	_____	+3	+2	+1	0	−1	−2	−3

B. About the Kind of Place Where I Will Work and the Things I Will Do

		Absolutely yes			Don't care			Absolutely no
1.	I can get to work easily.	+3	+2	+1	0	−1	−2	−3
2.	I may use public transportation to get to my job.	+3	+2	+1	0	−1	−2	−3
3.	The place where I work is separate from the place where I live.	+3	+2	+1	0	−1	−2	−3
4.	My house has a work program that is part of the program.	+3	+2	+1	0	−1	−2	−3
5.	The staff at my house provide transportation to and from my job.	+3	+2	+1	0	−1	−2	−3
6.	I will work with the same people I live with.	+3	+2	+1	0	−1	−2	−3
7.	I will work with coworkers who do not have disabilities.	+3	+2	+1	0	−1	−2	−3
8.	I will work with coworkers who have disabilities.	+3	+2	+1	0	−1	−2	−3
9.	My coworkers respect my opinions.	+3	+2	+1	0	−1	−2	−3
10.	My coworkers are friendly and helpful.	+3	+2	+1	0	−1	−2	−3
11.	My coworkers are as capable as me.	+3	+2	+1	0	−1	−2	−3
12.	The place where I work is in a safe area.	+3	+2	+1	0	−1	−2	−3
13.	The place where I work follows all government rules (like health and safety, wage and hour, and affirmative action regulations).	+3	+2	+1	0	−1	−2	−3
14.	The place where I work hires people of both sexes.	+3	+2	+1	0	−1	−2	−3
15.	The jobs I do where I work are important.	+3	+2	+1	0	−1	−2	−3
16.	My job does not require hard physical work.	+3	+2	+1	0	−1	−2	−3
17.	I work in a quiet area.	+3	+2	+1	0	−1	−2	−3
18.	My workplace is clean and orderly.	+3	+2	+1	0	−1	−2	−3
19.	I may, within reason, decide what I wear on my job.	+3	+2	+1	0	−1	−2	−3
20.	There is a place just for me to keep my personal things safe while I work on my job.	+3	+2	+1	0	−1	−2	−3
21.	My job has few changes in duties from day to day.	+3	+2	+1	0	−1	−2	−3
22.	My job has the same scheduled hours every week.	+3	+2	+1	0	−1	−2	−3
23.	I may, within reason, schedule my own work hours.	+3	+2	+1	0	−1	−2	−3
24.	I may, within reason, schedule my own vacation times.	+3	+2	+1	0	−1	−2	−3
25.	My work schedule will allow me to take part in social events and fun things at my house.	+3	+2	+1	0	−1	−2	−3

		Absolutely yes			Don't care			Absolutely no
26.	I will be protected from unkind remarks by other workers.	+3	+2	+1	0	−1	−2	−3
27.	Somebody at the place where I work knows how to give emergency first aid.	+3	+2	+1	0	−1	−2	−3
28.	Someone at the place where I work knows how to handle behavior problems.	+3	+2	+1	0	−1	−2	−3
29.	My supervisor has had special training to work with people with disabilities.	+3	+2	+1	0	−1	−2	−3
30.	My supervisor corrects my mistakes without humiliating or embarrassing me.	+3	+2	+1	0	−1	−2	−3
31.	My supervisor respects my opinions.	+3	+2	+1	0	−1	−2	−3
32.	My vocational teachers at the place where I work are employed over a long period of time; there is low staff turnover.	+3	+2	+1	0	−1	−2	−3
33.	My vocational teachers are well paid.	+3	+2	+1	0	−1	−2	−3
34.	The vocational teachers take part in regular inservice.	+3	+2	+1	0	−1	−2	−3
35.	_____	+3	+2	+1	0	−1	−2	−3
36.	_____	+3	+2	+1	0	−1	−2	−3
37.	_____	+3	+2	+1	0	−1	−2	−3

C. About My Pay and Job Benefits

		Absolutely yes			Don't care			Absolutely no
1.	The amount I am paid will depend on how much work I do, even if it is less than minimum wage.	+3	+2	+1	0	−1	−2	−3
2.	I will earn a salary that is the same that workers without disabilities get for doing the same job.	+3	+2	+1	0	−1	−2	−3
3.	I will be paid weekly on my job.	+3	+2	+1	0	−1	−2	−3
4.	I will be paid every other week on my job.	+3	+2	+1	0	−1	−2	−3
5.	I will be paid monthly on my job.	+3	+2	+1	0	−1	−2	−3
6.	I will have chances to work overtime and earn extra money on my job.	+3	+2	+1	0	−1	−2	−3
7.	I can control how much I earn so I don't lose my Social Security Disability Insurance (SSDI) benefits.	+3	+2	+1	0	−1	−2	−3
8.	I can control how much I earn so I don't lose my Supplemental Security Income (SSI) benefits.	+3	+2	+1	0	−1	−2	−3
9.	I will get help in planning to use my SSI benefits for special job-related expenses.	+3	+2	+1	0	−1	−2	−3
10.	I will have chances for advancement (promotions, raises in salary) in my job.	+3	+2	+1	0	−1	−2	−3
11.	I get help if I am laid off from my job.	+3	+2	+1	0	−1	−2	−3
12.	A community agency will help me find another job if my competitive job doesn't work out.	+3	+2	+1	0	−1	−2	−3
13.	My job will provide me with special insurance (disability/worker's compensation) in case I get hurt.	+3	+2	+1	0	−1	−2	−3
14.	My job will provide me with health insurance.	+3	+2	+1	0	−1	−2	−3
15.	My job will provide me with dental insurance.	+3	+2	+1	0	−1	−2	−3
16.	I have the same right to complain about things on my job that my coworkers without disabilities have.	+3	+2	+1	0	−1	−2	−3

		Absolutely yes			Don't care			Absolutely no
17.	My job will provide me with retirement benefits.	+3	+2	+1	0	−1	−2	−3
18.	_____	+3	+2	+1	0	−1	−2	−3
19.	_____	+3	+2	+1	0	−1	−2	−3
20.	_____	+3	+2	+1	0	−1	−2	−3

32 | WHAT IS VOCATIONAL REHABILITATION?

Perhaps you assume that state and federal education programs for your son or daughter end at age 22, the cutoff age for special education services. This is not the case for a large number of persons with disabilities. A nationwide federal and state system, *vocational rehabilitation* (VR), is in place. This program is designed to pick up where special education leaves off in the terms of vocational training and placement.

In Chapter 27 ("Why Should I Look at Employment Options?"), we describe how and why our culture places so much importance on work; people's jobs become, in large part, their identity. The VR service system is designed to provide people with disabilities the opportunity to become employed and therefore to enhance their self-identity and their contribution to society. VR offers a variety of services such as vocational evaluation, vocational counseling, education and training, and job placement.

THE HISTORY OF VOCATIONAL REHABILITATION

The first VR programs were established with the creation of the National Vocational Guidance Association in 1913. In 1916, the National Defense Act was passed by Congress. This act provided for vocational education and training for members of the armed forces. (The United States was about to enter World War I at the time.) In 1918, the Smith-Sears Veterans Rehabilitation Act provided for vocational training for veterans with disabilities, and in 1920 the Smith-Fess Act established limited vocational training, job placement, and counseling services for people with physical disabilities in general. By 1935, every state had some form of VR program.

The goals of the Rehabilitation Act of 1973 were: 1) to increase the number of federal service dollars going to the states, 2) to coordinate federal and state efforts to promote and expand employment opportunities for people with disabilities, and 3) to prohibit discrimination against people with disabilities in employment and promotion.

Federal VR offices were established under what is now known as the U.S. Department of Education. Specifically, these offices are under the management of the Rehabilitation Services Administration (RSA), which is part of the Office of Special Education and Rehabilitative Services (OSERS). Each state has its own program in operation. The programs are usually organized under state departments of education, social services, or human resources, and have branch offices throughout the state. (The

VR agency for each state is listed in Appendix 2, at the back of this book.) The money for VR services is provided through a federal-state matching program that provides 80% federal funds and 20% state funds.

The primary services provided by VR programs are vocational counseling and evaluation, vocational training, and job placement. VR is not an entitlement program, which means that all people with disabilities are not necessarily entitled to services. According to RSA's definition, services are provided when, in the judgment of the VR counselor, there is a reasonable expectation that a vocational handicap exists. The individual with a disability must have a significant functional impairment to employment and there must be a "reasonable expectation that vocational rehabilitation services will benefit the individual in terms of employability." "Employability" has been interpreted to mean a variety of things. It may describe the potential to do full-time competitive work, sheltered workshop work, home-based work, piece-rate work, part-time work, or any combination of these.

This chapter outlines the basic processes, methods and services that can help your son or daughter meet his or her vocational goals through VR.

ELIGIBILITY REQUIREMENTS FOR VOCATIONAL REHABILITATION

To qualify for VR services, your son or daughter must meet the following criteria: 1) the presence of a physical or mental disability which constitutes or results in a substantial handicap to employment, and 2) a reasonable expectation that he or she may benefit from VR services in terms of employability.

For the purposes of VR, a physical or mental disability is defined by Congress as a condition which "materially limits, contributes to limiting or, if not corrected, will probably result in limiting an individual's employment activities or vocational functioning." For instance, in Jolene Harris's case, the fact that she has mental retardation may materially limit her vocational functioning. The term "disability" is further defined as the presence of a continuing incapacity resulting from disease or injury. This means that if a single service (such as a herniectomy or appendectomy) is all that is necessary for rehabilitation, then the person would not be eligible for VR services.

A "substantial handicap to employment" is described as a physical or mental disability that impedes an individual's occupational performance by preventing him or her from obtaining, retaining, or preparing for employment consistent with personal capabilities and abilities. This determination is made on an individual basis. This means that VR services are available to persons who are presently working below their capabilities as well as to those who have never been employed.

VR regulations refer to "employability" as a determination that the provision of services is likely to enable an individual to enter or retain employment consistent with his or her other abilities in the competitive labor market. The VR counselor must determine that some potential for employment exists.

Federal law requires that first preference for VR services must be given to those persons with the most severe handicaps. Some persons with extremely severe disabilities (e.g., multiple sclerosis, severe mental illness, or cancer) may be found ineligible for service. There is a fine line between persons who are "most" eligible because of a severe disability and those who are ineligible because of a severe disability.

According to federal VR regulations, eligibility for services is based on whether or not a person with a disability has a "reasonable expectation that vocational rehabilitation services may benefit the individual in terms of employability." Every person who believes he or she may qualify for services has an absolute right to apply for services and arguably has a right to a preliminary diagnostic evaluation. There is no upper or lower age limitation. However, it is possible that government VR agencies could not reasonably provide services to a small child or an elderly person who would be incapable of benefiting from the service.

Although the law is not clear as to the right to a preliminary evaluation, it is reasonable to assume that before your son or daughter can be denied services, an evaluation of his or her potential to benefit from services must be made. If, after a preliminary evaluation, it is determined that he or she would not benefit, then justification exists for denying services.

Consider Jolene's situation. After her initial meeting with a VR counselor, and before the counselor decides what VR can do for Jolene, he or she will need information about Jolene's physical health, her physical and mental abilities, her potential in certain work-related areas, and, indeed, whether or not she is interested in working. A preliminary evaluation will answer many of these questions.

An applicant who has been determined eligible for services will go through further evaluation to determine the nature and scope of the services that are needed. This is called a *thorough diagnostic study*. The federal vocational rehabilitation regulations explain that a thorough diagnostic study includes:

> An appraisal of the individual's personality, intelligence level, educational achievement, work experience, personal, vocational, and social adjustment, employment opportunities, and other pertinent data helpful in determining the nature and scope of services needed. The study also includes, as appropriate for each individual, an appraisal of the individual's patterns of work behavior, ability to acquire occupational skill and capacity for successful job performance. (34 C.F.R., Sect. 361.32[b])

The nature and scope of services which Jolene will need to reach the goal of employment should take into account her total everyday needs and her present living situation. The VR counselor should work closely with Jolene's family and the special education program professionals at her school. Much of the information the VR counselor needs may be readily available through the evaluations and programs Jolene has participated in at school. Indeed, many of the vocational services Jolene needs may be available through the special education program. The *individualized education program* (IEP) developed for all students in special education can become a part of the VR program of services and vice versa. These two federal systems, Special Education and Vocational Rehabilitation, together provide a continuum of services for young adults with disabilities. The programs should not duplicate services, but, in fact, should provide appropriate complementary services in order to ensure that all needs are being addressed. This is accomplished by developing what we will term an *individualized transition program* (ITP), a written plan that oulines the programs and methods that will be used to help Jolene move from special education services to adult service programs. (By checking with the state agency responsible for VR services in your area, you can find out if ITPs are mandatory in your state and, if so, what procedures are involved in drawing up a mandatory ITP.) The VR counselor will also develop an *individualized written rehabilitation program* (IWRP) that will prescribe the scope of VR services Jolene will receive. The IWRP is developed jointly with the person who will receive the services. It takes into account the evaluation, strengths, needs, and vocational goals of the person.

WHAT SERVICES ARE AVAILABLE
THROUGH VOCATIONAL REHABILITATION PROGRAMS?

In the case of Maria Rodriguez, much of the preliminary diagnostic evaluation and determination of eligibility would not be necessary. Maria, presently employed full-time, clearly meets the employability criteria. Why would Maria want rehabilitation services?

Even though Maria is presently working full-time, she is only making minimum wage. Maria's dream is to have her own apartment. She understands budgeting and realizes that it is not possible to cover the costs of an apartment in Los Angeles by herself on a minimum wage income. She is also concerned about living on her own. She knows that it costs a lot more, but she doesn't really know what all the expenses are. She has never had to draw up her own budget, and she has never lived away from her parents. It is both a frightening and exciting prospect for Maria.

With more training, Maria feels she could get a better-paying job, possibly with health insurance and other benefits. In Maria's case, the VR agency may decide to develop an IWRP in the following service areas: residential living evaluation, additional vocational training, further education (possibly at the junior college level), and classes in budgeting and family living.

Once the objectives of the IWRP have been established jointly by the counselor, the person, and, if appropriate, his or her parent or guardian, the specific services needed to facilitate and implement the plan will be determined. In order to decide which services will be provided, it must be determined that the service is necessary to the implementation of the IWRP.

The broad scope of VR services reflects the variety of needs. Federal regulations require each state to assure that the following 15 categories of services are available to persons with disabilities as needed and appropriate:

1. Evaluation

Evaluation of every individual's VR potential is provided. This evaluation includes diagnostic and related services incidental to the determination of eligibility. Every one who meets the basic eligibility criteria will go through the evaluation process.

2. Counseling and Guidance

Each person will receive counseling and guidance through personal contact and interaction with a VR counselor. This is required in order to fulfill VR's "obligation of intake, eligibility determination, evaluation, IWRP development, protection of personal rights, case management, placement and closing of a case." Some people may require specialized counseling from an outside source, such as a psychiatrist or psychologist. In Maria's case, the counselor will help her determine which programs will benefit her.

3. Physical and Mental Restoration Services

Physical and mental restoration services are provided as necessary to correct or substantially modify a physical or mental condition which is stable or slowly progressive. The timing of the request for restoration services is critical. The Rehabilitation Services Administration has taken the position that federal VR funds should not be used to pay for restorative services for people with an incapacitating, progressive disorder until a thorough evaluation has been made. The purpose of the evaluation is to determine the person's "capacity for significant life work" should the services be approved.

If the only service needed is to address a temporary condition which may be remedied through surgery with no lasting effects, the services should be not be provided. (Examples include hysterectomy, hemorrhoidectomy, and cholecystectomy).

The following physical and mental restoration services are available if appropriate within the framework of the IWRP: medical or corrective surgical treatment; diagnosis and treatment for mental or emotional disorders by a certified psychologist or licensed psychiatrist; dentistry; nursing services; necessary hospitalization in connection with surgery or treatment and clinic services; convalescent or nursing home care; drugs and supplies; prosthetic, orthotic, or assistive devices (including hearing aids) essential to obtaining or retaining employment; eyeglasses and visual services; podiatry; physical therapy; occupational therapy; speech or hearing therapy; psychological services; therapeutic recreation services; medical social work services; treatment of acute or chronic medical complications associated with or arising out of physical and mental restoration services; special services for treatment of end-stage renal disease (transplantation, dialysis, artificial kidneys, and other supplies); and other medically related services (art therapy, dance therapy, music therapy, and psychodrama).

4. Training, Vocational and Other

Vocational training and other training services, including personal and vocational adjustment programs, are provided. Books, tools, equipment, and other training materials are provided as needed. Personal and vocational adjustment training is provided to improve attitudes toward work, to help an individual adjust to a recently acquired disability, and to strengthen work habits. Prevocational training is provided to supplement or enhance academic or basic training programs. The persons receiving services must maintain satisfactory performance and a good attendance record in order to continue to receive training services.

For Jolene Harris, personal and social adjustment and prevocational training are probably appropriate, whereas Maria Rodriguez would require a traditional adult vocational education program at a vocational training center or community college.

5. Maintenance

Maintenance payments covering an individual's basic living expenses are provided when living expenses increase because of the rehabilitation program. The purpose of maintenance is to assure that the person will be able to receive the full benefit of a VR service. Maintenance payments are not meant to serve as general relief or public assistance.

For instance, Maria may have to reduce her work hours in order to participate in training and evaluation. In this case, it would be appropriate for Maria to receive maintenance income to help her meet her basic living and transportation expenses.

6. Transportation

Transportation and related expenses are also covered for the purpose of supporting and maximizing the benefits of other services. Maria and Jolene would most likely qualify for transportation assistance to and from education, training, and evaluation programs.

7. Services to Family Members

Services to family members are designed to assist the people in an individual's family when it is deemed necessary to his or her vocational rehabilitation. Services to family members parallel those services available to the client. The person must show that these services are necessary to implement the IWRP. An example might be counseling and guidance services for a parent or guardian to enable him or her to understand and support the ward or child during training or education programs. For instance, Maria Rodriguez's traditional Mexican-American parents might not agree initially with their daughter's plan for independent living. A counselor could explain the financial and emotional benefits of such a plan and help Maria's family understand and support her goals.

8. Interpreter Services for Persons with Hearing Impairments

Interpreter services are available at all stages of the VR process from intake through closure. Anyone with a hearing impairment, including individuals who also have visual impairments, has a right to a qualified, competent interpreter.

9. Reader Services for People with Visual Impairments

Reader services include rehabilitation teaching services, note-taking services, and orientation and mobility services (cane training and independent living skills training) for people with impaired vision.

10. Aids and Devices

Telecommunications, sensory aids, and other technological aids and devices may be provided. Examples of these are computers, voice command wheelchairs, reading machines, and environmental control systems. Specialized devices must be prescribed or fitted by licensed or certified professionals and must satisfy engineering and safety standards.

11. Recruitment and Training Services

Recruitment and training services are designed to provide new work opportunities in the fields of rehabilitation, health, welfare, public safety, law enforcement, and other appropriate public service employment. This program is in keeping with the prohibition of discrimination in employment against people with disabilities in federal and state programs as outlined in Section 504 of the Rehabilitation Act of 1973.

12. Placement in Suitable Employment

Job placement is provided by the counselor or a professional placement specialist. Most programs encourage and require active participation by the person in the job search. One goal is to allow the individual to develop job-seeking skills. This is perhaps the most critical part of the process.

There are six basic criteria for determining if a placement is suitable:

1. The employer and the prospective employee are satisfied.
2. The person is maintaining adequate interpersonal relationships and acceptable behavior in the job environment.

3. The job is consistent with the person's capacities.
4. The individual has acceptable skills to perform and continue the work satisfactorily.
5. Working conditions will not aggravate the person's disability, and his or her disability will not jeopardize the health or safety of himself or herself or others.
6. The employment is regular and reasonably permanent, and the person receives wages commensurate with those paid to others for similar work under legal requirements.

13. Postemployment Services

Services may be provided after someone has obtained employment and his or her case has been closed. These services are available if needed to maintain the goal established in the IWRP, and are provided for a reasonable time after the case is closed. An economic needs test must be administered before most services are provided. However, evaluation, guidance and counseling, referral, and placement services do not require a needs test.

14. Occupational Licenses

Licenses, permits, or other written authority required by a state, city, or other governmental unit before one enters an occupation, begins a small business, or uses tools, equipment, and supplies, may be provided by a VR agency.

15. Other

The broad category, "Other," is a catch-all that allows the VR counselor to assist people with a variety of special needs. The regulations indicate that other goods and services may be provided that can reasonably be expected to benefit people with disabilities in terms of employability. Individual needs determine the appropriateness of the service. Examples include home modifications to improve accessibility and independence, and modifications to a vehicle to allow workers to drive or ride to and from employment and community resources.

HOW IS VOCATIONAL REHABILITATION FUNDED?

Think back to the Stuart family, who were introduced earlier in the book. Steve Stuart, age 17, has severe mental retardation. Would VR be appropriate for Steve?

As we indicated earlier, there is a fine line between persons who are "most" eligible for VR services and those who are ineligible because of a severe handicapping condition. Steve has severe mental retardation, is nonverbal, uses a walker, has some hearing loss and mild behavior problems, and is seizure-prone (although his seizures are controlled with medication). Through preliminary diagnostic evaluation, it is determined that Steve functions at the intellectual level of a 4-year-old. Can VR help him?

Let's assume Steve has been found eligible for services. The question now becomes, "What types of services will be provided?" Many direct services do not require the use of individually allocated service dollars. These include guidance, counseling, referral, and placement. Other services may be made possible by funds and programs from other federal or state agencies (see the example illustrated earlier of the coordination of services with VR and Special Education). These are defined as funds "available under any other program to meet, in whole or in part, the cost of vocational rehabilitation services." Examples are Medicaid, Medicare, individual or group insurance benefits, grants and scholarships, and workers' compensation. Some of these funding options are discussed in Section II of this book (Chapters 9–16).

A traditional VR approach to Steve's vocational needs may be an IWRP designed to prepare him for placement in a day activity center. You may recall the description of this program from Chapter 29 as a program for persons with severe and multiple disabilities who typically are viewed as unemployable. The program emphasis is usually on prevocational skill development, with the goal of movement into paid employment.

Further assume that Steve is working with a new VR counselor, John, a young man just graduated from a master's program in rehabilitation counseling, and Marge, John's supervisor, a woman in her early 50s. When Marge suggests that Steven enter a day activity center, John interrupts her, saying, "How about a trial placement with that new on-the-job training program here in town? It's a grant program funded through J.T.P.A. [Job Training Partnership Act] funds and it's designed specifically for severe mental disabilities. I attended a seminar on it last month. The company receives half the cost of wages and in turn provides what they call a 'job coach.' This is a coworker who teaches and who would supervise Steven's work for as long as is necessary. I hear it's working really well with other people who have a disability as severe as Steven's. I'd like to give him a shot at it. It's paid for by J.T.P.A., so there's no drain on our funds. The job coach will fade out if Steven can handle the work. If he can't, then the coworker will continue to work with him, and supervise him. The company agrees to hire Steve after a certain period at time. I think it might work for Steven."

Marge is not convinced, but agrees to give it a try.

In this case, Steve is not only eligible for VR services, he is also eligible for a program funded by the U.S. Department of Labor (J.T.P.A.). In addition, he may meet the eligibility criteria for assistance from Medicaid and Medicare and Supplementary Security Income (SSI) when he reaches the age of majority.

Federal regulations require the state VR program to give full consideration to any similar benefits available to an individual with a disability. The VR counselor is responsible for searching for alternative funding sources. If other sources are identified, the person who is eligible is required to apply for the services offered by them. This does not mean that VR counseling, guidance, referral, and placement services will stop. The VR counselor is responsible for helping the person apply for other services and for coordinating the provision of services through VR and other agencies.

SUMMARY

The VR system in your state is charged with providing valuable services for eligible people with disabilities. Eligibility is determined on a case-by-case basis. Given this approach, it is not possible to list specific criteria that are used to determine whether your son or daughter will be eligible. The case-by-case approach allows VR personnel to exercise considerable latitude in dealing with people with disabilities. You should also bear in mind that the regulations governing VR services in each state are constantly changing.

The trend, however, appears to favor a continued effort by VR agencies to serve more people with more severe disabilities. We urge you to investigate VR services in your area. In the chapters that follow, we discuss adult services agencies and informal contacts as potential sources of vocational placements for your son or daughter. We encourage you to explore these alternative sources only after VR services have been sought and eligibility has been established. Employment options that may be identified in existing adult service agencies may be obtained through VR. In some communities, VR agencies work closely with adult service agencies, and often refer people for placement in adult service agencies that operate vocational programs. In other communities, VR agencies may not make appropriate referrals to adult agencies. When referrals are not made, it is especially important for you to search for other options on your own.

If all the families planning for the future sought VR services, then the existing needs of people with disabilities would be documented. The federal VR program must be made aware of the lack of adequate vocational opportunities for people with disabilities. Even if you have been denied services in the past, we strongly recommend that you contact the VR agency in your area again. Remember, eligibility criteria change, and your son or daughter may now be eligible. If you discover that your son or daughter remains ineligible, you will be documenting continued need. You will be saying, in effect, "I had a need a year ago and I still have a need. When will help become available?"

33 HOW CAN I USE ADULT SERVICES AGENCIES TO HELP MY SON OR DAUGHTER?

As used in this chapter, the term *adult services* encompasses a wide range of programs and agencies. Comprehensive nonprofit agencies providing residential, employment, and recreational opportunities that vary from state to state and community to community are included in this category. These agencies may be supported to varying degrees by federal, state, and local funds (for example, county funds specifically intended for adult services for people with disabilities). Some of these agencies depend on nongovernment sources of funding either totally (for example, client fees, insurance payments, United Way allocations, or donations from other charitable and philanthropic organizations), or to augment government assistance.

Adult services agencies also vary as to the range of programs they offer. Many provide for comprehensive adult needs (for example, residential, vocational, recreational, transportation, and continued habilitation programs). Some agencies provide services for people with specific disabilities only (such as those with vision or hearing impairments or people with physical disabilities only).

Other programs exist which are funded by federal or state grants. Among these are Project Transition II in Vermont, Project EARN in Illinois, The Employment Training Program in Washington, D.C., and Full Citizenship in Kansas. After the grant funds designated to establish and initially support such projects' efforts expire, some programs continue providing services by charging a fee for service or by other arrangements. Often, special projects like those mentioned above are administered or affiliated with state or private universitities or colleges.

It is important to note at this point that while the various adult service programs may be sources of potential jobs for people with disabilities, the vocational rehabilitation (VR) system described in the preceding chapter remains the best starting point for entry into the world of work. If your son or daughter does not qualify for VR services because he or she is judged "unemployable," you will find yourself in a situation in which you need other services. The purpose of this chapter is to help you find those needed services.

Likewise, if you or your family member choose for one reason or another to bypass VR, this chapter can be of assistance to you. It may be helpful even if you have used VR. The job acquired through VR may have failed to meet the needs and preferences of your son or daughter, or your family member's needs and preferences may have changed over time and a new job may be in order.

*   *   *

The Stuart family provides a good example of the changes the VR system is experiencing. Jack and Rose Stuart had initially sought VR services when Steve became 17 years old. After an initial consultation with a VR counselor, Steve was deemed ineligible because of "the poor expectation of deriving benefit from services." The school program Steve attended provided a half-day vocational placement in a local sheltered workshop. Steve participated in this arrangement, but did not seem to enjoy it.

Jack, Steve's father, was very dissatisfied with the sheltered workshop as well. He would periodically stop in at the workshop when Steve was there. Jack's job had a flexible schedule, so he was able to view the total workshop operation over the course of several visits. He shared his concerns with his wife.

"I was there again today for about a half-hour and it was just like always. Rose, they don't do anything there. Steve and several other young people were just sitting in front of empty work benches. The supervisor said it was break time—it's always break time there. They have no work contracts."

The sheltered workshop was experiencing many problems. The contracts it had were few, and they paid poorly. Steve "worked" (or at least spent time there) about 15 hours a week. In the first 4 months he was there, he earned a total of $117, or about 48¢ per hour. Jack felt strongly that this was not the best situation for his son. When Steve's individualized habilitation program (IHP) meeting was held at the end of his first year at the workshop, the situation came to a head.

The workshop supervisor suggested that Steve spend the summer working full-time in the program. Jack controlled his anger and merely asked, "Doing what? There are no opportunities here for Steve. Besides, he doesn't like coming to the workshop."

"Now, Mr. Stuart," the workshop supervisor said, with an edge in his voice, "Steve is a very, very handicapped child. He needs to learn that work is important. Perhaps he gets his negative attitude about our workshop from you. Mr. Stuart, believe me, Stevie could not possibly work outside our workshop—no, no, no—this is best for the boy."

The anger within Jack subsided. The workshop supervisor had just convinced Jack of the action he must take. He was freed, and it felt good. Jack looked directly at Herb Clark, the supervisor, and in a calm, measured voice took charge of the meeting.

"First, Herbie, my son's name is Steven. I sometimes call him Steve. He doesn't like the name Stevie, never has. Second, Steve is not a very, very handicapped child, he is a young adult with some disabilities. Third, his, as you call it, negative attitude is caused by the workshop, not me or his home. He is bored here. Fourth, Steve will find a job elsewhere. This meeting, sir, is over. Good day!"

As Jack rose and turned to leave, Mr. Clark stammered and stuttered, but finally managed to blurt out, "Mr. Stuart, you, you're wrong. And, and, you'll be sorry. Now just settle down and reconsider . . . "

Jack quietly closed the door behind him, muffling Mr. Clark's harried voice as he left. "I don't know how," he thought aloud, "but Steven will get a job he likes. He will."

Jack and Rose made another appointment with the VR regional office. The rules had changed and now it was determined that Steve was eligible for all services. After an extensive evaluation and determination of Steve's preferences, a job was found in the cataloguing section of the library at a private college in Salina. The VR agency hired a trained job coach to assist him. Steve continues to make steady progress and thoroughly enjoys his new job.

FINDING ADULT SERVICE AGENCIES THAT OFFER EMPLOYMENT OPTIONS

Think back to the process described in Chapter 21 for locating residential options. The process for identifying adult service agencies that provide employment options is similar. You need a place to start, a springboard into the world of work. Initial contacts will lead to other possibilities. As with residential options, you are interested at this point in identifying as many vocational possibilities as you can.

Local Resources

The VR agency in your state is the best place to begin your search. This is true for two important reasons. First, this agency can provide a thorough evaluation of your son's or daughter's vocational needs, preferences, skills, and deficits. If you have not already done so, you may want to read the previous chapter on VR to understand the services that are available. Second, even if this agency cannot provide vocational training and maintenance services for your son or daughter, it can provide information that may enable you to locate alternative vocational training programs and opportunities. In Appendix 2, at the back of this book, you will find the address of the VR agency in your state.

Other sources that were helpful in the search for residential options may be helpful in this search as well. Local Association for Retarded Citizens chapters, community mental health agencies, and local school district personnel (for example, guidance counselors, special education teachers, transition specialists, and administrators) may be able to provide leads.

It is also possible that programs that address the vocational needs of people with disabilities may be operating at a university or college in your community or state. If this is not the case, university-affiliated professionals can often direct you to appropriate resources.

WHAT INFORMATION SHOULD I GET FROM THESE AGENCIES?

Your initial contacts have already begun, and using some type of master list will help you keep names, phone numbers, and descriptions of services in order. The master list at this stage need not be complicated. Figure 33.1 is the organization sheet that Eloisa Rodriguez developed when she began to look into vocational options with Maria.

As you begin receiving the information you requested, you may find an organizational system very helpful. You can use file folders or large envelopes to keep information from different programs and agencies separate. You can jot down notes on the inside covers of the folders or on the outside of the envelopes. Different people have different systems that work best for them, but the goal is to organize your search in a manner that will make the process work for you.

Specific Information to Request

Many programs that provide vocational opportunities will have brochures, pamphlets, and other written materials available describing the services they offer. However, you may want to ask some specific questions during your initial request for information. You will find this detailed information very valuable as you begin evaluating individual programs and decide which to visit and, later, which to investigate further.

The following list includes questions you may find useful in your initial evaluation of vocational options:

> What types of employment programs do you provide (e.g., sheltered work, competitive employment)?
> Do you provide vocational evaluations for people?
> Are there costs associated with any evaluation?
> Do you serve people with all types and levels of disabling conditions?
> Do you have programs to teach specific skills that people may need to acquire and keep a job?
> Is there a waiting list?
> What are the procedures for initiating an application for services?
> What is the cost of services?

These questions are just a small sample; you will probably think of other specific issues that are important to you. Your search for employment options will undoubtedly turn up ones that are unsuited to the needs of your son or daughter. At this point, your goal is to identify as many possibilities as you can. The next phone call you make may indeed connect you with the ideal employment option. With this thought in mind, we offer one last suggestion about questions and how to ask them: If a contact you made does not offer the services you seek, this is not necessarily a dead end. End all contacts, both promising and disappointing, with a final question: "Do you know of any other agency or program that might provide employment opportunities?" A contact that appeared to be a dead-end street could well lead to a four-lane highway.

HOW DO I GO ABOUT EVALUATING AGENCIES BEFORE VISITING THEM?

An initial review of the information you have gathered on potential employment should be directed at weeding out obviously inappropriate programs. You should also rate the options so that you can decide which are worth exploring further. The axe you wield as you clear a path to a good job placement should not cut too wide. Options that are clearly inappropriate will be evident, but those that do not immediately strike you as being poor may warrant continued investigation.

What makes a job inappropriate? The answer will be individually yours. You, your son or daughter, and others involved in the planning have unique preferences as well as needs. You and others may decide that a job is inappropriate on a number of grounds. A particular job may not offer the income desired, a work site may be too dangerous, perhaps there is no potential for advancement, a job program may be too segregated, or your son or daughter may not want to do the kind of work associated with a particular option.

After your initial review of potential vocational placements, you will perhaps

Name of Program	Date First Contacted	Contact Person	Phone #	Services Offered
Onward and Upward	11/01/87	O. I. Folks	555-2239	Voc. Ed., training in applications, sheltered work.
Work with Industry	11/03/87	M. E. Johnston	555-6846	Supported work, day activities

Figure 33.1. A form that Eloisa Rodriguez developed to help her and her daughter, Maria, investigate vocational options for Maria.

have identified some that show promise. You may find it helpful at this point to rate the options. There are many ways to do this. You may find the method that was used by the Hughes family helpful.

*   *   *

Lowell and Barbara Hughes made an appointment with the VR office in Indianapolis to have Brian evaluated. As Lowell and Barbara suspected would happen, Brian was found ineligible for services because of his low employability potential. His parents were determined to find some program that would provide for Brian's vocational needs, however.

The counselor proved very helpful. She directed the Hughes family to three agencies in the Indianapolis area that specialized in providing a range of services for people with severe disabilities. After contacting the three agencies, and a fourth one that was identified during this initial search, Lowell and Barbara organized the information so that they could evaluate their options.

Forward, Inc. provided a large packet of information and the social worker at the agency had been helpful in answering many questions over the telephone. Forward, Inc. operated only vocational programs for people with developmental disabilities. The programs consisted of two large sheltered workshops employing more than 100 people.

Independent Living Services provided vocational training, placement in community job settings, and follow-up support, but it served only those people who were eligible for VR assistance. It was obvious, at least at this time, that this was not an option for Brian. Barbara Hughes wrote a thank-you note to the agency in which she asked that she be contacted if the eligibility policy changed in the future. Lowell and Barbara continue to receive the agency's semi-annual newsletter. Lowell recommended the agency to a friend who has a daughter with a disability, and she is currently employed as a result.

Sunshine Enterprises was a program operating in a neighboring county. The scant information this agency sent by mail made one fact crystal clear: The extent of its "vocational services" was a day activity program lasting 2 hours per day Monday through Thursday. The pamphlet read, "Emphasis is placed on teaching clients a variety of board and table games (checkers, dominoes, cards), as these teach excellent prevocational skills. Each client will also work on a crafts project (either a strung hot pad or an ashtray) and will have a finished product at the end of the year—just in time for Christmas!"

Barbara shook her head and said to her husband, "Brian hates board games." Lowell added, "How can they claim they are providing a vocational service? And that crafts project. One ashtray or one pot holder a year?" They agreed that this agency would not meet Brian's needs or preferences at all.

The last agency, Partners in Business, was a coalition of merchants who provided jobs in their own businesses for people with disabilities. The agency worked closely with the state VR office but did not require that all applicants be VR-eligible.

The idea of Brian working in a community setting was something Lowell and Barbara had never considered. As Barbara pondered, one thought kept returning again and again—"Why not?" Although Lowell remained skeptical, both decided to look at Partners in Business more closely. Forward, Inc. also seemed to warrant closer inspection.

Having narrowed their search, the Hughes family could concentrate their efforts. At the same time, the doors remained open to consider other options still to be identified. The Hugheses considered Brian's preferences as well as their choices (the value of a real job versus day activity) in their evaluation. This is but one example of how to do an initial review of the options. There are perhaps as many other methods as there are families.

34 HOW DO I DETERMINE WHICH VOCATIONAL AGENCY IS BEST FOR MY SON OR DAUGHTER?

WHAT DO I DO WHEN VISITING AN AGENCY?

The next step in the evaluation process is to visit your potential choices. As we stressed in the chapters on residential selection (Chapters 20–26), a written description of a program may be deceiving. The management and staff of most adult service agencies will gladly meet with prospective consumers of their services and with interested family members.

At this point you might ask, "Who should visit these potential work sites?" Any family member(s) or friend(s) involved in the planning should visit, but most important, your son or daughter should visit the potential workplaces.

Observing the way your son or daughter reacts to a vocational environment can help him or her, as well as you and others, decide if a particular option is, in fact, appropriate. If capable and interested, your son or daughter should be encouraged to ask questions while visiting different job sites. You and others who come along on your visit may want to direct questions to your family member to better assess personal feelings and impressions. These questions should be specifically about job duties and responsibilities. Some examples:

Would you like to work making plastic cups like the other people here do?
Do you think there is enough light in this building?
Is the workroom too warm for you?
Could you take orders from the boss and follow her instructions?

Make sure you schedule your visit at a time when the work site is at its peak of activity. Visiting during the lunch hour will provide little information on things such as overall noise and activity levels. Also, be prepared to dedicate at least 45 minutes to an hour to your visit. This amount of time can give you a fuller understanding of an environment than a 15-minute walk-through.

WHAT QUESTIONS SHOULD I ASK?

Many families identify four general areas of concern relating to vocational placements: *wages, safety, job-related benefits,* and *relationships with coworkers.* You may share similar concerns and should feel free to ask the questions that will provide the information you need to assist you in further planning.

The items you or your son or daughter identified as being important in the employment checklist provided at the end of Chapter 31 (pp. 263–266) can also serve as a guide for evaluating an adult service agency during your visit. The preferences noted by your son or daughter can help you formulate specific questions you may want to ask during a visit to a potential work setting. For example, assume that Anna Levine and her parents competed the following checklist question in Part A as follows:

9) I may work in a place where nobody smokes.

$$(+3) \quad +2 \quad +1 \quad 0 \quad -1 \quad -2 \quad -3$$

During a visit to a potential job site, Anna or her parents may ask specific questions relating to her preference for a smoke-free environment, such as "What are the company's smoking policies?," and "Is a smoke-free area available to your employees?"

Some very different questions may be prompted by Item 16 on the checklist (from Part C):

16) I have the same right to complain about things on my job that my coworkers without disabilities have.

$$+3 \quad +2 \quad +1 \quad 0 \quad -1 \quad -2 \quad -3$$

Some of these questions might be:

> Is there a union here?
> When will I be eligible to join it?
> What are company grievance procedures?
> Who do I see if I am having problems on my job?

Questions relating to salary, safety concerns, and fringe benefits might include:

> How will my son or daughter be paid? By the hour, the task?
> How much can a person earn during a week here?
> What is the average for a worker here?
> Who will be the supervisor?
> What is the extent of the supervisor's experience in working with people with disabilities?
> What are the emergency procedures in the event someone is hurt on the job?
> Do other people with disabilities work here now, or have any worked here in the past?
> How do you view the role of a job coach?
> How are absences or illnesses handled?
> Do workers earn vacation time?
> What benefits are associated with this job?
> What happens if my son or daughter starts work here and for some reason fails at the job?

Many questions will come to mind as you visit work sites. If the person showing you around cannot answer your questions, you may want to ask to speak to someone who can. Some people find it helpful to bring a notebook when visiting possible employment sites. Taking notes can help you remember unanswered questions as well as important information you may want to add to your planning records.

Some people recommend that other workers in the job setting be interviewed during a visit. On first thought, this may sound like a good idea—talking with those who work in the setting should logically provide useful information. However, there may be drawbacks to questioning the employees regarding their impressions of their jobs and coworkers. Such a tactic may inadvertently accentuate the perceived differences between people with disabilities and those who do not have disabilities.

Think of the possible reactions other people in a workplace may have to some of the following questions:

How do you like working with people with disabilities?
Is there ever any trouble between workers with disabilities and those who do not have disabilities?
Do both types of workers interact with one another?

The other workers may wonder if people with disabilities are sources of problems—if they aren't, then why is such emphasis being placed on relationships? Good intentions may backfire. It may be best simply to help your son or daughter adjust to a new job by supporting the development of positive relationships with other workers.

If a job site employs other workers with disabilities, asking the parents or other relatives of these workers their impressions may provide useful information. Some questions you may want to ask are:

How long has your son or daughter worked there?
Does he or she like the job?
Have there been any problems at work because of your son's or daughter's disability? If so, what was the problem?
How was it resolved?
How does your son or daughter get along with coworkers?
Is there anything my son or daughter should be particularly aware of concerning this job?

Other parents and relatives will often be eager to help you by sharing their own experiences. Having gone through the process before you, they can alert you to any pitfalls they encountered as well as identify their own successes. They can be valuable sources of support at a time you may find difficult and somewhat stressful for your family.

WHAT DO I DO AFTER A VISIT?

After you visit a work site, you may want to discuss your impressions with others. This can help you get input from others whose opinions you respect or whom you may want to include in further planning. You may want to add any additional information you obtain about a work site in this way to your file on that agency. If, after the visit, you identify questions you failed to ask during the visit, or if new questions have arisen, you can follow up by phone or schedule a second visit.

Perhaps your visit convinced you that the option is suited to the needs and preferences of your son or daughter, as well as those of other family members. In that case, you may want to initiate the application procedure at this point, expecially if there is a waiting list.

If you have identified other promising vocational options, you will want to visit them first. Seeing other employment programs can give you a basis for comparisons to programs you have already visited. A program that appeared impressive in isolation may lose some of its luster when compared to other programs.

There will always remain the possibility that new programs will be initiated, so any decision you may make at this point need not be considered permanent. Programs also change. An ideal placement today may evolve into one that no longer serves your son's or daughter's needs, just as it is possible that a person will grow and mature to the point where a new job opportunity needs to be considered. The key is understanding that transition is not a one-time event, but an ongoing, dynamic process. You and others are planning for transition both into and *through* adulthood.

35 WHAT ARE SOME INFORMAL WAYS TO FIND A JOB?

For many people, finding a job involves using their informal support network; relatives and friends often provide leads that eventually enable one to secure a position. For example, an opening may occur at the place where a friend works. Not only do you have inside information, which gives your son or daughter a jump on other job seekers, but your son or daughter also has the advantage of using your friend as a reference.

On other occasions, relatives or friends may own their own businesses where jobs may be available to people with disabilities. Talking about the vocational needs of his brother with a disability, one person gave the following account:

> My brother has always been fortunate in that area. My father runs a rather large construction business and as long as I can remember my brother has worked there. He is now a carpenter's helper, makes good money, has a good benefit package, and seems very happy. I don't think my brother has ever had a vocational assessment performed by any professional or agency. There was never any need.

You and your relative with a disability may choose to explore the informal sources of jobs. In this chapter, we offer some suggestions to assist you. The term *informal* is used here to describe options other than vocational rehabilitation (VR) and adult services agencies. It will quickly become apparent that your informal search can lead you to some established organizations. The means you use to locate the right job are not as important as the end result—the job itself.

HOW CAN FRIENDS AND RELATIVES HELP?

It is a good idea to inform your friends and relatives that your son or daughter is looking for work. You should explain his or her work preferences and job skills. An honest assessment of your son's or daughter's deficits should also be provided.

Discuss the issues of references and recommendations openly. A relative or close friend may wish to help you and your family with your search, but may not be willing to serve as a reference. Having a clear understanding at the beginning can prevent embarrassment or bruised feelings later. If a close friend or relative wishes to serve as a reference, that person will need as much information as possible to give a good recommendation.

Someone you know may be willing to serve as an informal job coach for your son or daughter. One adult service agency in Kansas, for example, has recently instituted a supported employment program based on a "friends network."

When this particular service agency initially decided to implement the supported employment model, there were more ifs than certainties. The agency professionals knew what they wanted to do, but did not know how to get started. One member of the agency staff, however, had a friend who worked in a lumber yard where there was job opening. The agency quickly contacted the business's owner and a placement for a young man with moderate mental retardation was soon secured. The agreement involved a 90-day trial period. The agency offered the services of a trained job coach to facilitate the transition.

After approximately 1 month has passed, during which the new worker and his job coach learned the duties and responsibilities of the position, a wonderful twist was added. The person who had first told the agency of the opening at the lumber yard announced that he wanted to take the new worker under his wing, teach him the ropes, and serve as both friend and coworker.

The results have been very positive. Two other people with disabilities have also secured jobs at the lumber yard. Other workers at the yard came forward and helped to train the new employees. The adult service agency was able to use its trained job coaches in other employment settings, thereby expanding competitive employment options. It all began with a friend.

WHAT ABOUT WANT ADS AND PLACEMENT SERVICES?

Scan the classified section of your local newspaper any evening. If you live in an average-sized town you may be surprised at the number of jobs available. Many are entry-level positions that require no previous experience. With support, many people with disabilities could fill these positions. Take, for example, the following newspaper ad:

> Help Wanted. No experience necessary, we will train. Flexible hours to meet your schedule, above minimum wage, good benefits. Apply in person. Bud's Drive-In, 811 W. 6th St.

What types of support might a person with a disability need to compete for jobs in the community? The support needed could be minimal. Perhaps assistance in completing the application or help during the interview is all that is required. Once the individual has secured a position, getting to and from work may require family assistance. The employer may also be approached to work out a specific on-the-job training program to maximize the potential for a successful placement.

Some people may require a great deal of support to obtain and hold a job. Close supervision by a person who is sensitive to your son's or daughter's individual strengths and weaknesses may be required. Such situations require cooperation between the employer, your son or daughter, and anyone else who may be involved. The needs of the employer must be considered just as important as those of potential workers with disabilities. If the employer cannot make a profit, jobs will not be available.

If people with disabilities and their families work closely with potential employers, the result could be more people with disabilities working in truly integrated community settings. The employers would also benefit. Many entry-level jobs in the food service and entertainment industries, for example, are left unfilled. Fast-food operations report high employee turnover. As the labor pool (traditionally teenagers) continues to shrink, the expanding fast-food companies have started exploring new options. Their willingness to try new approaches to hiring and retaining dedicated employees could meet the needs of your son or daughter.

Many communities have job placement services. The ones operated by the state agency responsible for human resources do not charge for their services. Job placement counselors at these agencies match employer needs to potential employees' skills. A visit to a local work placement agency may be rewarding. The person with a disability can be placed on a list if there are no immediate openings, and he or she can be contacted when new positions become available.

WHAT ABOUT OTHER APPROACHES?

A friend recently shared an exciting experience which confirms that employment opportunities can be found in nontraditional areas. Mark is 20 years old and has mild mental retardation. He graduated from high school and has been employed for 2 years in a sheltered workshop. He was not satisified with his work placement, but could not find the support he needed to get other work. He lived with his sister after his mother died, and although his home life was happy, his sister was unaware of alternatives to the workshop.

Mark made friends with a supervisor at the workshop, a young man named David. One day David announced that he was going to join the Army. David was scheduled to take the Army entrance test and invited Mark to join him. Mark met with the recruiter and made arrangements to take the entrance test, too. He failed to pass the test by a narrow margin, but he was far from discouraged. As he put it, "I now know what to study."

With the help of his friend David and others, Mark worked hard to bone up on his skills. A few months later, he again took the entrance test, and passed. He entered the Army, successfully completed basic training, and is currently stationed at a post in Texas. A mechanic, Mark works on the myriad of vehicles the Army maintains. He now talks of making the military a career. Time will tell whether he remains in the service, but he is happy, makes a good living, and is proud that he did it "for myself."

The military is not the answer for everyone, but some people with disabilities may find this a challenging, rewarding option. The various branches of the armed forces have different requirements. Depending on the rate of enlistment and staffing needs, these requirements periodically change. A visit to a local recruiter will provide the necessary information.

Another area seldom tapped is the civil service. Because there are many vocational positions within various federal, state, and local government agencies that are suitable for people with disabilities, the opportunity exists to match a specific employment preference with a specific job. The written tests required to obtain some of these jobs vary as to difficulty. But, as was the case with Mark, these tests can be retaken if a person fails to qualify the first time. Once someone knows what to study, his or her chances for success will greatly improve.

Perhaps the time is long overdue to ask the same question of your son or daughter that is continually asked of people without a disability: "What do you want to do for a living after you finish school? You want to be a nurse's aid? Fine. Here is what is required . . . You want to be an auto mechanic? Fine. Here are the requirements." No matter what your son or daughter wants to be, the requirements can be determined and a plan of study and training can be developed so that he or she has a shot at achieving specific goals.

Vocational placements represent important decisions for your son or daughter, yourself, and others involved in future planning. Specific service systems and agencies exist which are charged with providing assistance in securing such placements. Some of the systems described in the preceding chapters may meet your needs, while others will not. Individual preferences will dictate the approaches that suit you and your son or daughter best.

ADVOCACY

You and other parents and family members are interested in securing the best possible package of services for your son or daughter. People often discover that there are parts of the total package of services that are weak. Perhaps some component of a residential program does not fully address your son's or daughter's preferences. Your son or daughter may not be happy with a job for some reason.

You have four options when addressing program weaknesses:1)Accept things as they are. The weaknesses may disappear, but more likely they won't. In this case, nothing changes and the package remains less than ideal. 2) Withdraw your son or daughter from those services that are not meeting individual needs and preferences. However, alternative services may not be available. The end result is an incomplete spectrum of services. 3) You may choose to advocate changes in the services that will eliminate identified weaknesses. 4) You may find it impossible to effect changes within an existing service or program and decide to advocate other options to meet your son's or daughter's individual needs.

The three chapters in this section deal with advocacy. In Chapter 36, we suggest ways of effectively advocating specific changes within a program. In Chapter 37, we describe efforts to advocate the establishment of alternative options when existing ones fail to meet needs and preferences. In Chapter 38 we describe self-advocacy—people with disabilities speaking for themselves. Self-advocacy is an important skill, in that it empowers people with disabilities to exert greater control over their own lives.

Advocacy is an outcome of the decision-making process we described earlier in the book. You identify a weakness in a program—there is a problem. Advocacy of change represents the other steps of the decision-making process—it is taking action. During the evaluation process, if you discover that your actions did not improve the situation, advocating outside the system is but another action in the decision-making process.

Self-advocacy can be coupled with the advocacy efforts of parents or others who seek change. Such a coupling acknowledges that your son or daughter should be a part of any decision-making process. In the chapters on guardianship, we introduced the concept of concurrent consent. Combining the efforts of your son or daughter, yourself, and others is a parallel to concurrent consent. Think of it as concurrent advocacy to achieve results that will benefit everyone involved.

36

HOW CAN I ADVOCATE WITHIN ESTABLISHED PROGRAMS?

Like most parents, you probably have concerns about the quality of your son's or daughter's program—whether it is a high school, a residential program such as a group home, a vocational program such as a sheltered workshop, or a recreational program in the community. Your concerns may center on whether your son's or daughter's preferences are being met. If they are not, your family's preferences probably are not being satisfied either. You also may have concerns about whether your son or daughter is getting the kind of training and support that will enable him or her to do his or her best. If you have these concerns, you need a critical skill—knowing how to advocate. To advocate is to represent the interests of your son or daughter in dealing with people who influence how programs are carried out.

In this chapter, we apply the steps involved in decision-making that we discussed in Section I to a process for your advocacy efforts. This process has six parts: *defining the problem, brainstorming, evaluating and choosing alternatives, communicating the decision to others, taking action to resolve the problem,* and *evaluating the outcomes of your action.*

DEFINING THE PROBLEM

Your son or daughter probably will encounter a variety of problems in a program. For example, a high school program may not provide relevant training for life in the community; a residential program may ignore personal preferences for socialization and recreation; a job may be boring and stigmatizing. If you can define the type of problem and how serious it is, you will be better able to resolve it.

We encourage you to try to see problems from the perspective of your son or daughter as you identify his or her preferences by using the Preference Checklist (see Appendix 3). It is necessary to involve your son or daughter in identifying preferences to the greatest extent possible. You can do this through direct communication or with the Shoes Test. It is also important to understand that being attuned to your son or daughter's preferences is a continual process, necessary to the creation of the kind of life-style appropriate to your son's or daughter's preferences. You can use the Preference Checklist to monitor or check on how things are going for your son or daughter at regular intervals (for example, every 3–6 months), when your son or daughter expresses concerns, or when you suspect that problems are occurring. When a significant gap exists between your son's or daughter's preferences and his or her social/interpersonal, community life, residential, and vocational options, then a problem exists and needs to be defined. Thus, your beginning point for defining problems is the continued use of the Preference Checklist.

A barrier often faced by the parents of children with severe disabilities is that their son or daughter cannot directly communicate concerns or frustrations. You may perceive that your son or daughter is having problems, but you may also sense that these problems show up more when you are not present. For example, you may suspect that the residential supervisor in your son's or daughter's group home has a communication style characterized by sarcasm and negativism. A complicating issue may be that, because the supervisor communicates with you in a more positive way, you cannot document what you suspect.

You might use several strategies to identify or verify the problem, such as unannounced visits to the program, talking with other people with disabilities who participate in the program and who have more advanced communication skills than your son or daughter, talking with other parents who have sons or daughters in the same program, and talking with staff members in other components of the agency's program who may have some firsthand information they might share. Some of these strategies may appear to be snoopy, but you may find yourself in a situation where you might need to do some detective work to know for sure if a problem exists.

Assume you can determine what the problem is. Now, what do you do? One key to defining problems is to state them directly and constructively. The checklist lets you know what is most important to your son or daughter. If something important (a high preference item) is not being addressed, your problem has been defined.

There may be occasions where your son or daughter may be encountering several different problems, but it is impossible to address all of them at the same time. Choosing the problem with the highest priority can enable you to start your advocacy efforts where you are likely to have the greatest payoff.

Up to this point, we have considered only the "problem-definition" step from your son's or daughter's perspective. That is a necessary point of view, but it probably should never be the only point of view. After all, many families have members with different and sometimes conflicting preferences. Thus, one of the problems may be that your son's or daughter's preferences may not be yours; or, if they are yours, they may not be those of another family member. It may be necessary to define the problem by determining whose problem it is, and whether that person—your son or daughter, other child, spouse, in-law, parent, etc.—can have the problem solved in a way that is agreeable to other family members. A whole-family approach certainly can complicate future-planning. But would any of us want to take the perspective of only one person? In the rest of this chapter, we take the easy approach: The problem of the one person with a disability is a problem for the whole family.

*   *   *

Let's pick up with the Stuart family and Steve's job, which we discussed in Chapter 33. As you might recall, Rose had insisted to Jack that they take Steve to the vocational rehabilitation (VR) office to have him evaluated. Rose had attended a conference on transitional planning sponsored by the state developmental disabilities planning council and she had learned that vocational rehabilitation would cover the cost of job coaches. It took Rose and Jack a while to get up their courage to try to get services from yet another system—vocational rehabilitation (VR). They were discouraged and frustrated when the VR counselor met with them only to say, "We're sorry, but Steve has too severe a disability. We believe he can't be successful in competitive employment, and that he'll always need a sheltered workshop."

Although the parents of the other students in Steve's class seemed resigned to the sheltered workshop as the only option for their children, Rose and Jack were convinced that the right thing to do was to integrate Steve into a workplace; segregation wasn't for them. Steve clearly preferred to work alongside people both with and without disabilities—he had grown up in a family and lived in a community where he had always been included with everyone else. Official designations concerning disabilities played absolutely no role in Steven's perception of his world. The people he liked were simply his friends.

It also bothered Rose and Jack that the sheltered workshop in their community always seemed to get such glowing praise from the local newspaper, and that everybody in town thought it was so wonderful that people with mental retardation were working there. They were bothered because the facts did not justify the image. Rose had learned from a program sponsored by the local Association for Retarded Citizens that the average wage for the clients with severe disabilities was 31¢ per hour. To make things worse, at the transitional conference she attended, Rose saw a videotape of people with disabilities like Steve's working in food service in other places around the country, earning minimum wage and more. She just wondered why it wasn't happening in her community. When she made inquiries at the VR agency, she was told to go to the workshop and ask the director if he could arrange a supported employment placement for Steve. The Stuarts defined their problem this way: Family preferences for competitive employment are not being satisified. Steve wanted to be employed with coworkers who did not have disabilities, and Rose and Jack wanted the same.

Jack and Rose knew they had a long row to hoe because Steve had been attending the sheltered workshop half days for the last 2 years of school. At the two meetings they had with the director and the vocational coordinator, they were told about Steve's problems and how "he is fortunate to even be given a chance in Work Activity, Level 1, which is the lowest program." They know that the people who enter this program stay there for years, and their chances ever to work in a regular community program are very slim.

"Rose," Jack said, after one of their meetings with the sheltered workshop director and the vocational coordinator, "it's a simple bottom-line matter. The bottom line isn't money, although Steve could earn more outside the workshop. And it isn't that I'm looking for a fight . . . the 'convenience' approach is appealing. No, the bottom line is our values. We have made them clear by keeping Steve home and having him be part of this community. We're not about to segregate him now!"

"You're absolutely right," Rose said, enthusiastically. "I heard someone at that future-planning workshop quote a professor named Lou Brown. She said this Dr. Brown once said that 'prevocational means never.' You know, once you start in prevocational, you never leave it to go to real work for real money."

"Yes," Jack said. "And the move-through model the director told us about is bunk. 'Move-through' means 'never leave.' Rose, we can't do that to Steve. We've got to fight the segregation, exploitation, and hypocrisy."

They knew they were fighting an uphill battle, and they had to get the best ideas possible if they were going to convince the administrators at the sheltered workshop that Steve could be a candidate for supported employment.

BRAINSTORMING

Brainstorming means thinking of as many solutions as possible to a problem. Brainstorming is valuable because it can uncover new ways of approaching problems that are likely to be successful. Before you brainstorm, identify family members, friends, or professionals who are creative and who have an understanding of your son's or daughter's problems. Encourage them to think with you of many different ways to approach your problem. As you think together, it is important for everyone to feel free to suggest every possible alternative, even those that might sound ridiculous at the outset. Often, ideas that initially may seem unusual will have the uniqueness that may provide a special solution.

* * *

Jack and Rose Stuart invited their friends, the Wilsons, over for Sunday dinner. In choosing this time, they considered that their daughters would be there too, to hear it all. They could find out what the girls thought. After dessert, Jack leaned back in his chair and told everyone that he and Rose and their daughters needed their help because they had some hard work to do to promote Steve's preference for a real chance at a real job. Here are some of the ideas they came up with in that Sunday afternoon brainstorming session:

> Find out if any of the employees at the workshop had been placed in supported employment and, if so, what had brought about their placement.
> Call the director of the state developmental disabilities agency and ask that person to send some written material about competitive employment that they could share with the workshop director.
> Contact the vocational rehabilitation services office in the state capital to ask for help with developing supported employment.
> Set up a meeting with the chairperson of the board of directors of the workshop to ask for a chance to talk with the board members about supported employment.
> Start their own supported employment training program with Steve during weekends and evenings to teach him to wash cars and windows, and then help him get some jobs from neighbors and friends.
> Have Jerry Wilson talk to his employer at the plastics company where he worked about hiring Steve if the sheltered workshop would provide a job coach.

After everyone left, Jack chuckled as he told Rose, "It must have been something you put in the roast. I've never known us to come up with so many good ideas in such a short time."

Rose's answer went straight to the point. "No, dear. It's not the food. It's just that we put our resources together, namely family, friends, our commitment to Steve, and good ideas. And some of those ideas . . . Well! It's amazing what you can come up with if you look outside the narrow tunnel of tradition . . . you know, the tradition of school or workshop."

EVALUATING AND CHOOSING ALTERNATIVES

After your brainstorming is completed, your next task is to evaluate each alternative and decide whether you think it would help resolve the problem. You might consider such factors as how long it will take you to implement the alternative, whether any financial costs will be associated with implementation, how much resistance you may encounter from the school, workshop, or other service providers, and whether there will be any repercussions for your son or daughter if you implement the alternative. Usually, each alternative will have some benefits and some drawbacks, and you will need to weigh these to determine which alternative will be in the long-term interests of your son or daughter and other family members. Ultimately, you will need to choose a plan of action that you believe will be the most effective in resolving the problem.

* * *

Later that evening, Jack and Rose reviewed their list of alternatives and talked about how successful each might be. The one that gave them the greatest hope, and even excitement, was Jerry Wilson's offer to talk to his employer about hiring Steve. Steve idolized Jerry; this alone would likely mean that Steve would do his best, and Jerry could even stop by to see Steve and encourage him. It seemed so natural. Jack had gotten his first job through a friend from his church. Friends always help friends get jobs. Why shouldn't this work for Steve, too? If it didn't, there would be a lot of disappointed people . . . Steve, Jack and Rose and their daughters, the Wilsons, the plastics company, and maybe even other families.

"You know, Jack," cautioned Rose. "Some people will say we're just plain foolish to try this with Steve. Can you imagine what they're saying at that workshop? But there's another group who want us to succeed . . . all those families who are beginning to hear about schools without walls, about community-based instruction, about supported work, and about integration, productivity, and independence. So much is riding on this. We've got to succeed!"

COMMUNICATING THE DECISION TO OTHERS

In many cases, you will not have to communicate your decision to some of the people affected by it, because they will have helped you reach it, as in the Stuarts' case. Most times, however, you will have to tell others what you have decided. The Stuarts will have to tell Steve what lies ahead of him—new places, people, tasks, and skills. They will have to tell Steve's teachers, the workshop director, VR counselor, and family friends.

If the Stuarts had made the conventional decision to proceed from special education to the workshop, they would not have had to explain their reasons, or at least they would not have had to do so in detail. Any one of these explanations would have been sufficient: "We just did what everyone else did," or "It's suited to Steve," or "It's convenient, and we're getting older," or "Steve's too disabled for anything else," or "We're afraid to take a risk, and there's not much risk in doing the usual thing."

Because the Stuarts decided to do something different, they would probably want to explain in detail what they decided, why, how, and with whose advice and help. They might also want to explain how they planned to carry out their decision. For them, as for you, what you say to people, whom you choose to communicate with, and how you announce your decision can have a big impact on your decision's acceptability within your family, among professionals and service providers, and ultimately to your son and daughter. In the Stuarts' case, Jack and Rose decided to tell "the whole world."

"Jack," Rose said, "We've always relied on our friends, and we've built a good network of support for Steve. Those people we took in and regarded as family are entitled to be told, like family."

"I don't know, Rose," said Jack. "What if we don't succeed? What if Steve fails? It's a matter of our privacy, and our pride."

"You never quit," Rose answered. "And you never learn. If we want Steve to succeed, we'll need our friends. And if the idea doesn't work—and it's not that Steve or we will fail, because some of us may fail him or some aspect of the plan may fail us— we'll need our friends even more. So, we'll tell them all—and we'll do it now. As for the teachers and workshop, they'll have to know, too. Let's be reasonable, polite and uncritical of them. We may need their help, and whether we do or not, we should be as cordial to them as we'd want them to be to us."

Communicating your decision requires you, like the Stuarts, to think about whom to tell, what to say, how to say it, and when to disclose. These are important decisions, and necessary ones. Good communication is a prelude to action, and it can help you carry out your plan.

TAKING ACTION TO RESOLVE THE PROBLEM

Our best advice on taking action is to do so with gusto and determination. In our experience as advocates for people with disabilities, we have found that taking action requires perserverance and a strong commitment to your goal. You are likely to encounter some teachers, program administrators, residential house managers, vocational counselors, or other professionals who will welcome your assistance in resolving problems, just as you will find others who will strongly resist your ideas and involvement. (Although early childhood and school programs for students with disabilities have long encouraged parent involvement, many adult program personnel are unsure of how to work with parents and are uncomfortable when parents get involved in trying to resolve problems.) If you encounter resistance, it is important for you to know that other parents have had the same experience and that the collective wisdom of parents is that your son's and daughter's needs must guide your efforts.

As you go about the tasks involved in taking action, a style that is usually effective is to be persistent, steady, firm, and even-tempered. The more positive and constructive you can be in your communication, the greater the chance you can influence the professionals in the program to respond to your efforts in a positive manner.

You should keep several other considerations in mind. As Rose and Jack know, "the lone wolf is easy prey." That's the first consideration. If you try to take action alone, you will probably not be as successful as if you gather the support and interest of others, especially those who may be experiencing similar problems. Consider establishing a network of other interested families, adults with disabilities, and interested fellow citizens to address the problems that concern you.

The second consideration is that you must be willing to "play hard ball" if necessary. In many instances, merely making a request will not bring about a solution or even change one aspect of the problem. Sometimes you may need to file a formal grievance, initiate a due process hearing against the public school system, write a letter to the state agency that has responsibility for the program from which your son or daughter receives services, contact the protection and advocacy office in your state (see Appendix 2 for names and addresses of these agencies), or ask the news media to call attention to the nature of the problem experienced by your son or daughter. It is usually a good idea to use the least drastic means possible to resolve your problem, but be willing to resort to more drastic means when necessary. In Appendix 5 you will find descriptions of books that provide helpful information on strategies for taking more drastic action.

*   *   *

Jack and Rose first scheduled a meeting with the vocational coordinator at the sheltered workshop and Steve's teacher to tell them that they had learned about supported employment and that they thought this option would be best for Steve. Jack and Rose said that their friend, Jerry Wilson, who works at the Starr Plastics Company, had offered to talk to his employer about finding a job for Steve if a job coach could be provided. Jerry had done this and found his employer very receptive. The employer said that he basically believed that "everyone deserved a chance to work." He liked the idea of the job coach and said he wished he had had something like this last year when he had to let a Vietnam veteran with a physical disability go because he simply did not have the personnel to provide the necessary training.

   With excitement over what they considered a "golden opportunity," Rose and Jack asked if either the school or workshop would be able to provide a job coach. They even added that they would be willing to pay for the job coach if necessary. Steve's teacher agreed to have the paraprofessional working in her class serve as a job coach for Steve at the plastics company.

   Jack and Rose were thrilled with this arrangement, and Steve was proud to have a chance to work at the same place as his good friend, Jerry Wilson. Steve worked 2 hours a day for several months until the end of the school year, and he improved his productivity from 30 minutes of idle time per hour to 2 minutes of idle time per hour by the end of 3 months. Jack and Rose thought this was a fine reason for a celebration and held a cookout in Steve's honor. All his friends came to congratulate him.

   But the storm clouds started gathering again as summer began. When school was out, the plan was for the sheltered workshop to provide the supervision for Steve's employment over the summer. But the workshop director was unwilling to keep Steve at his job at the plastics company because the workshop did not have enough staff to dedicate a job coach exclusively to Steve. Jack and Rose thought that would be easy to take care of when they offered to pay for the job coach. They had been saving their money to send the girls to college, and they thought it was only fair that they invest some money in Steve's education as well. The vocational coordinator and the director, however, didn't respond positively. "We're just too busy to fool with supported employment for someone with a severe disability like Steve's. You've got to face it: Steve just won't ever be able to make it in the real world," one of them said.

   Jack and Rose were shocked to hear this, because everything they had heard about Steve's supported employment placement had been encouraging. Now they were hearing a different story. Whom should they believe? The staff at the workshop discounted the reports from the job coach about Steve's work attitude and habits. "We're just certain Steve has behavior problems," they asserted. "The job coach from the high school just didn't want to seem unsuccessful, or to disappoint you." Meanwhile, the workshop director and the vocational coordinator placed Steve back at the workshop. There his productivity level immediately dropped and behavior problems started occurring at least several times a week. It was upsetting and scary to see Steve become increasingly dependent, lonely, lethargic, depressed, aggressive, and self-injurious.

Jack hit the nail on the head one night when he said to Rose, "Steve's behavior is a problem, no doubt. But all that behavior modification isn't helping much, and I doubt that it will. The real problem is that he just doesn't like the workshop. Maybe Steve's trying to tell us something, and maybe we aren't listening. I bet Steve isn't the problem. I bet the place is the problem."

"That's what I've been thinking," Rose said. "And, you'll be happy to know, that's what many professionals think, according to my contacts at the state planning council."

In response to the Stuarts' continual requests to have Steve placed back at the plastics company where he had succeeded, the workshop staff said Steve would not be able to leave until he could prove that he could work hard and behave well in the workshop. Jack asked what would happen if Steve could work hard 4–6 weeks without any behavior problems, and he was told that the staff might interpret that to mean that Steve really liked the workshop and should stay there.

Jack was dumbfounded once more at how uncommon common sense had become. He despairingly said to Rose, "Can't they see the bind they're putting our son in? If Steve succeeds in the workshop, he gets to stay; and if Steve fails in the workshop, he gets to stay."

After a couple of months of dealing with the sheltered workshop so often that it seemed like they were eating, sleeping, and breathing advocacy, Jack and Rose were more than discouraged. The workshop was the program that people were saying Steve should enter after high school. Yet they knew that, if Steve went into this program, he probably would never find a job in the community. If students like Steve could succeed at real jobs in other communities, why couldn't Jack and Rose find a real job here at home? "Jack," said Rose one night, "I'm fed up. Mother once told me that the end of the rope is the end of the rope, no matter how long the rope seems. Well I'm at the end of my rope. We've tried everything, and nothing works. Steve is stuck, his behavior is bad, he's very depressed, the workshop won't change, and behavior modification is missing the cause of his behavior. Where do we go from here?"

Jack's answer was puzzling. "Are you sure we've tried everything? Could it be that we haven't thought about all of our choices?"

EVALUATING THE OUTCOMES OF ACTION

The best way to evaluate the outcomes of your action is to go back to the problem definition and ask yourself if the problem has been adequately resolved. If the problem has been resolved to your satisfaction and that of your son or daughter, you can give a positive rating to the outcome of your action and move onto other issues that concern you, or even take a break from advocacy for awhile. If the problem has not been resolved, the approach you should consider is to repeat the brainstorming process in the hope of identifying new alternatives that might be more successful. Essentially, you can recycle through this problem-solving process so that you can continue to work on the problem in new ways.

It is important to recognize when your actions are sufficient and when to retrench and try another way. We have been in situations ourselves where our first, second, or even third alternatives were unsuccessful, and we needed to keep trying new approaches until we found one that worked. At some point you will probably be in that situation, too. The key is to not give up or get discouraged, but to persevere to the point where you succeed in solving the problem.

Rose and Jack had never been so frustrated in their lives. First of all, they had never worked as hard for anything for Steve as they had worked to get him a regular job at the Starr Plastics Company. When they looked back at their efforts, they realized how many times they had met with the school system and sheltered workshop officials. It seemed that the school always referred them to the workshop, and the workshop always referred them to the school. They began to get the idea that the transition from school to work really means that "the buck never stops" because each agency pointed to the other one, rather than taking responsibility itself.

Rose commented to Fran Wilson, "I feel like a ping-pong ball. The school system hits me to the workshop, and the workshop hits me back over to the school. I go back and forth, and the game seems to never end."

As Jack and Rose saw Steve's behavior deteriorate, they themselves became increasingly depressed. Steve had more behavior problems in the workshop that summer than in all his other years combined. Jack and Rose knew that they could not stand by and watch their son go downhill.

Evaluating the outcomes of their actions, they decided that their efforts had been unsuccessful, in spite of how hard they had worked and how much they had wanted to resolve the problem that they initially defined—finding Steve employment with coworkers who did not have disabilities.

Jack was watching television one evening when he heard someone say, "No matter how far down the wrong road you go, it's never too late to turn around if it is the wrong road." This hit Jack like a bolt of lightning. At that very moment he resolved to prevail and he called Rose into the room.

"Honey, we're wasting our energy. Steve is never going back to Starr Plastics by our efforts to work with the sheltered workshop. We're going down the wrong road, and the wrong road can only take us in the wrong direction. Let's turn around, and we'll find a way. But it'll be a different way. It'll be *our* way."

You have seen the frustration the Stuarts encountered attempting to change the system to meet Steve's needs. It appears that they will have to leave the existing system to reach their goal—a frightening prospect. Other families may be dissuaded from considering efforts to change conditions for their sons or daughters because they learn of failed attempts by families like the Stuarts. If we could eavesdrop on the conversations of some of these other families we might hear some interesting comments:

> "You can't fight city hall and you can't fight the system."
> "It's just the way things are and we have to accept them."
> "Look what happened to Jack and Rose Stuart. They disagreed with the workshop and Steve lost his place there as a result."
> "Maybe things aren't really that bad—they could be worse. Leave well enough alone."
> "That's the way things are done. They've always been done that way."

Yet, we must keep in mind the saying—if there are no complaints, then things must be fine. Changes come as a result of people complaining about problems. The Stuarts are learning a system, but should we view their action as a failure? Does their inability to achieve change mean other families in similar circumstances should not advocate for their sons or daughters? We believe the answer to both questions in a resounding "NO!"

Sadly, the system failed Steven Stuart, but systems differ just as individual needs and preferences differ. Advocacy remains the key to continuing positive changes. Look at another of our families, the Levines, and briefly follow their advocacy efforts, which ended very differently . . .

For months, Anna Levine had asked her parents to allow her to get an apartment of her own. Many of her friends were living away from home and she too wanted "a place of my own." Ben and Ruth resisted at first, but finally agreed to give it a try if Anna agreed to live in a program that was supervised by professionals who were trained to support people with mental disabilities. They found an adult service agency in a nearby suburb which operated semisupervised apartments. After a few weeks of completing forms, making in-house evaluations, and taking care of other administrative necessities, the big day finally arrived and Anna moved into her apartment.

A couple of months passed and Anna seemed to be doing beautifully. There were the expected adjustment problems, but the program staff worked closely with Anna and her family and the future looked bright. On a visit to their daughter's apartment one day, Ben and Ruth were surprised to hear Anna announce that she wanted to return home because she was not happy in the apartment anymore. Ben's first reaction was typical of him:

"No problem, baby—your home is always there for you. Come on, get some things together and we'll go home. We can get the rest of your things later."

Ruth, however, knew that the situation presented an opportunity for Anna to learn.

"Ben," she said, "sometimes you act as if you'd placed your brains in neutral. If you ran your business like you sometimes run your personal life, you'd have been a pauper years ago. Anna," she continued, "let's sit, talk, find out what's wrong. You were so happy here, now you say you want to leave. Anna, most things that happen to us in life have reasons. If you can identify the reasons maybe you can change them. But if you don't even try—then life controls you."

"Well," Anna said, "I really do like my apartment, but some things I don't."

Anna and her parents will use the same decision-making process that the Stuarts used. As you will see, the problem in this case is very different from that which confronted Steven Stuart and his family. The outcome for Anna will also be different.

HOW DID THE LEVINES DEFINE THE PROBLEM?

After a brief review of Anna's life in her apartment, it became clear that for the most part she was quite happy and that her stated desire to return to her parents' home was a hasty reaction to certain small aspects of her situation. Anna said she was not allowed to do certain things in her apartment, which frustrated her. Questioning by her parents soon identified the key issues.

"What kind of things, Anna?," her mother asked.

"Things, some important things," Anna replied.

"Look at this room," continued Anna with a sweeping motion of her hand toward the walls of the living room.

"It's a nice room," said Ben. "You do a fine job of taking care of this place."

"No, pictures, they don't let me hang pictures on the walls. Only in my bedroom, and then they say I can only use the two nails that are already there. It's not fair," Anna said.

"They don't let you—who's they?," Ben asked.

"The people, the agency that runs these apartments. My caseworker, she says they have rules," Anna replied.

The problem was identified. Agency rules prevented Anna from hanging pictures on her walls and she was not happy. Anna had many framed portraits of family members and friends and she had always displayed them in her room when she lived with her parents. The portraits and other prized pictures were important to her. Without them, her life was less than she wanted it to be.

HOW DID THE LEVINES BRAINSTORM?

Having identified the problem, Ruth asked that everyone consider possible solutions. Some interesting possibilities were mentioned.

> Have Anna defy the rules and hang the pictures, daring the agency to take action (Ben's defiant suggestion).
> Look for another residential program that would allow Anna the freedom to have pictures, portraits, and so forth.
> Have Anna return to her parents' home.
> Discuss the regulations with agency staff to determine if they could be changed.
> Accept the situation as it is, accepting that regulations are regulations.

HOW DID THE LEVINES EVALUATE AND CHOOSE AN ALTERNATIVE?

Anna rejected the idea of returning home or looking for another apartment. She had friends living near by and did not want to move. She gently chided her father for suggesting that she break the agency's rules. She reminded him that he had always taught her to respect authority and rules. This left two options, and it was Anna who chose the one she wanted to pursue.

"Mother," she said, "if you don't try nothing changes. Would you and dad go with me to talk to my case manager about changing the rule against pictures?"

HOW DID THE LEVINES COMMUNICATE THE DECISION?

Ben suggested that he, Ruth, and Anna all be present for a discussion of the agency's policy. He also suggested that besides Anna's caseworker, they request that the director of the agency be present. Ben wanted someone at the meeting who had the authority to make immediate changes. "Go to the top," he said, "deal with those in charge. That's the way to get results."

Ruth offered to contact both the caseworker and agency director to arrange a meeting. Anna and Ben agreed, and Ruth used her daughter's phone then and there to set a meeting for the following day. Ruth explained clearly why a meeting was requested and did not demand any concessions over the phone. The stage was set for negotiations the next day.

HOW DID THE LEVINES TAKE ACTION?

Ruth, Ben, and Anna arrived at the agency director's office the following afternoon. The director, Ms. Groski, and the case manager welcomed the Levines warmly. After some brief small talk, Ms. Groski opened the meeting.

"Perhaps we should get down to business. There seems to be some problem with our policy on hanging pictures on the walls in Anna's apartment. Let's see if we can clear up this issue," Ms. Groski said.

"Why," Ruth spoke up, indicating she would be spokesperson, "can't Anna put up her pictures and other things?"

"Mrs. Levine, the reason is simple," answered Ms. Groski. "That is the agency policy."

"Why?" Ruth asked.

"Because, it was decided, well, some time ago."

"Why?"

"Well, because . . . to keep people from destroying the walls, of course."

Taking a deep breadth, Ruth took the initiative, "Tell me, Ms. Groski, do you rent an apartment?"

"Yes I do," she replied.

"Do you hang things on your walls?," continued Ruth.

"Yes, but that's different," Ms. Groski said, adding, "my apartment is my home."

"And what do you think Anna's apartment is?," Ruth asked.

"Of course, but I don't destroy my walls," Ms. Groski retorted.

"And you are sure that Anna would?," Ruth said, trying to keep her anger from showing.

Ms. Groski became quiet, and her face flushed with embarrassment. She realized she had said some illogical things. She apologized to Anna and then to Anna's parents. She asked that everyone work on finding a solution. The agency policy did not respect a person's preferences, and Ms. Groski wanted to find a way to protect Anna's rights while ensuring that the agency's residential units would not be misused.

It was Ben who suggested the solution that was finally adopted. The agency would begin treating Anna and others as landlords treated renters—as competent adults. Anna would pay a damage deposit. If Anna left her apartment and if there was excessive damage to the walls, she would forfeit part or all of the deposit, depending on the situation.

HOW DID THE LEVINES EVALUATE THE OUTCOME?

Anna was pleased with the outcome. She decorated her apartment as she wanted it. Other problems arose, but the source of her original discontent had been eliminated. Anna learned to solve other problems as they surfaced using the process she and her parents had used. The issue of hanging pictures may not strike some as significant, but for Anna it was important. Resolving it added a degree of happiness to her life and that, we would all agree, is important.

37

HOW DO I ADVOCATE NEW PROGRAMS FOR MY SON OR DAUGHTER?

Sometimes you will find yourself in the Stuarts' situation. No matter how hard you try to meet your son's or daughter's needs through established programs in your community, you may find that those programs take all of you down the wrong road. If that happens, your best option may be to do as the Stuarts have done—turn around and find another road.

One reason for these "wrong roads" is that the philosophy and nature of model adult services are changing so rapidly that the kinds of services that seemed most appropriate 2 years ago might be outdated today. Progress is constantly being made toward creating new possibilities and removing the limitations placed on people with disabilities.

WHAT CAN I DO WHEN THE PROGRAMS IN MY COMMUNITY ARE UNRESPONSIVE TO THE NEEDS OF MY SON OR DAUGHTER?

If programs in your community are not responsive, consider the problem-solving process we described in the last chapter. This six-step process involves *defining the problem, creatively brainstorming, identifying and evaluating alternatives, communicating your decision, taking action,* and *evaluating the results.* Essentially, your problem is that no programs in your community are tailored to your son's or daughters needs. You could follow the steps of the advocacy process to come up with an action plan to help create new programs and opportunities. Perhaps your first response to this idea is like that of many parents, which is that you do not have the time, energy, and expertise to create programs. Many parents feel that they are too tired, when their sons and daughters are adolescents or adults, to invest themselves in program development. But Jack and Rose Stuart were surprised to learn that sometimes it is far easier and less time-consuming to create new programs than it is to change entrenched programs that follow traditional practices. So, although it may seem more difficult to start a new program, you may find that it is easier than some of your other alternatives.

HOW DO I DEFINE THE PROBLEM?

If you have already decided that you are headed down the wrong road, you have already defined the problem that faces you. That problem is that a significant gap exists between the preferences of your son or daughter and the nature of the established programs available to you. The next problem is to establish new programs that respond to your son's or daughter's preferences and that will increase his or her satisfaction with life-style options.

As part of the process of defining the problem, you should take every opportunity to learn as much as you can about state-of-the-art services for people with needs similar to those of your son or daughter. Knowledge is power. The more you know, the more power you will have to establish quality programs. You may want to think carefully about all the sources of information available to you. Here are some likely sources:

> The books and other printed materials listed in Appendix 5 are filled with relevant information. Ask your public library to order some of these resources, suggest to the local Association for Retarded Citizens that a library be set up for parents on state-of-the-art programs, and consider, if possible, spending some of your own money to purchase the materials that seem most relevant to you.
>
> Contact the departments of special education at the colleges and universities in your area and ask to speak to a faculty member who specializes in the education of students with mental retardation and the transition from high school to adulthood and adult services. Tell that person you are embarking on developing a new program, and ask for advice and suggestions concerning resource material and helpful individuals.
>
> More than 50 parent information and training centers are funded by the U.S. Department of Education. The names and addresses of these centers are included in Appendix 2. Their purpose is to assist parents with advocacy efforts, and they have knowledgeable staff members who can be a helpful resource for you.
>
> Every state has a developmental disabilities planning council (similar to the one that sponsored the conference Rose Stuart attended, where she first learned about supported employment), a department of education, and an office of vocational rehabilitation. You can request literature from them on quality programs and the names of people who may be able to help you with consultation.
>
> Organizations such as the Association for Retarded Citizens, the American Association on Mental Retardation, and The Association for Persons with Severe Handicaps have long advocated quality services in the community. You can go to local, state, and national leaders to ask for their assistance in helping you develop a new program.
>
> Several clearinghouses offer information to parents and other advocates interested in developing community-based programs for people with disabilities. These clearinghouses are listed in Appendix 2.

Your major commitment will be to ensure that your efforts toward developing new programs are directed at developing the *best* programs possible—that is why knowledge is a source of power to you.

*   *   *

Jack and Rose made a commitment to find another road to help them develop job opportunities for Steve. It was a bold step to decide to withdraw him from the adult service program at the end of his high school program, just as he was needing some security for the future. In the small town where they lived, Jack and Rose knew that when they withdrew Steve from the program, they would and could never go back. In fact, the director of the sheltered workshop was shocked when Jack and Rose met with him to tell him their decision to start their own program for Steve. His response was, "What's going to happen when you fail?" If Jack and Rose had not been so strong in their values and so determined to make their dreams come true, such a question might have really scared them. Jack replied, "We're not going to fail. And that's not a threat, that's a promise." After they left the meeting, they decided to celebrate being "free at last, free at last." They did not know what the future held, but they did know that it hurts to beat your head against a brick wall, and they did not want to keep having such a headache.

They immediately began to read everything they could find about supported employment and how to go about starting it in their community. They contacted the Kansas Developmental Disabilities Planning Council and received a packet of helpful information. From their local office of vocational rehabilitation, they learned that some model programs were being developed in Wichita, Lawrence, and Hays, Kansas, and they decided to call the people in those programs to find out what they were doing. Rose asked Fran Wilson if she would like to come along on a trip to Lawrence to find out about a new program, Full Citizenship, Inc. The two of them drove to Lawrence, visited with some of the members of the executive committee, and picked up all the literature they could get their hands on about this new effort. They knew then that they were not alone. Some other parents, aided by value-driven professionals backed by a strong data base, had started down a new road, too.

HOW DO I BRAINSTORM?

When seeking ideas for starting new programs, you can follow the brainstorming process of involving creative and knowledgeable people and being sure to discuss all ideas. Let's review a couple of points particularly relevant to starting new programs.

First, the people you select to help you brainstorm are critically important to the ideas that will emerge. Also, the people you invite to brainstorm might very well be the nucleus of a new board of directors for a nonprofit organization charged with developing a program consistent with your goals and dreams. Thus, you may want to think about inviting people with different backgrounds and interests. For example, you could include other parents with similar values who have a son or daughter with a disability, your own son or daughter, or other adolescents or adults with disabilities who can share their own perspectives, professionals who work in the area of the program that you want to develop and who have values similar to your own, members of the community who have access to resources and who influence public opinion, and people who have been successful in starting other human service organizations. You will have an opportunity to find out about their interest in being involved in planning and implementing new programs. You do not have to gather every single person together for brainstorming. You might have several groups of people involved in thinking about possible directions for a new program, and you may even talk with some people individually if they are unable to meet with others or if they would be more comfortable sharing ideas outside of a larger group.

Starting a new program is so overwhelming that people tend to limit possibilities from the outset. As we stated earlier, it is particularly important to avoid censoring any ideas. We even encourage you at this point to believe in the impossible. You have no idea how many parents have set out to start a program that is truly consistent with their son's or daughter's preferences, and how many of them have been success- ful. We are inspired by their success, and we know that almost anything is possible for people with similar goals and the willingness to work hard. Thus, in your brainstorm- ing process, try not to fall into the trap of saying things like, "Yes, it would be ideal if my daughter could live in her own condominium, but we have to be realistic in recog- nizing that such independence is impossible for people with mental retardation." Avoid the "Yes, but . . ." trap. If owning a home is desirable for your son or daughter, we can assure you that it is possible to consider this option. Remember what Robert Kennedy said: "Some people see things as they are and ask why. Others see things as they might be and ask why not." We encourage you to ask and ask again and again, "Why not?"

When starting a new program, you will want to brainstorm about many dif- ferent aspects of program development. Some of the most important things to consider are the different types of programs you might develop. (You could focus on residential or vocational; or, within the vocational area, you could focus on competitive or sup- ported employment.) You can also brainstorm about the process that you might follow in developing programs, discussing whether to establish a nonprofit organization, join the effort of a public or private agency already established to encourage them to move in a new direction, or pursue a private effort for your son or daughter only. You can consider where you might get funds for program development and personnel. Again, the key in brainstorming is to be as creative as possible in considering many different ideas. You will need to think about what program you want to develop and how you want to do it.

*   *   *

After their trip to Lawrence, Rose and Fran got together with their husbands, two parents of other young people with disabilities who will graduate from high school in the next couple of years, their minister, and a social worker from the local mental health center, to talk about the possibilities of starting a new program in their commu- nity. They reviewed the articles of incoporation of Full Citizenship, Inc., and decided that they were interested in a very similar organization. Rose and Fran excitedly told everyone about some of the job sites they had visited in Lawrence, where even people with severe disabilities were working successfully at the University of Kansas. If such jobs were possible in Lawrence, they wondered why they couldn't approach the Wheatland Community College and ask if such employment opportunities would be possible there.

Their minister also suggested that some jobs might be available taking care of church property. He added that jobs might also be obtained through some of the mem- bers of the congregation. He volunteered to talk with some of the church members about jobs that they might be able to provide for people with disabilities.

Mr. Hubert, the social worker from the mental health center, kept urging the group to consider going to the director of the sheltered workshop and asking if a new component could be added to the workshop, rather than start a separate organization. He argued that the workshop very much needed to move in this direction, and maybe this group could be a source of motivation in that direction. A lot of time was spent in the brainstorming session talking about whether it would be advantageous to start a new program or to try to modify the one that already existed. It became clear that the majority opinion was that a fresh start was needed.

The "Stuart brainstormers" (as they now called one group) also focused a lot of attention on whether they should address only vocational needs, or whether they should take on the full range of responsibility, as Full Citizenship, Inc., had done, in the areas of social relationships, community living, and both residential and supported employment. They recognized how important it was for every member of the group to have a chance to think about this, because they wanted to address the important needs in their community. But they did not want to get bogged down by taking on too much responsibility.

HOW DO I EVALUATE AND CHOOSE ALTERNATIVES?

The purpose of brainstorming is to open up a number of different possibilities, and the purpose of evaluating and choosing alternatives is to make wise selections among options. At this point, you should begin to define more precisely the kind of program that will best suit your son or daughter. Then you can begin to consider the best process for achieving your goal. Recently, we ourselves were involved in the process of developing a new program in our community. At the point of evaluating and choosing the most important alternatives, we spent a lot of time writing down the values that we wanted to guide our program development efforts. By writing and refining these values, we were able to move toward a consensus statement among a group of six people with a shared interest in program development advocacy. This statement of values became the basis for the articles of incorporation of Full Citizenship, Inc., a new nonprofit organization that is directed toward starting social, community living, residential, and vocational options in our community (see Appendix 6).

You should review these Articles of Incorporation carefully. The major point is that, as you begin to write down your values and translate them into a code that will guide program development, it will become easier to evaluate and choose alternatives.

* * *

Jack and Rose, working with their friends, found what a time-consuming process it can be to brainstorm and then evaluate and choose alternatives. They must have met five or six times over a 3-month period before they finally arrived at the alternatives most important to them. It was hard for Rose, particularly, to spend this much time in discussion, because her main objective was to get her own son into a job as soon as possible. She kept saying, "His clock is ticking, and we can't just sit around and let him waste all this valuable time." But she also knew how important it was to decide carefully on the alternatives to pursue. After more discussion than they would like to recall, the final decision was to develop an organization called, like the one in Lawrence, Full Citizenship, Inc., and to use articles of incorporation very similar to those of the organization in Lawrence. They decided, however, to limit the Wheatland Full Citizenship, Inc., to employment options for 2–3 years before deciding whether to develop programs in other areas, such as residential options. They also decided that they wanted to work on many kinds of employment opportunities and that they would pursue jobs at the community college as well as in every other business in their community where someone expressed interest. After the last meeting, when they signed their articles of incorporation, Jack and Rose could not believe how much fun they had had. What a change it had been from the past, from tension, the discussion of problems, and negative reports about Steve, who was now totally out of the old-style workshop. Now their efforts would be to create something positive and constructive, something that could work for people with needs like Steve's and offer them hope for the future. For the first time, they really believed that Steve had a future worth planning for. Believing in what might be was one of the most uplifting experiences they had ever had. "That Bobby Kennedy," Rose said, "sure was right to advise thinking about what might be and asking, 'why not'!"

HOW DO I COMMUNICATE MY DECISION?

Whether you are advocating within existing programs or to create new ones, there comes a time when you have to tell others what your decisions are. The same rules for communicating your decisions apply to both situations. You will have to tell your son or daughter what your decisions are. You will need to tell the people who will provide services to your son or daughter, as well as family friends and your allies in the new program.

Because you are taking a different road, you will be asked many more questions than if you had followed the usual road. You will want to prepare to answer them by focusing on who will be walking down that road with you, what road you have chosen to follow, where you plan for it to take you, when you will start your journey, how long you plan to be on it, how you plan to find the road and the journey's end, and why you have chosen to take a different route. Remember that there are other major considerations as you announce your decision: Whom to tell, what to tell (the who, what, where, when, how, and why), and how you communicate.

Telling those who need and want to know, and being confident (but not over-confident), enthusiastic (but not "hyped"), and desirous of their advice and help, will help you build a network of allies—an informal support system that will be available when you need help, make mistakes, get depressed by the difficulties or angry at the failures, and that will be there when you not only have little successes, but hit the grand slam that carries you all the way on your journey. To make your decision accept-able or defensible is the minimum you want when you communicate your plan; to make it so appealing that you earn a colleague is the most you can hope for.

"Rose," said Jack, "we're probably fools for doing what we want to do, and our friends and Steve's teachers and counselors will know we are when we tell them our plans. But, fools or not, I don't give a hoot what people think. It's Steve's life, and ours, and the heck with the nay-sayers!"

Rose, always the fence-mender, always the diplomat, and always Jack's public supporter, demurred. "Jack, I know just how you feel. And sometimes, I feel that way, too. But I don't show it as much as you, so why don't you let me tell folks. You know the old saying about trapping more flies with honey than with vinegar. Well, let me use the honey."

HOW DO I TAKE ACTION TO RESOLVE THE PROBLEM?

As we stated in the last chapter, you need to take action with gusto and determination. Sometimes it is too overwhelming and scary to think about the many responsibilities associated with starting new programs. We once heard someone talk about the "salami technique"—recognizing that a large salami in its whole and total form is unmanageable and impossible to eat, but knowing that, when it is thinly sliced, it becomes quite manageable and enjoyable. You can think of the total program development as being a huge salami and your task as being one of taking very thin slices, one by one, as your time and appetite permit, so that you eventually proceed through to the last slice. As you take action, your ability to take a slice at a time is critical to seeing the entire project through.

Another suggestion is to be ever mindful of the important role that personnel play in the success of any program. Invariably, excellent programs have highly competent and committed staff; inadequate programs have staff of questionable competence and commitment. Many factors must come together to create excellence, but the hub of the program will be the people who run it. Thus, as you think about personnel issues, make no compromises on the quality of the people you hire. Try to make certain that they too are "why not" types rather than "yes, but" types. This means that you should strive to develop a salary scale that will enable you to attract top talent.

In the vocational component of the Full Citizenship, Inc., program in which we are involved, we were surprised to find how readily available the resources were to put together a quality supported employment program. We were able to combine funds from the school system, university, VR, and private foundations to create a program nucleus with a genuine capacity to grow. Essentially, we found that the resources were available in various places, but they had not previously been pulled together and organized in a systematic and comprehensive fashion. Thus, taking action means getting into funding streams that will enable you to accomplish your goals. We found that the various agencies which contributed money were receptive to a new organization that was willing to assume responsibility for developing a quality supported employment program.

HOW CAN I EVALUATE THE OUTCOMES OF MY ACTIONS?

When it's time to evaluate outcomes, you will want to consider whether your son or daughter's preferences—the ones that led to you to determine that a new program was needed in your community—have been satisfied by the program you have developed. Has your son or daughter been able to achieve through the new program what he or she was unable to achieve without it? If so, it is likely that your actions have resulted in successful outcomes; if not, you will need to refine the new program to ensure that it does accomplish its goals. At times you will find that you are only partially successful. Also, as time passes, the preferences and needs of your son or daughter might change, and issues may emerge that were not present when you started your planning. Thus, there is a continual need to monitor your own efforts to ensure that you are, indeed, headed down the right road.

*   *   *

At this point, Jack and Rose, along with 18 other people from their community who have joined the board of directors of Full Citizenship, Inc., are well underway toward organizing supported employment. They have applied for a grant from the Office of Vocational Rehabilitation in the state capital, Topeka, to fund a supported employment specialist for 1 year. In addition, they heard that the Dole Foundation in Washington,

D.C., gives grants to projects to help them provide employment for people with disabilities. A committee of the board has been authorized to submit a proposal to the Dole Foundation for funds to hire an executive director whose job will be to put together other resources. Meanwhile, the best news of all is that Steve is working productively again at the Starr Plastics Company and is able to maintain a productivity level that people never thought would be possible for him. He looks forward to getting there every day, takes pride in his work, and was thrilled beyond words when his coworkers planned a surprise birthday party for him one lunch hour.

*   *   *

How do Jack and Rose Stuart evaluate their efforts, now that it has been about 10 months since they started this new program? Jack says it's just too early to tell. He and Rose know, however, that they have never been as satisfied with Steve's performance as they are now—he is bringing home a bigger weekly paycheck than he was able to make at the sheltered workshop in a 2-month period, and his sisters and friends are extremely proud that he is in the mainstream of community life. They realize that there is a great deal of work yet to be done, but the most important thing is that they are convinced that they are headed down the right road and that the time and energy they invest in program development will result in benefits for Steve and for others with similar needs in their community. Jack says, "I would do it again in a minute, but my only regret is that we wasted so much time. I know better than to travel the wrong road, and it won't happen again. That's not a threat, it's my promise!"

38 | HOW CAN MY SON OR DAUGHTER BECOME A SELF-ADVOCATE?

Ludwig Bismark fidgeted with his fingers as he paced back and forth across his bedroom. He hated his nervous habit of picking at the skin around his fingernails—already, he had drawn some blood on his left index finger. As much as he disliked the habit, he found himself doing it whenever he faced stressful situations.

Ludwig had been invited to a dance being sponsored by a group of people he knew, People First of Himshoot. The members were people with mental retardation and People First was a national organization that promoted self-advocacy—people standing up and speaking out for themselves. Ludwig wanted very much to go to the dance and he wanted to learn more about self-advocacy.

As Ludwig paced, he thought about his life and relived some of his experiences. A constant in his life had been that few people had ever really listened to him. Sure, there were many who talked with him, and these he considered as his friends. Yet when he tried to express his desires and preferences, too often people tried to influence him. He remembered last week when he wanted to stay overnight at a friend's house—he felt anger as he recalled his conversation with his parents:

"Papa, Max Pflum, the choir director, asked if I could stay at his house Saturday night. We would go to church the next day early, then work on painting the pastor's house."

"Luddy," his father replied, "Max Pflum doesn't have room for you."

"Yes, he does."

Well, even so, what do you know about painting?"

"I know a lot. I've done it before."

"No, Luddy," his mother interjected, "you don't like to paint."

"You stay home," his father added. "You'll be safe here; get these silly ideas out of your mind."

Things like that were always happening—people telling him what he liked or didn't like, what he needed, and what he should do. It made no sense, how could somebody else know what he wanted? He was the best person to understand his likes and dislikes, why wouldn't others listen to him? He made up his mind then and there that he would tell his father that he was going to the dance. He also decided to learn more about the People First group. He was 40 years old, he was not a child, and he did not want to be treated as one. Adults make decisions for themselves and Ludwig was determined to be an adult.

He went downstairs and found his father sitting at the kitchen table. He swallowed hard, took a deep breath, and began the conversation.

"Papa, there is a dance this Friday in town. I want to go to it, papa, I want to go to this dance."

"But Luddy," his father started, "a dance, it will be late, you will be tired."

"No, papa, I am going."

WHAT IS SELF-ADVOCACY?

If an experienced member of a self-advocacy group were asked to explain what self-advocacy means, he or she might say, "Self-advocacy is knowing our rights and standing up for them." Or, "It's helping each other make our own choices," or, "It's speaking for ourselves." What exactly do these things mean?

We'll begin with the concept of *advocacy*. Advocacy usually means one person asserts the interests of another person, the way a lawyer does for a client or a citizen advocate does for a person with a disability. The Association for Retarded Citizens of the United States (ARC-US) is an example of a nationwide organization of family members and professionals who advocate on behalf of people with mental retardation. In contrast, self-advocacy means people with disabilities asserting their own rights and interests, usually without others' help. It can mean that they do not allow others to do things for them which they are capable of doing for themselves.

Self-advocacy rests on several assumptions. One is that all people with disabilities have innate potentials that have either been untapped or underused. Accordingly, self-advocacy involves seeking ways to tap or use these underdeveloped resources. Self-advocacy is also based on the assumption that dependence causes continued dependence, but independence leads to even greater independence. Self-advocates do not attempt to formulate one definition of independence; rather, they believe that individuals must be free to define independence for themselves. Third, self-advocates assume that, by taking greater control of their lives, they will add to the overall quality of their lives. Finally, self-advocates assume that they are their own best teachers.

That final assumption explains the emphasis placed on self-advocacy groups. The members of these groups learn from one another by undertaking a variety of group activities, ranging from recreation to community education and political involvement. Self-advocacy groups may vary considerably as to their goals, but what defines them is that their activities emerge from a consumer-dominated process of decision-making. The consumers, the people with disabilities, determine the activities for the group and carry them out. In this way, they learn from each other, increase their capacities to exercise choice in other aspects of their daily lives, and acquire the confidence to do so by being in an environment that is supportive and nonjudgmental.

A key member of any self-advocacy group is the advisor. This is usually a person who does not have a mental disability. The advisor is chosen by the group and works for the people within the group, serving at their pleasure. While many advisors today are professionals in the various fields associated with developmental disabilities, there are advisors who have little professional knowledge prior to joining a self-advocacy group. Most groups have more than one advisor and the vast majority of advisors are volunteers.

The advisor's main responsibility is to gently guide a group through a decision-making process so that the members do as much for themselves as their individual capabilities allow. This means the advisor must know when to pull back. The group may decide to engage in an activity that the advisor may feel will not be productive—for example, starting a letter-writing campaign to have a municipal government finance transportation for people with disabilities. The advisor may understand that revenue sources for such a major project are currently not available. Thus, the advisor may be tempted to urge the members to become involved in a different project, one with a greater likelihood of success.

The sensitive advisor will understand, however, that success is relative. In choosing a project and working through it, the members of the group are realizing success in other important ways—for example, choosing and controlling a situation. This alone is a measure of their empowerment, for their success is unrelated to eventual outcomes. While certainly clichéd, the adage, "We learn from our mistakes," concisely expresses the point.

The issue of risk-taking is another pressing concern for advisors. When should risks be taken? What are acceptable risks and what are not? There is never an easy answer. Believing that moderate risk-taking is a prerequisite to personal growth can be a helpful guide for advisors. Facing risks and working to overcome them increases self-confidence. After all, empowerment is a valued goal of self-advocacy.

HOW DID THE SELF-ADVOCACY MOVEMENT GET STARTED?

The roots of the self-advocacy movement are the social clubs established by people with mental disabilities in Sweden in the early 1960s. Those clubs were run by members who elected officers and developed decision-making and other organizational skills, and sought to support each other. The clubs organized regional meetings to share ideas and experiences with members of different groups. These activities culminated in two successful national conferences in 1968 and 1970.

The Swedish experience inspired people with mental disabilities in Great Britain to organize a national conference in 1972. In 1973, self-advocates in British Columbia held a regional conference. The Canadian conference was attended by consumers from Oregon, who promptly organized the United States' first statewide self-advocacy conference in 1974.

Another self-advocacy group was given a giant boost in 1973 when Drs. Gunnar and Rosemary Dybwad (who were recognized national leaders in the ARC) led the Association for Retarded Citizens of Massachusetts (ARC-Mass.) in sponsoring its first self-advocacy conference. For the next decade, ARC-Mass. continued to sponsor annual state conferences. The Oregon and Massachusetts initiatives have been followed by others in many additional states. The notion that people with disabilities could themselves organize and run a conference inspired people across the country, and provided the impetus for the growth of local self-advocacy. Today, there are hundreds of local self-advocacy groups in the United States and around the world.

National coalitions continue to exert influence as well. People First and United Together are two national networks of affiliated local self-advocacy groups. Efforts to increase communication between international self-advocacy movements resulted in the First International Self-Advocacy Conference, held in 1984 in Tacoma, Washington. Consumers from the United States, Canada, Great Britain, Australia, New Zealand, and the Cook Islands participated.

The movement's growth indicates that people with disabilities are determined to take an active part in shaping their own destinies. They will continue to assert themselves and demand that their voices be heard and heeded.

CAN A SELF-ADVOCACY GROUP BENEFIT MY SON OR DAUGHTER?

In this section, we present several examples—some from real life, others involving the families in this book—of how your son or daughter can benefit from a self-advocacy group. Gary Brunk, an advisor to a local self-advocacy group, tells a true story about the potential power of the self-advocacy movement. Gary was doing training sessions with two local self-advocacy groups. One group, associated with a sheltered workshop, told him about a county commissioner who time and again had demonstrated insensitivity to disinterest in the needs of people with disabilities. The group's frustration led it to organize and recruit friends in a campaign to get out the vote in the next county election. The group interested several hundred people who otherwise might not have voted, and, by a small margin, the county commissioner failed to be re-elected. As the members of the self-advocacy group told their story, Gary could see the pride in their faces and hear it in their voices. They had found success in exercising their right to vote, and their collective voice "made a difference."

That same evening, Gary met with the other, very different group. The meeting was held behind the locked doors of a cottage on the grounds of a state institution. As the members of this group talked about self-advocacy, it became clear that they had difficulty comprehending such basic concepts as individual rights and the responsibilities which accompany these rights. Gary realized that it was difficult for these people to understand the basics of freedom when their own world was limited by locked doors and "security screens" stretched across their windows.

The contrast between the two groups illustrates the impact of expression of choice on people's lives. The consumers at the sheltered workshop were managing to carve out a place in their daily lives for dignity and self-respect through their exercise of the rights of citizenship. The members of the other group were struggling to understand the very concept of self-advocacy, and what choice, dignity, and responsibility could mean in their own lives. Yet, the members of this latter group were taking the first steps to assert control over some part of their lives. The level of sophistication of this group was far less than that of the first group, but the potential for growth was great.

Self-advocacy groups do not follow a corporate blueprint. Instead, they reflect the needs, strengths, and weaknesses of the individual members. Self-advocacy groups also experience continuous change, reflected in both the membership as a whole and in individual members. There are not set membership criteria for these groups. Most people with disabilities can and do benefit from involvement in self-advocacy activities.

Now, take a look at some of the young adults from some of the families we introduced earlier in this book to see how involvement in self-advocacy can be beneficial.

Maria Rodriguez had joined a self-advocacy group at the invitation of her friend, Jaime Alvarado. At first, Maria looked at the group as a social club whose activities she thoroughly enjoyed. Soon, however, she found herself assuming positions of leadership in the group, and learned that she had talents never before tapped.

She served as the coordinator of her group's fund-raising committee and did an outstanding job. With considerable initial help from the group's two volunteer advisors, she organized strategy and brainstorming sessions. She contacted the organizers of an annual neighborhood festival and arranged to have her group operate a vending booth at the event, where they sold soft drinks and popcorn. More and more, she took the initiative in preparing for the festival. She negotiated a fair price with local soft drink distributors and managed to have them agree to donate all the popcorn. After the 2-day festival, Maria proudly reported the fund-raising committee's receipts at a monthly group meeting. Net profits from sales and contributions were just over $375. It was a very successful and enjoyable endeavor.

At a later group meeting, Maria and other members were discussing strategies for dealing with personal problems. Maria mentioned the problems she was having with her brother concerning her boyfriend, Ramon. "My brother Geraldo is such a fool," she moaned. "He hates my boyfriend, Ramon, and he's ordered me to quit seeing him. He can't do that. It's my life, ¿qué no?"

Several members nodded in agreement as she went on. "I'll show him. Ramon and I will get married and then Geraldo can't do anything. Everything will be fine after we're married."

With an edge of fear in her voice, one member asked, "Maria, do you know what you're doing? Have you thought about this?"

"It's my life," Maria snapped back.

Soon the 15 members were arguing and taking sides. One of the advisors asked if he could speak. "Maria," he began tentatively, "if you want, we can help you think through this."

After Maria grudgingly consented to the group's help, the advisor continued. "My friends," he said, "let's help Maria, and at the same time we can learn something we can use in our own lives to solve other problems. We will use a method called problem-solving. Here are the steps." The advisor wrote the six steps on the portable blackboard at the end of the room:

1. Defining the problem—what exactly is the problem?
2. Brainstorming—what are some things that could be done to solve the problem?
3. Evaluating and choosing alternatives—what are the pros and cons of the possible solutions, and what should you do?
4. Communicating the decision to others—announce your decision.
5. Taking action—do it!
6. Ongoing evaluation—how well does the solution work, and are there problems with what you have done?

The group eagerly jumped into the process, having fun while they all learned valuable new skills. What follows are the group's collective efforts.

1. Defining the Problem

Maria at first insisted that her problem was how to marry Ramon, but after some group discussion she and her friends determined differently. Her problem, it seemed, was that Geraldo did not feel Ramon met certain "standards" and had, therefore, ordered Maria to end the relationship. With the group's help, Maria identified the characteristics of Ramon that Geraldo found offensive. In short, Ramon had a history of trouble with the law, used marijuana and sometimes cocaine, was unemployed, and, Geraldo insisted, was merely "using" Maria. Maria countered that they truly enjoyed each other's company and that Ramon had pledged his undying love to her.

2. Brainstorming

The advisor reminded the group that at this point they needed to identify as many possible solutions as they could. There were no right or wrong ideas; the evaluation phase would come later. Several solutions were suggested by the group, and one member listed them on the blackboard:

> Tell Geraldo to mind his own business.
> Threaten Geraldo.
> Have Maria's mother talk to Geraldo.
> Get married. Then, Geraldo could not interfere.
> Sneak around to see Ramon.
> Have Ramon talk to Geraldo.
> Have Ramon beat Geraldo up.
> Plead with Geraldo to change his mind.
> Have the police or an attorney explain Maria's rights to Geraldo.
> Have members of the group talk to Geraldo.

3. Evaluating and Choosing Alternatives

The group thought it was now time to evaluate the ideas, but one member said they had missed one other possible solution—Geraldo may be right. Perhaps Maria *should* break off her relationship with Ramon.

The group began their evaluation with this last item.

"Does he use drugs, Maria? Is that true?" asked Jaime.

"Well, yes, sometimes. But he says it's okay because everyone does it," Maria said.

"I don't," said one member.

"I don't either," said another.

"Me neither."

"Maria, do you use drugs?," one person asked.

"No, of course not!," Maria responded angrily.

"So Ramon is wrong," another friend said. "Not everyone uses drugs."

"Even if everyone did, it's against the law," someone else interjected.

"Maria, he doesn't work. Where does he get the money to buy the stuff?," someone asked.

"I don't know," she said.

"Does he steal money to buy it?"

"See," Maria said, "you don't like him either. Now you're all calling him a thief. Sometimes he borrows money from me. Maybe that's how he buys it. See, you're all wrong!"

"Maria," asked a friend, "how much money have you lent him? Does he pay it back?"

"Not much," Maria snapped.

"How much, Maria?"

"Well, maybe $40, that's all," Maria answered.

"Only $40, Maria? Are you sure?"

"Well, about $40 a week," Maria said, tears welling in her eyes.

"Maria, $40 a week! How much have you lent him by now?"

"Almost $300," she sobbed.

"Does he pay you back? When will he pay you back?" a worried friend asked.

"He hasn't, not yet. He can't afford to. He doesn't have a job. But he will, I know he will," Maria said.

"Maria, you always talk about the wonderful dates you have with Ramon," Jaime said, his voice full of concern. "Movies, going out to eat. How can he afford to do those things if he can't pay you back?"

Maria remained silent.

"Maria . . .? Maria, how?"

"I pay for those things, too," Maria confessed. "But he loves me," she sobbed.

"Maria," asked another friend, her voice filled with concern and pity, "does he love you or your money?"

"Me," Maria responded quickly. "He's proved that. After all, he said he is going to break up with Angela and start seeing only me. That proves his love for me." Maria's voice indicated she did not really believe this.

"Maria, I know Angela," Jaime said, "and I found out he borrows money from her, too. And Angela doesn't know Ramon is seeing you, but he's seeing another girl I know named Serafina. He told Angela that to prove his love, he'll break up with Serafina and see only Angela. Maria, how many true loves does Ramon have? He doesn't need to work—he lives off you and the others."

Maria was now crying and her friends, the other self-advocates, came close to comfort her. Maria was important to them all.

After a few minutes, Maria's sobs subsided to a few muffled sniffles and hiccoughs. Dabbing her eyes with a handkerchief, she said haltingly, "I called Geraldo a fool. *I'm* the fool. And to think I wanted to marry that jerk, Ramon."

4. Communicating the Decision

Maria made up her mind. She had been fooled by Ramon and her actions had caused problems with her brother. With the help of her friends in the self-advocacy group, she was now prepared to announce that she was making a change in her life. First, she communicated her decision to the group members who discussed with her the other people who needed to know her decision. She would tell Geraldo and then Ramon. Later that evening, after the group's meeting, she had a long talk with her brother and explained everything to him. He consoled her; she was such a beautiful person and he cared for her so much. Geraldo offered to speak to Ramon the next day, to tell him Maria's decision. Maria thanked him for his offer but said it was her responsibility. "Besides," she added, "I want to see his face when I tell him I know all about his many girlfriends!"

5. Taking Action

Maria met Ramon at the small corner diner the next evening. She felt a great sense of pride. She was taking charge of her life; she was about to make a move that she knew was in her best interest. After Ramon arrived, Maria calmly but firmly told him of her decision. Ramon tried to change her mind.

"Maria," he said, "look, you're not going to be able to find a better boyfriend than me."

"A boy you are," replied Maria, "but you have no idea what it means to be a friend."

Well, if you break up with me," Ramon responded angrily, "I'll never repay the money I borrowed from you."

"You never were going to anyway," Maria said. "Goodbye Ramon."

She stood up and walked toward the door. A contented smile of success and reassurance covered her face. She was Maria Rodriguez and she controlled her own life.

6. Ongoing Evaluation

Ramon tried twice to get Maria to see him again, but to no avail. The second time he called she was getting ready to go to a movie with friends. With a hint of irritation in her voice she explained that she was much too busy with her friends and personal interests to continue the conversation. The absence of Ramon from her life did not present a problem. She easily filled her social life with people who really cared for her, and for whom she cared. Wishing Ramon a nice life, she firmly said goodbye and hung up the phone. Ramon knew she meant it—she heard no more from him.

Because self-advocacy groups like Maria's deal with real life problems, individual members learn everyday living skills. The groups mix learning with leisure and recreational activities. As much as possible, the advisors stay out of group decisions, to ensure maximum direction and participation by the consumers. Note the absence of the advisor during the resolution of Maria's problem.

At this point, you may be thinking that a person such as Maria may indeed be able to benefit from self-advocacy, but what about someone with more severe disabilities. Take a look at Brian Hughes's experiences with the self-advocacy movement.

When Marilyn Ramsey, an occupational therapist at Brian's school, first approached Brian's mother about the possibility of self-advocacy involvement, Barbara was very skeptical. After all, Brain had severe disabilities and limited mental capacity, and Barbara felt that he would not be able to understand the concept of self-advocacy. Marilyn, who served as a volunteer advisor to a local self-advocacy group, pressed Barbara. She said Brian could benefit and asked that he be allowed to give it a try.

Brian started to attend the group's meetings. The other self-advocates went out of their way to make him feel welcome. Two members, Jeff and Brenda, took a special interest in Brian. While neither had severe disabilities like Brian's, both were less capable in many life areas than most of the other group members. Jeff and Brenda felt great pride and a sense of achievement by being there to assist someone. It helped them realize that they were more capable than they had thought.

Brian obviously enjoyed the self-advocacy meetings and the group's other activities. Perhaps it was the group's attention to the rights of everyone to make his or her own choices that most benefited Brian. Although he was unable to speak, he expressed his likes and dislikes in other ways. Through various combinations of body posture, gestures, facial expression, verbalization, laughter, and tears, Brian articulated his preferences.

Whenever Brian tried to communicate his feelings, other self-advocates would immediately respond. For example, on one occasion the group had organized an outing to a local lake. Soon after the group arrived at the beach and set up their "camp" (beach umbrella, blankets, the mandatory cooler and boom box), people started heading for the water.

Marilyn told Jeff and Brenda that she would help them get Brian into the water.

They began coaxing Brian to the water's edge, but he planted his feet and refused to move.

Marilyn took the young man's hand and said, "Come on, Brian, you'll love it."
Brian replied firmly, "No, no water."

When Marilyn started pulling on his arm, Brian let out a piercing shriek. Jeff snapped into action.

"He doesn't want to go," Jeff said.

"Oh, Jeff, once he's in the water, he'll like it. You'll see," Marilyn insisted. "He's just afraid, that's all."

"No, he doesn't want to go in," Jeff insisted.

Marilyn froze. So Brian did not want to go into the water. That, after all was the purpose of the self-advocacy group, to help its members express their choices. She had just been treating him differently because he had fewer abilities than the rest of the self-advocacy group.

"Brian," she said, "so you don't want to go into the water. I'm sorry. You don't have to go if you don't want to."

She stopped her attempts to persuade Brian. He immediately became calmer, and his smile seemed to possess his entire face. His preferences had just been met. No matter how small the matter may have seemed, he had just experienced control over a situation, and therefore control over his life. He spent the rest of the day happily watching his friends and others on the beach. He enjoyed himself completely. Another self-advocate commented, "Brian's a landlubber, but he's having more fun today than any of us."

Brian continued to attend the group's meetings and was involved in many of its activities. There were some he chose not to join, and his friends in the group never tried to press him. Most of the group members became very sensitive to Brian's sometimes subtle expressions of his likes and dislikes, and respected them. Brian began to gain greater control of his life, learning that his preferences could and often did affect what happened to him.

IS SELF-ADVOCACY HERE TO STAY?

Maria and Brian benefited in different ways from their involvement with the self-advocacy movement. Other people gain in still other ways. People with disabilities will continue to need the voices of others around them to advocate quality services, but the voice of the self-advocate must be heard and incorporated into the total movement.

In spite of the growth of self-advocacy, it is still a very fragile movement. It is fragile because, almost by definition, self-advocates are people with few resources and are therefore somewhat isolated. All over the country there are self-advocacy groups with no idea of how many other such groups exist in their area, state, or region. That isolation is debilitating.

Self-advocacy is also a fragile movement because it depends on advisors, and advisors come and go. Historically, one pattern emerges—if the advisor leaves the group and if there is not a replacement, the group often tends to wither away and die.

Another threat to self-advocacy is inconsistent funding. Competing interests vie for limited funds. The situation is made even worse during times of budget restraint on the state and federal levels. With limited resources available, self-advocates often find themselves losing the funding war to professionals and other advocacy groups such as parent organizations.

To better understand the need for self-advocacy, we must first understand more vividly the daily experiences of people who become self-advocates. These people speak often of the stigma of disability, and its results are evident to many professionals and family members. In our society, people with disabilities are seen as different from the rest, as less than whole. It is extremely difficult for an individual with a severe disability to overcome that stigma, because such a breakthrough requires both departing from a category to which one is assigned by society, and recognizing the reality of the category and accepting it as valid at some level.

A strong self-advocacy movement can help shape the nature of services, and effectively demand accountability from service providers, policy planners, families, and society in general. The end result can be programs that respond to the real needs of people with disabilities.

Jesse Davis is president of United Together, a national network of self-advocates. Davis lived most of his life in an institution in Arkansas, and only since 1986 has he been allowed to live in the community. He often says, "I'm free now, but I'm not forgetting the people I left behind; I'm not forgetting my friends in the institution." It is that declaration of the dignity of helping each other that is affirmed by self-advocacy. Davis's statement does much to explain the growth of the self-advocacy movement and to confirm its necessity.

Richard Lovelace wrote, "Stone walls do not a prison make, nor iron bars a cage." A prison is any place we may find ourselves where we do not want or do not deserve to be.

39 | SEVEN FAMILIES—A SUMMARY

We have followed portions of the lives of seven families through this book. They are not real families in the sense that you could go to one of their hometowns, find them, and speak with them. Yet in another sense, these are very real families in that they represent people who could easily be your friends, neighbors, or relatives. Perhaps, certain aspects of family composition or personality, or the preferences and needs of the young people with disabilities, remind you of your own family. We hope this is the case because that was our intention. The families are a composite of the many families we know, have worked with in varying degrees, and, in all cases, from whom we have learned much. The families know who they are and we are deeply indebted to them for their contributions to this book. They are sharing, through the seven families, their insights, victories, defeats, and strengths, as well as the reality of living every day and moving toward tomorrow and the days that follow.

If the families came to life, the credit belongs to the many families we have known. Any failure of the families in this book to seem real is attributable to your authors' humble abilities, but we hope the information we have presented will help you plan for the kind of future you want for your unique family.

Transition is not a single event, but an ongoing, dynamic process. Transitions are lifelong events, and life itself is a transition. Individual transitions extend beyond the individual; also affected are family, friends, and society at large. The effects of what happened today to you, to your son or daughter, to your neighbor, or to someone you do not even know will not stop with the event itself. We believe that individual events ultimately affect all of us. People are unavoidably interdependent.

In keeping with our belief that every passing minute brings growth and change, this final chapter has two objectives:

1. We seek to provide a thumbnail sketch of the individual families for your easy reference. In a sense, this is meant to be a portrait and a summary of how each family functions, a guide to understanding and learning from the families.
2. We attempt to project the families beyond the "today" of this book, because we understand that transitions are continual. We offer some hint of what may or may not await the families. Plans made in the previous pages are subject to continuous changes brought on by time, changing needs, and changing preferences. Will Jolene marry? Will Werner sell the farm? Will

Maria's parents move, leaving her alone in Southern California? Will she want to stay? Will Arnold succeed in his profession, and what if he doesn't? Will some families experience divorce? What about death? What if . . .?

These are our intentions. We summarize, but do not presume to conclude this book. Conclusions will be individual; they'll be found in your life and that of other families. We wish you success in all your transitions.

THE BISMARK FAMILY

The Bismark family includes:

> Werner (father), age 74
> Maya (mother), age 70
> Otto (Werner's brother), age 66
> Member with a disability: Ludwig ("Luddy"), age 40
> Herman (brother), age 49
> Uta (sister), age 45

Luddy was born after a difficult delivery during which doctors suspect his brain suffered oxygen deprivation. He developed slowly, until mental retardation was confirmed by the family physician when he was about 6. Luddy never attended school. He lived a protected and isolated life on the family farm, but became adept at many complex farm chores. In particular, he always showed an amazing ability to deal with animals. After his brother, Herman, left the farm, Luddy assumed more responsibilities. As his father's health steadily deteriorated, he gradually found himself taking on even more responsibility.

Ludwig, although never formally tested, probably has mild mental retardation. His mother taught him to read, he has excellent verbal and physical skills, and with a little help can manage money and do other arithmetic tasks. Upon meeting him, people might comment that he acts immature for his age. This may be more the result of his isolated childhood and adolescence than of his mental disability.

Family Economics

Werner and his wife, Maya, own 380 acres of fertile farmland, their house and the various farm buildings, some livestock and poultry, and assorted farm machinery. Even after falling land prices are taken into account, and considering rising farm debts, Werner and his wife have a sizable estate. Both have always been frugal and have managed to save a tidy sum, although they have not invested it wisely—bank interest on a savings account only amounts to so much.

Werner and Maya do not realize it, but they own many desirable antiques. Most of their furniture would command top prices from collectors, as would their assorted glassware, bric-a-brac, and collectible vintage farm items. Like Werner's mother, Maya never threw anything away and the large attic is packed with an antique dealer's dreams.

The family has not made financial arrangements. Given the extent of their potential estate, they are in a precarious situation. Werner does not have a Will and his family has no idea of how his estate would be divided in the event of his death and what would happen to Ludwig. Werner's small life insurance policy has Ludwig listed as the sole beneficiary, which may not be in Ludwig's or Maya's best interests.

Family Dynamics

Werner's father immigrated to the United States many years ago from Germany. Although Werner has lived most of his life in Iowa, he has resisted Americanization. While acknowledging that the political system in the United States is vastly superior to what he knew in the Old Country, he remains distrustful of governments in general. This is why he never investigated government entitlement programs for his son.

Werner's brother Otto owns a hardware and feed store in the rural community of Himshoot. Werner's oldest son, Herman, is a partner in his uncle's business. Herman's sister, Uta, also lives in Himshoot. She and her husband have three children of their own while Herman and his wife have four children and are expecting another soon. No one in Werner's immediate family is interested in taking over his farm, and he expresses bitterness mixed with sadness over the situation. The farm has been his life, and the prospect of it slipping from family hands distresses him. Werner continues to insist that it will pass on to Ludwig, in spite of his concerns that Ludwig may not be able to handle the many responsibilities associated with agribusiness.

Despite the independent paths the individual members have taken, the Bismarks could be described as a close family. They are all devoutly religious, and participate in the many activities of the local Brethren (German Baptist) Church. Uta, Herman, Otto, and their families are frequent visitors at the Bismark farm. Werner, Maya, and Ludwig often visit their "city" relatives also. A frequent topic of conversation at recent gatherings has been Werner's failing health, the status of the farm, and Ludwig's future.

Discussing the future is painful for Werner, and inevitably he withdraws from such conversations. His relatives, however, have discussed the situation among themselves and have decided to pursue the issue until Werner understands the need to act. They have enlisted the help of the pastor of their church, Pastor Schaefer, realizing the great respect Werner has for this man. Pastor Schaefer shares the anxiety everyone else feels and understands the importance of planning.

Ludwig, although he grew up in an environment that allowed him few opportunities to express his preference, has started to assert himself more in recent years. A number of factors can be identified that may have had a role in Luddy "finding his voice." His father has become more dependent on Ludwig to manage the everyday farming operations. Ludwig has learned that he has abilities in many areas and this has added greatly to his self-confidence. Dealing with other farmers and a variety of merchants has given him the opportunity to practice decision-making and social-interpersonal skills.

A second influential factor has been Ludwig's close friendship with Gus, who works at the Heidlemann farm. Over the years, they have become very close friends, sharing personal aspirations and providing each other with material and psychological support. Largely because of this friendship, Ludwig gradually learned that his own fears and desires were in many ways no different from those of other people. With his friend's help, Ludwig has been able to clarify in his own mind the type of future he wants and the things he will need to do to achieve it.

A third factor in Ludwig's growing assertiveness is his relationship with Helena. Helena is the sister of Paulina, who is engaged to Gus. A strong emotional bond exists between Ludwig and Helena that is approaching what some would call love. They have tentatively started talking about their combined futures, and, have even discussed the possibility of marriage. Ludwig is proud of his relationship with Helena. He once told his brother that Helena's feelings for him are especially important because unlike his family she, an outsider, *chose* to love him.

We don't know if Helena has any disabilities and we contend that such a question is irrelevant. She and Ludwig provide each other with support and both have benefited from the relationship. They are carefully and slowly making plans, weighing the pros and cons of any actions they may take. They are both clearly engaging in sound, reasoned decision-making.

Future Planning

The Bismarks are in the first stages of planning. Family members disagree at this point as to what actions should be taken, but at least they are talking. Many families find it difficult to agree completely on many issues, especially early in the decision-making process. The Bismarks, like these other families, will find it necessary to make compromises if everyone's needs are to be met.

The inclusion of Pastor Schaefer in the planning process shows how the word "family" has different meanings for different people. The whole family approach we spoke of earlier suggests including all interested parties in the planning process. Significant people in your son's or daughter's life constitute the whole family. The members of the whole family are not determined by blood relationships only. The Bismarks have identified their key players, just as you will identify your planning team.

The Future

Werner's health continues to deteriorate, and as it does, other family members become more concerned about the slow progress of their planning efforts. Otto, Herman, and Uta continue to urge Werner to talk about the future. Pastor Schaefer proves invaluable in moving the process forward. He rallies the church's congregation to assist one of their own.

Church members contact the offices of the Social Security Administration in Dubuque, Iowa, and compile information on entitlement programs for which Ludwig and his parents might qualify. Another member who is an attorney investigates the law concerning the inheritance of farm property, and develops some strategies Werner could use to remain on his beloved land, lease part of his fields, and farm the remainder with Ludwig's help. Still another member gathers information on vocational rehabilitation programs which could help Ludwig learn skills and become more independent.

Pastor Schaefer presents all the information to Werner one Saturday, and they spend a grueling afternoon discussing the possibilities. Werner now farms a much smaller section of land, concentrating on vegetables he trucks to markets in nearby communities. Ludwig helps his father, but now has more free time, which he spends working for wages on the Notsula poultry farm. Gus marries Paulina and became a full partner in the farming operation. Ludwig continues to see Helena and the topic of marriage is discussed more often.

Werner is thinking seriously about drawing up a Will and discussing Trust arrangements for Ludwig. His family continues to gently prod him, but they know when to back off. They know Werner will act when he is ready. The pieces are starting to come together, but it will require more time. Given Werner's age and health, time for this family is an unknown quantity.

THE HARRIS FAMILY

The Harris family includes:

> Odessa (mother), age 35
> Owen Weeks (Odessa's brother), age 42
> Aunt Jewell (Odessa's aunt), age 59
> Eula Mae Weeks (Odessa's mother), age 72
> Alvin Weeks (Odessa's father), age 71
> Reverend Davis (The Harris family's pastor)
> Member with a disability: Jolene, age 17

Jolene has Down syndrome and a congenital heart condition that requires regular monitoring by a specialist at a nearby medical center. Jolene has moderate mental retardation but, as is the general case, her abilities in different areas vary. She has excellent verbal, motor, and social skills. She is very outgoing and enjoys working and being around younger children, as well as people her own age.

Her family has always included her in all its activities, providing an environment that has enabled her to develop her potential to the maximum. She understands her medical condition but does not consider herself different from other adolescents. At times, she resists her family's efforts to restrict her physical activities because of her heart condition, but has never had behavior outbursts resulting from a desire to be on the go when others thought she should slow down.

Family Economics

Odessa comes from a black family that has lived in Georgia's Chattahoochee Valley for generations. She married Joseph Harris, and for years moved with him to the various duty stations where his career as a noncommissioned officer in the U.S. Marine Corps took him. Joseph was killed in Vietnam. Odessa currently holds a supervisory position in one of the many textile mills in the valley, making about $20,000 annually. She receives a small widow's pension from the federal government, and her daughter continues to receive medical and other benefits as well.

Odessa owns her modest home outright and has a small savings account. Her practicality has enabled her to live comfortably and to see to her daughter's medical and personal needs while maintaining financial stability. The members of the Harris family freely share their skills and goods among themselves, and this form of support has an important place in Odessa's financial picture.

Family Dynamics

Odessa was living in Havelock, North Carolina, close to the Marine air station, when her husband died in combat. Her daughter was 2 years old at the time of her father's death and never knew him. Odessa returned to her home in West Point, Georgia, where she was warmly received. Her brother, Owen, has assumed the role of father for his niece and the two have a strong, loving bond. Owen graduated from Georgia Southern University on the GI Bill, and now works as a social worker in Columbus, Georgia, an hour's drive from Odessa's home in West Point. He is not married and spends many weekends with Odessa and other family members back home.

Jolene sings in the choir and is actively involved in every aspect of her church's activities. Odessa attends church services on Sunday with her sister Jewell and her own parents, but is not religious. Her attitude was once a source of intense family strife, but Reverend Davis intervened, explaining that everyone develops a unique relationship with God. The role of any church, according to Reverend Davis, is to support its members and leave the judging to the Lord.

Odessa's family is very close, and Aunt Jewell regularly keeps an eye on Jolene after school. Odessa has started to date recently, and her family encourages her to find another person who might fill the void left by Joseph's death. She has no immediate plans to remarry, feeling that her daughter is at an age where her mother is most needed. Odessa has become somewhat depressed recently, worrying about her daughter's future. Her close family continues to be a major source of emotional support.

Like the Harris-Weeks family, many families find strength within themselves. While social support networks can provide coping mechanisms for their members, the family support network is a crucial component of an individual's inner stength. Families are often sources of needed material and financial support as well.

Future Planning

Owen has played a key role in planning for Jolene's future. His position with the Georgia Human Services Department enables him to be a source of information on options for people with disabilities. There are times when his views clash with Odessa's about what is best for Jolene. Odessa feels strongly that Jolene wants to remain in West Point so she can continue to be close to her family and her own friends. Odessa has convinced Owen that any plans for Jolene must respect her personal preferences.

After much evaluation of her own motives, Odessa decided it would be in her daughter's best interest to have a guardian after she reached adulthood. With Owen's help and help from the Georgia ARC, a guardianship arrangement was developed. Odessa will be her daughter's personal guardian while the state ARC will manage Jolene's financial affairs. Jolene's financial future was planned using a Trust package that Owen and the ARC helped develop. In her Will, Odessa designated that upon her death personal guardianship should pass to Owen.

Jolene continues to live at home and attend her special education program. She works part-time at the day care center run cooperatively by local community charities. She enjoys her work and has indicated that she wants to remain in a job where she can help others. Odessa and school personnel are working together to plan an education program that will allow Jolene to gradually work more hours in the day care setting. Many people are concerned that the work requirements, coupled with the extended work hours, will be far too taxing on Jolene's health. They have asked Jolene's physician to be involved in future individualized education program (IEP) meetings, and she has agreed.

The Future

Jolene continues her day care work after leaving school. Because of her health, she works only 20 hours per week. When not at work, she attends a day activity program where she continues to receive instruction designed to improve her self-help skills. She lives at home and will continue to do so for the foreseeable future. This arrangement is both her wish and that of her mother. This is not an unusual situation, but one that many families prefer. Residential needs may be met by the family while adult service agencies provide for other adult needs.

Owen remains unmarried and moves to Atlanta, where he is now a section supervisor in his agency. He sees less of Jolene now but remains intensely interested in her affairs. He is considering his own need to plan for the future and has asked Odessa to help him think through the different financial plans he is considering. They will talk when he visits at Thanksgiving.

THE HUGHES FAMILY

The Hughes family includes:

Lowell (father), age 45
Barbara (mother), age 40
Abby (half-sister), age 13
Member with a disability: Brian, age 17

Brian developed normally until he contracted encephalitis at age 4 and suffered brain damage. He now attends a special education program designed for students with moderate mental retardation. Brian has excellent motor skills and is involved in many sports activities, his favorite being softball. At the International Special Olympics Games held in the summer of 1987 in South Bend, Indiana, he won two gold medals and a bronze. He had them framed, and they proudly hang in the great room of the Hughes home.

Family Economics

The Hughes family enjoys an upper–middle-class life-style, with a combined annual income of nearly $100,000. Lowell is an executive vice-president of a large bank and his wife is a senior real estate broker. They have made many astute investments and are on the threshold of realizing handsome returns. Despite the ups and downs of the stock market, their income next year should nearly double.

Family Dynamics

Brian's biological father deserted his family when Brian was 2 years old. Barbara met and married Lowell about a year later. Lowell subsequently adopted Brian and, like his wife, was devastated by his son's illness. A daughter, Abby, was born during the very difficult period when Brian was recovering from encephalitis and it was becoming apparent that permanent damage had occurred. The bond between Barbara and her husband was cemented at that time. Neither could have survived the ordeal without the other's unlimited love and support.

Abby is very protective of her brother and has gotten into trouble at school as a result. Recently, a classmate made crude remarks about her brother and, outraged, Abby sought retribution. She actively pursued the classmate's boyfriend and succeeded in disrupting that friendship. The manner in which she pursued the boy, however, led her teachers to call Abby's parents to a school conference. The teachers were concerned about Abby's overt sexual advances toward the boy. Abby's actions are not unusual. Many times, brothers and sisters will come to the rescue of a sibling with a disability with actions that seem inexplicable at first glance.

Lowell is actively involved in the arts, especially because his daughter is very talented in music and dance. Barbara is involved in local advocacy groups and served as the chairperson for her community's United Way campaign last year. She is also vice-president of her county's chapter of the Association for Retarded Citizens (ARC). Lowell thinks his wife is overprotective of Brian and they have quarreled often in the last few years over this issue. Lowell has shifted more of his attention to Abby in an attempt to defuse the tension in his marriage.

Future Planning

When Lowell first started talking with his wife about making plans for Brian's future, Barbara was uncooperative. She insisted that Brian was still "just a boy," so planning could and should wait. After some self-evaluation, she identified the reasons for her attitude. She had taken primary responsibility for her son and found that she resented her husband's intrusion into her self-defined area of responsibility. At the same time, her marriage was being buffeted by her resentment over Lowell's apparently declining interest in Brian. Such a situation is a paradox that many families experience. Once Barbara understood her hidden agenda, she found it easier to adjust her thinking and actions.

As Barbara and Lowell cooperatively planned, both sources of her resentment faded away. Lowell truly loved his adopted son and his renewed attention to him did not affect Lowell's close relationship with Abby. Lowell's expertise in financial matters nicely complemented Barbara's efforts to make plans to meet Brian's diverse adult needs. Barbara worked closely with Brian's teacher and therapists, and together they identified Brian's vocational skills and interests. Brian's IEP goals were established to emphasize preparation for a job. He would be placed in a variety of work situations so that he could become better acquainted with employment options while learning his new skills.

Lowell, working with banking colleagues, assembled a creative financial package that would enable Brian to own his own home. Barbara's knowledge of real estate was a valuable asset to the family in the complicated financial planning. The result would be a home for their son that would enhance his total integration into his home community.

The Future

The dream of home ownership did come true for Brian. He moved into a three-bedroom house across town from his parents and rented one bedroom with house privileges to another young man with disabilities. Brian receives vocational, case management, and other support services from a local adult service agency. Lowell became very proficient at developing creative financing packages, and now helps other families investigate possibilities for home ownership by people with disabilities.

Barbara and Lowell continue to have periodic disagreements over the risks Brian should be allowed to take. She worries about her son's ability to keep his current job as a utility maintenance worker at a local motel. She would prefer that he work in a sheltered workshop that the local ARC operates. Yet, as the weeks pass and Brian's work skills improve with his social skills, Barbara's fears subside somewhat. She is not unlike other parents who may react skeptically at first when a son or daughter begins to work in a job in a community setting. Too long have parents been told that sheltered employment is the only option for many people with disabilities.

Abby's talents also blossom. She is cast in a leading role in a production of "The Nutcracker." Two members of the design crew of the dance theater company have disabilities. Seeing the success these people are enjoying helps Barbara deal with her fears about her own son's employment. As more and more people with disabilities start to work among their fellow citizens, fears will disappear and attitudes will change. Success in the community will foster future success for others.

THE LEVINE FAMILY

The Levine family includes:

> Ben (father), age 55
> Ruth (mother), age 48
> Arnold (brother), age 25
> Saundra (sister-in-law), age 25
> Member with a disability: Anna, age 19

Anna has mild mental retardation. She is a strikingly pretty young woman who successfully completed high school along with her friends without disabilities. She is extremely shy but not withdrawn. When Anna is with close friends, her wit and personality glow and she is "one of the gang." Her best friend, Zillah Miller, grew up with Anna and to this day questions the evaluation that put a label on her friend. Anna's parents also fought the initial determination. They sought second opinions, taking their daughter to a variety of experts, trying an array of "cures," hoping that the next professional they consulted would assure them that everything would be okay.

Ben and Ruth, like many other parents, received conflicting prognoses. It is easy to call their situation a typical case of denial. We now know that the Levine experience is far from unusual. Searching for a cause and a means to reverse that cause is not uncommon. It seems to be a behavior all people use to adjust to unwanted experiences. But it is unfortunate and grossly unfair that relatives of people with disabilities are, at times, singled out and accused of being unrealistic—they are often admonished to accept, overnight, situations that require time to define and accommodate. There are people who speak of "stages of accepting," listing these sequences by numbers— Stage 1, 2, and so forth. The truth is that adjustments are like transitions—lurches forward followed by slips toward yesterday, steps into tomorrow that leave fresh footprints in the past.

Family Economics

Ben's scrap metal business has become very profitable, and Ruth has had great success as a buyer for one of Chicago's most elegant department stores. They now enjoy an annual six-figure income supplemented by returns from investments, stocks, and bonds. They recently had their financial situation thoroughly appraised with an eye toward early retirement. The assessment gave them a clear idea of how best to proceed with making financial plans for themselves and their family.

Family Dynamics

The Levines reside in an affluent Lake Shore suburb of Chicago, and recently purchased a second home in Florida where they plan to live after retirement. Anna does not like Florida, and has said she would rather remain in the Chicago area. Ruth and Ben are involved in the activities of different Jewish charities, but neither are deeply religious. Their son, Arnold, graduated with honors in political science from the University of Chicago and chose to study law. He recently graduated from the School of Law at Northwestern University.

Childhood sweethearts, Arnold and Saundra married soon after she received her master's degree in business. Arnold maintains close ties with his family, but Saundra has found it difficult to fit in and often feels ill at ease around her in-laws. Close in age to Anna, Saundra has tried to involve her in social activities and they are starting to form a friendship. Ben was mildly disappointed when Arnold showed no interest in taking over his business but now is very proud of his son's career. Like her brother, Anna has also shown little interest. Anna works part-time in a small art studio and shows promise in the medium of clay. She started at her job doing various maintenance tasks, moved up to finishing rough molds, and now is starting to help in designing. She has also tried her hand at the glazing process.

Anna would like to find an apartment of her own and leave school to pursue her job full-time. Her parents have been hesitant and have sided with her teacher, who thinks Anna should continue in her special education program at the private school she attends. Anna is becoming unhappy with the situation and conflicts are starting to arise. Arnold sides with his sister, which adds to the family conflicts.

The Levines are representative of many families in which ideas sometimes conflict. The whole-family approach stresses considering individual needs and incorporating the views of individual members. Problem-solving within the context of the whole family can identify compromise solutions that serve everyone's needs.

Future Planning

Ben is anxious to make plans for his daughter to protect her future. He realizes that, although she has only minor disabilities, Anna will need some ongoing support to be successful. Ben, like his wife, looks forward to moving to Florida and a more leisurely life. With the help of his business attorney and son, he established a Trust for Anna that will protect her and allow Ruth and him to move from the area. Anna moved to her own apartment and receives support from the adult service agency that operates other supervised apartments in the area. After some initial adjustment problems, Anna appears to be doing very well.

The agency that supervises her apartment program at first wanted Anna to be involved in its supported employment and leisure programs also. Because of the advocacy efforts of her parents as well as her own self-advocacy, the program staff relented, realizing that Anna needed support in only one area of adult life. Supported living arrangements must be tailored to individual needs, as in Anna's case. Further, as in Anna's case, the total package must be flexible enough to meet changing needs.

The Future

Ben sells their scrap metal business, and Ruth retires from her job. They make changes in Anna's Trust and their own Wills to reflect their changed financial situations. They move to Florida, but make frequent visits to Chicago, as Ben says, "to maintain contacts with the three most important things in life: family, friends, and the Cubs, in that order." Anna visits her parents in Florida but has no intention of moving there.

Anna remains somewhat shy but forms her own circle of friends, which includes people with and without disabilities. She does not yet show an interest in wanting a family of her own but does date. Arnold and Saundra eventually divorce. Their transition affects others in their families and there remain many adjustments the individual members must make. Anna continues to feel her loyalties split between Arnold and his former wife and she continues to see a counselor to cope with her feelings. She and Saundra still see each other, but far less frequently.

The Cubs have another dismal season, but the fans already dream of the glories that will accrue next year. Plans for the future may not always work out, and will often require adjustments. But, as we have said throughout this book, there are foundations for the future upon which a total structure can be built that will accommodate the changes.

THE RODRIGUEZ FAMILY

The Rodriguez family includes:

Luis (father), age 55
Eloisa (mother), age 50
Geraldo (brother), age 24
Member with a disability: Maria, age 26

Luis and Eloisa emigrated from Mexico 27 years ago, and have since become U.S. citizens. Both children were born in the United States. The family has always lived in a solidly Hispanic community, and the children did not learn to speak English until they started school. Maria had a very hard time adjusting to the new culture she found at school, and began falling behind her peers at an early age. Yet, in her own community she had fewer problems and found herself, in effect, leading a double life. This caused her much stress, and she reacted by lashing out at a world she could not understand.

Trouble at school led to evaluations, and at age 10, Maria was classified mildly mentally retarded and placed in a special education program. Geraldo is convinced that his sister was culturally deprived and that her diagnosis was a gross error. Her parents believe that professionals must have known what they were doing and never questioned the decision.

Family Economics

Luis has been employed for 25 years as a longshoreman and his wife now works part-time for a catering service. Their combined annual income is $35,000. They recently paid off the mortgage on their two-bedroom house in an Hispanic neighborhood in Los Angeles. They both plan to live there when Luis retires in 10 years. Given Social Security and a union pension, Luis looks forward to a fairly secure future, but worries about his daughter.

Family Dynamics

The Rodriguezes are a close family, but Geraldo has chosen to live in another part of Los Angeles. He recently started as a reporter with the *Los Angeles Times*, which has given him a broader view than that of his parents. Luis and Eloisa gain strength from their friends and relatives who live in the tight barrio community, and often find themselves disagreeing with their son's positions in regard to Maria.

Maria works as part of a housekeeping crew through a sheltered workshop and is very dissatisfied. Luis insists she keep her job, while Maria continually expresses her displeasure. Maria has made many friends who encourage her to assert herself with her father. She has dated a lot, much to her father's displeasure. Recently, her choice of boyfriends has been a major source of family discord. Both her father and brother have questioned the backgrounds and intentions of her male friends.

Maria again feels trapped, as she did in school. She has withdrawn, and at times finds herself in heated arguments with her family. She loves them as deeply as they love her, but believes they are not allowing her the freedom she both wants and feels she can handle. When she mentioned that she was considering moving to an apartment with a friend, her father became furious. Her mother, who had usually intervened on her side, supported her husband's position on this issue.

With the best of intentions, Maria's parents are inadvertently adding to her problems. Fear of change and potential harm may lead some families to hold on to their present situation. But dignity includes the right to take measured risks. Planning for the future should include providing opportunities for people to express their preferences and to act on them. Support services, properly arranged, can enhance independence within safe parameters that allow failure but not injury.

Future Planning

Geraldo continued to advocate greater freedom for his sister and succeeded in gaining concessions from his parents. Maria quit her job at the workshop and found employment as a laboratory assistant at the state university in Los Angeles. Geraldo used his friendship with a professor at his alma mater to get his sister the job. Luis agreed to the arrangement only after he extracted a promise from Maria that she would return to the sheltered workshop within 3 months if her new job did not work out.

Maria succeeded beyond her father's expectations and her life improved in other ways. She joined a self-advocacy group and started asserting herself in ways that did not anger her parents. As she gained more self-confidence, she felt more self-respect. She ended her relationship with a boyfriend who was clearly using her and has since found other interests.

Maria continues to talk about eventually moving to an apartment, and now her parents are less adamant that she remain at home. Her father recently said he might agree if she found an apartment in a safe area close to her parents. Maria has started looking at the classified ads and getting leads from friends.

Maria enrolled in a driver's training course and someday would like to own her own car. She continues to have money management problems, but gets informal help from a friend. Although her caseworker from the sheltered workshop periodically contacts her, Maria is proving her ability to be almost totally independent in most aspects of her life. The caseworker is also helping Maria search for a suitable apartment.

Luis had a Will drawn and now feels more secure about his own future as well as that of his children. Should he die soon, the legal arrangements he has made will provide for his wife and will augment his daughter's income in a manner that will enhance the quality of her life. He was pleasantly surprised by the financial options his small estate afforded him.

The Future

Maria is still living at home, although she has not abandoned the goal of having her own apartment. It's just that now she enjoys freedom in many areas of her life, and feels less of a need to assert herself in every area. Geraldo marries, and his wife and Maria become good friends. Geraldo is anticipating a move to San Francisco to accept a position with a newspaper in that city. Maria and her parents are anxious over the possibility of Geraldo being so far from them. Another transition looms, as is always the case for most families.

Maria fails her driving test, but learns much from the experience. She plans to try again after some more experience driving with her father. Eloisa, who has never driven, enrolls in the driver's training program her daughter took. Maria is now helping her mother study at home after work. Problems and setbacks will inevitably re-emerge, but Maria is learning and growing. Her growth affects those around her as well, and transitions continue to come, be met, and be mastered.

THE STUART FAMILY

The Stuart family includes:

> Jack (father), age 45
> Rose (mother), age 40
> Emma (Rose's mother), age 72
> Sally (sister), age 16
> Theresa (sister), age 12
> Jerry and Fran Wilson (friends)
> Member with a disability: Steve, age 17

Steve has severe and multiple disabilities. He is nonverbal and has considerable difficulties understanding others, although there are many indications that he reacts selectively to people around him. That is, around certain people he seems more responsive than when he is seen around other people. Steve may, in fact, be communicating strong preferences by ignoring people or situations he does not like, and by ignoring directions to do things he prefers not to do. Steve needs a walker to get around, but is remarkably agile. He has autism and behavior problems. Rarely self-abusive, he has, however, attacked others and destroyed things in his environment.

Steve attends school in a self-contained classroom. His parents have started to question this setting, and advocate its change. Steve was recently recommended for placement in a sheltered workshop after it was determined that his continuation in a supported work setting at a large light-industry plant in the local area was inappropriate. He is doing poorly in his work placement. His productivity is low, he appears agitated when at the workshop, and his behavioral outbursts are becoming both more frequent and severe.

Family Economics

Jack is a skilled finish carpenter who works for an established construction company. Rose is employed part-time as the coordinator of the continuing education program sponsored by the parish of Good Shepherd Church. The family's combined annual income is about $40,000. Because Jack and Rose are intent on providing their daughters an opportunity to attend college, they have established a college fund at their savings and loan. As Steve approaches maturity, Rose has begun to question the wisdom of providing for Sally and Theresa while not planning for Steve.

Finances are often strained, and Jack is often preoccupied by money problems. He too wonders what will happen to his son. The family home, purchased on a 30-year mortgage, is modest. But because of Jack's craftsmanship, it is probably worth much more than its insured value. Jack has excellent life and health insurance. He also has a valuable collection of carpentry tools, many that he received from his father, also an excellent carpenter. Like many people, Jack has never reviewed his assets and does not know his family's net worth.

Family Dynamics

The Stuarts live in the farming community of Wheatland, Kansas, population about 42,000. Jack's family, in his words, "have always lived in Wheatland." While he has many relatives in the area, he does not maintain strong ties with them. Rose's family also has a long history in central Kansas. Rose's mother, Emma, continues to live in the old house near the center of town where Rose spent her childhood. Emma's husband, H. O. Siddenfadden, operated his family's appliance sales and service business successfully for years before selling it shortly before his death. Emma intends to leave part of her medium-sized estate to her favorite daughter, and favorite (and only) son-in-law.

Jack and Rose have a strong relationship. All aspects of their lives are shared. Communication has been their strongest ally in dealing with the ever-changing challenges they have faced. They have not always agreed with each other, but each always knew where the other stood on an issue. Compromise always came easy. Recently the pattern has changed, and neither is happy with the prolonged periods of silence they both have noticed.

The Stuarts are experiencing the stress associated with multiple, concurrent family transitions. Sally is maturing, dating, gaining independence, taking her first tentative steps into her own adulthood. Her parents sometimes find the process overwhelming. Emma recently had a mild stroke, and Rose now spends much of her time helping her mother slowly recover. Jack had a serious injury this past year and his wrenched back has yet to fully recover—he wonders if it ever will. Theresa is entering puberty and life is changing for her, influencing the changes in her family while changes in her family influence her. As a pebble tossed into a pond causes ripples that affect objects that in turn change the ripples, change is affecting the Stuarts even as they themselves are creating change. They are not alone—the same is true for you and other families.

Future Planning

Rose and Jack tried to work within the system to get the services their son wanted and needed, but found that the options offered were unresponsive to Steve's needs and preferences. After many months of trying, hoping, failing, trying again, and failing again, they decided the time had come to leave the regular system and create new options. They investigated vocational rehabilitation (VR) and secured a job coach for Steve. Steve got a position in the library of the local community college, working in the new acquisitions and circulations section. That was 2 years ago—he's still there, and the job coach was phased out. Now, other employees can provide the support Steve needs. This arrangement, incidentally, does not reduce the overall efficiency or effectiveness of the library.

Sally is now a freshman at Purdue University, where she intends to major in speech therapy. Her goal is to help people without voices speak their dreams so that those with voices may stop, listen, and hear. It is not unusual that brothers or sisters with a disability contribute to the lives of their siblings in this way. While Sally chose to help others who have needs similar to her brother's, other siblings choose careers not directly related to people with disabilities. Yet, we find that the positive contributions of family members with disabilities can have profound influences on siblings. The myth that all brothers and sisters are adversely affected by a sibling with a disability is fading—let's hope for its quick demise.

Emma died suddenly 6 months ago. She had always spoken of how she wanted to leave her estate to others, but unfortunately she never drafted a Will. Her estate remains in probate. No one knows when the matter will be resolved. Jack and Rose finalized their Trust for Steve after getting advice from their lawyer. It's a modest trust, but Steve's life is more secure now. Jerry and Fran Wilson, close friends, agreed to be named Trustees. If one or both of Steve's sisters indicate at a later date that they want to be Trustees, Jack and Rose may change the arrangements. They did not want to give their daughters a responsibility without their consent. Sally and Theresa had input into the decision on the Trust and, for now, everyone agrees it is in everyone's best interest.

The Future

Emma Siddenfadden's Will remains in probate because of liens on the estate and other legal technicalities. The seemingly endless process continues to trouble Rose. She wants to distribute personal items from her mother's estate to various family members. Emma had talked about having this done, and Rose longs to carry out her late mother's wish. No one who knew Emma will ever forget her, but the legal wrangling prevents some of them from moving forward in their individual grieving processes. Emma had always been a careful planner; she would plan so that she could be in charge of her life. If only she had known that her sudden death would wrest control from those she loved most.

Even as their mourning for Emma continues, another tragedy devastates the Stuart family when Sally, driving home from Purdue University on spring break, is killed in a head-on collision with a drunk driver. Steven, who appeared to accept and understand his grandmother's death, becomes extremely withdrawn following Sally's funeral. Fran and Jerry Wilson play an important role by trying to comfort their brutally jarred friends. Rose seeks solace in her belief in a purpose directed by her Lord, but Jack curses a God who would allow such a horror.

Unavoidably, less of the Stuarts' concentration and energy will be directed toward Steven for the foreseeable future. But fortunately, the Full Citizenship group in Wheatland is able to step in and provide the support Steven needs. Full Citizenship at this point is an established service program, and its members realize that they must expand the scope of the services they offer. To help people like Steven cope with some of the emotional crises involved in life's transitions, Full Citizenship hires a professional counselor skilled in working with people with disabilities.

THE WEBER FAMILY

The Weber family includes:

Henry (father), age 67
Lillian (mother), age 58
Gary (brother), age 32

Susan (sister), age 28
Member with a disability: David, age 17

David was born with hydrocephaly. He had a shunt in infancy to relieve pressure and drain excess fluid. Operations related to the shunt kept him in the hospital for much of his early life—a situation that put considerable financial stress on the family. Kidney failure requires dialysis four times a day. Because his body destroys red blood cells, he requires weekly blood transfusions. Through these, he has been exposed to the AIDS virus, although at this time he does not exhibit any symptoms of active AIDS.

David has limited speech and some behavior problems. Lillian is convinced that his episodes of self-injurious behavior are directly tied to physical pain. David can walk only a few steps at at time before he becomes so tired he literally collapses. He has been in a homebound school program for 3 years because of his chronic health needs.

Family Economics

The Weber family has a modest annual income of less than $25,000. Henry's health insurance policy helps pay for David's large medical expenses. Henry has a small life insurance policy, payable to his wife, worth $20,000. Lillian has no life insurance. The Webers own their modest home—value about $40,000. They have no further assets.

Family Dynamics

The Webers, of German-Swedish background, live in a modest neighborhood in Jamestown, a town of about 35,000 in the rolling hills of southwestern New York State. Henry was an over-the-road trucker for 30 years, but for the past 7 years has worked as a dispatcher for the same firm for which he drove. He makes considerably less as a dispatcher, and is bitter about the situation. He is in failing health and may be forced to retire soon.

Lillian worked as a licensed practical nurse for many years before David's birth. Her professional training has made it possible for her to take care of her son's needs. Lillian has always had primary responsibility for David. She, like her husband, has no close friends. Her one outing each week is to attend Sunday services at the Lutheran Church. For the brief time she is gone, Henry watches David.

Son Gary lives in California. He joined the Marine Corps when he was 18 and has never returned to visit. The last contact from Gary was more than 5 years ago. He called to say that he and his wife had had a child. No one knows if he is still married, what his career is, or, for that matter, if he is still in California. What is known about Gary is that he resented the attention he was denied after his younger brother was born. Gary's insubstantial boyhood relationship with his father may partly explain his detachment from his family. Henry was often on the road, and when he was home he spent almost no time with Gary.

Susan, recently divorced, is a flight attendant based in Miami. She shows little interest in David, and maintains minimal contact with her family. She last visited during the winter holidays about 2 years ago, although she calls for brief chats about once a month.

Future Planning

The Webers did not make any plans until Lillian took action. Given the extent of David's chronic health needs, life for the Webers seemed to have settled into a routine of dialysis, transfusions, around-the-clock care, and monthly trips to see an assortment of health care professionals. It is easy to see how this family developed a "one day at a time" strategy.

Lillian and Henry drew up a Will to meet their family's needs. They had some initial difficulty finding a lawyer to draw up the Will. They found that some attorneys, although thoroughly competent in dealing with routine family Wills, did not always understand the unique needs of people with disabilities. Fortunately, the first law firm they contacted directed them to another firm that specialized in disability issues.

They prepared all the necessary paperwork to enable David to start receiving all the various government benefits to which he was entitled. The caseworker from the Social Security office was very helpful in this matter. The contacts with the caseworker produced an unexpected side benefit—Lillian learned that an agency in the community provided respite care services for families that had members with chronic health problems. The Webers qualified for the services and now, once a week for 4 hours, Lillian receives a much-needed break from her responsibilities. Lillian hopes to have the respite care time increased in the future. Both Lillian and Henry are still learning about the intricacies of the adult service system, but the planning they have done so far has given Lillian a sense of accomplishment. She is beginning to explore employment options for David. She feels an inner peace that gives her the extra energy to continue her planning efforts.

The Future

Henry continues to play a peripheral role in the plans for David. Lillian finds herself becoming frustrated because her husband is not as involved as she wants him to be. After thinking about the situation, she realizes that planning is one of her strengths, and that her situation is not an uncommon one. Families adopt decision-making strategies that suit their individual styles. Some families proceed with total commitment by both parents, while others find this contrary to their established style of making everyday decisions. Lillian had taken the lead in making decisions throughout her marriage, so continuing to do so now is not out of the ordinary.

Henry retires earlier than expected because of his deteriorating health. Subsequently, he becomes more withdrawn and finds the free time heavy on his hands. Because he has started to drink heavily, Lillian helps him find a self-support program for people with drinking problems, which Henry sporadically attends. The recent events in the Webers' lives illustrate that transitions continually occur. David's transition to adulthood is occurring at the same time that the family is coping with changes brought on by Henry's transition to retirement. For many families, periods of multiple transiton are not uncommon.

Gary remains absent from the family, but Susan has increased the frequency of her contacts. She plans to make an extended visit during her winter holidays. She has asked that her mother explain some of the plans that have been made for David while she is home. She also plans to talk with her father about his adjustment to his life in the hope that she can persuade him to tackle his problems more directly. Her renewed interest has already had positive results on her parents; they are looking forward to her visit.

appendix one
GLOSSARY

adjudication   Legal procedure by which a court determines if an adult is mentally incompetent to make some or all decisions for himself or herself.

administrator/administratrix   Someone appointed by the probate court to administer the estate of a deceased person when no executor has been named in the deceased's Will. *Administrator* is the male form, and *administratrix* the female form, of this word.

adult foster care   Residential option in which people, usually families, take adults into their homes to whom they are not related. The foster care providers receive reimbursement from various government sources.

beneficiary   Any person or legal entity (e.g., a corporation or charitable institution) to whom property is given. Any person or legal entity capable of holding title to property may be a beneficiary of a trust or a Last Will and Testament. Basically, any person has the capacity to be a beneficiary.

boarding homes   Residential options that provide living space, meals, and limited training programs to people with disabilities.

Codicil   An addition to a Last Will and Testament to change, explain, or add to its provisions.

collective guardianship   A nonprofit corporation appointed by a court to be a personal guardian (the guardian of a person) or a financial guardian (the guardian of a person's property). The corporation is specifically organized for the principal purpose of serving as a guardian for a person with disabilities.

compensation of the Trustee   A Trustee under a Trust has a right to be compensated for services to the Trust, but may waive this right and serve without charge. For the Trustee to receive compensation, it is not necessary that this compensation be expressly provided for in the Trust. If the Trust fails to create a provision for compensation, the Trustee will be awarded a reasonable fee for services, with the amount set either by court order or by statute. If the Trust is administered by co-Trustees, the total compensation usually is divided among them according to the services each has performed.

A court will award the Trustee a reasonable fee for services, taking into account the time and effort involved, special skills that the Trustee used, the market rates for similar work, the success or failure of the Trustee, the amount of income and principal involved, the risk and responsibilities the Trustee incurred, and other relevant factors.

The court may reduce or refuse compensation if the Trustee is guilty of a breach of trust.

competitive employment   A vocational option in which people with disabilities obtain work by virtue of being qualified (usually with special help) for a position. These people may continue to receive assistance from adult service agencies to meet their vocational and other needs, for example, residential programs and leisure programs.

concurrent consent   A combination of direct and substitute consent. Involves people arriving at a joint decision to give or withhold consent.

consent   A legal concept referring to a person's action in approving or disapproving of some action in which he or she is involved, or that will affect him or her.

decedent   A deceased (dead) person.

de facto   Based on particular circumstances (in fact); a legal concept referring to a situation in which a person acts in a manner that indicates his or her mental incompetence.

de jure   Through the law; a legal concept referring to a court determination that an adult is mentally incompetent (see *adjudication*).

direct consent   Approval or disapproval for some action, given directly by the person immediately affected.

discretionary Trust   The name of this type of Trust derives from the fact that the Trustee has the power under the Trust to act according to his or her own discretion. For example, a Trustee under a discretionary Trust can give the beneficiary of the Trust some benefits, or nothing at all. Another characteristic of a discretionary Trust is that, prior to the Trustee's decision, a creditor of the beneficiary cannot compel the Trustee to act.

distribution   The act of a probate court, executor, or Trustee to distribute and apportion property of the decedent according to the decedent's Last Will and Testament or Trust according to the laws of intestate succession.

duties of the Trustee   The Trustee must perform his or her duties with ordinary care, unless a different standard of care is stated in the Trust instrument. The more common duties of a Trustee include:

duty of loyalty   The Trustee must administer the Trust in the best interest of the beneficiary and not let a third party's interest or the Trustee's own interest interfere with the administration of the Trust.

duty of administration   The Trustee must administer the Trust upon his or her acceptance of the Trust. This duty is required even though the Trustee may not receive any compensation for services.

duty to account   The Trustee must keep and report accurate accounts with respect to the financial condition of the Trust and his or her administration of it.

duty to inform   The Trustee must furnish the beneficiary complete information upon request. The Trustee must also permit the beneficiary or a person authorized by the beneficiary to inspect the Trust property.

duty to make productive   The Trustee must determine what funds are available for investment, what investments should be made, and what should be done in managing land or other income-producing property.

duty to earmark   The Trustee must separate Trust property from all other property. The Trustee must not commingle Trust funds with his own, or with other people's funds. The Trustee must mark bonds and notes as being held as in Trust.

duty not to delegate   The Trustee may not delegate to others those acts that he or she can reasonably perform. The Trustee can, however, delegate other acts. To determine which acts may be delegated, the Trustee should consider the following factors:

1. amount of discretion involved
2. value and character of property involved
3. whether the property is principal or income
4. remoteness or proximity of the subject matter of the Trust
5. if the act requires professional skills or facilities that the Trustee may or may not possess.

duty of impartiality   If there are two or more beneficiaries of a Trust, the Trustee must deal impartially with all of them. Under some Trusts, and depending on their terms, a Trustee may, however, have the discretion to favor one beneficiary over the other.

estate   1. The property in which a living person has legal rights or interests. 2. The property left by a deceased person.

execution   1. The fulfilling of any and all legal requirements necessary to make a legal document valid. 2. The enforcement of a legislative or judicial decree or judgment.

executor/executrix   A person named in the Will to oversee the distribution of property listed in the Will. If male, known as the executor; if female, as the executrix.

fiduciary   A person who handles another's money or property in a way that involves confidence and trust.

general guardianship   A legal arrangement in which a person (the guardian) has the power of the guardianship of the person (the ward) as well as the guardianship of the estate, on behalf of a person adjudicated to be incompetent (the ward).

gift   The transfer of property from one person to another without any contract or consideration (exchange of money, goods, or services).

group home continuum   A spectrum of residential options that provide living and training arrangements designed to meet individual needs. The continuum of programs within this option includes the following:

1. *supervised group living:* residential facilities serving a varying number of people with disability in which paid staff provide training and 24-hour-a-day supervision to meet the individual needs of the people living in the residence.
2. *semi-independent living:* a broad range of residential options. The physical structure of these options varies greatly. The common characteristic is that staff do not live in the residences occupied by the people with disabilities. Staff are available to provide supervision and assistance as needed by the individuals living in these residences.

guardian ad litem   Someone who serves as a guardian for another person for the purpose of a court hearing (e.g., a hearing to determine competence). The court usually appoints the guardian ad litem, who usually is a lawyer.

guardianship   A legal relationship; a method by which the law deals with the issues of mental incompetence and consent. A court determines if the person in question has complete or partial mental competence, or complete incompetence. If the court finds the person has partial competence or complete incompetence (the finding is called an adjudication), a competent person (a guardian) is empowered to give or withhold consent on behalf of the adjudicated person (the ward).

guardianship of the estate   A legal arrangement in which a person (the guardian) has authority to give or withhold consent on behalf of another (the ward) in decisions relating to the ward's financial matters.

guardianship of the person   A legal arrangement in which a person (the guardian) has authority to give consent on behalf of another (the ward) in decisions relating to the ward's choices of where to live and where to work, among other personal choices.

implied consent   A legal doctrine which is the basis of the assumption that a person who is mentally incompetent would give or withhold consent to certain action if he or she were competent to do so. Implied consent usually applies to emergency medical treatment, although it may apply to other actions or services.

income beneficiary   An income beneficiary is a person or other legal entity entitled to income from the Trust property. An income beneficiary receives income for life; upon his or her death, the principal of the Trust passes to another person (called the remainderman).

independent living   Residential options in which people live in their own houses, apartments, etc. These people require only limited assistance from adult service agencies.

individual guardianship   The appointment of one individual by a court to serve as guardian for another person (the ward). The guardianship is "individual" because an individual, not a corporation (collective guardianship), is appointed.

intentional communities   Residential option in which people with disabilities and without disabilities choose to live together. The actual residential arrangements vary from community to community. L'Arche homes and CampHill villages are examples of intentional communities.

intermediate care facilities for the mentally retarded (ICFs/MR)   Residential facilities funded under the federal Medicaid program (Title XIX of the Social Security Act). The number of people who live in a given ICF/MR varies from facility to facility. Guidelines for operation depend on the type of facility. Two types of ICFs/MR exist.

1. *small ICF/MR:* serves 15 or fewer people
2. *large ICF/MR:* serves 16 or more people

intestate   Someone who dies without a Last Will and Testament or whose Will has been invalidated by a probate court. Someone who dies without a Will dies *intestate*, and his or her estate is distributed under the *intestacy laws* of the decedent's state of residence.

irrevocable Trust   A Trust that may not be revoked or changed once it has been created.

joint guardianship   A situation in which the court appoints two or more persons or corporations to serve as guardians for a ward; also called coguardianship.

joint tenancy   The ownership of property by two or more persons, all of whom have the right to succeed automatically to the ownership interest of a joint tenant who dies.

life estate   The right of a person to use property for the duration of his or her life or for the duration of another's life.

limited guardianship   A situation in which a court recognizes that a person (the ward) has partial mental competence in one or more areas of decision-making and can thereby consent to some kinds of decisions. The court gives the guardian authority to give consent on the ward's behalf only in those areas in which the ward is determined mentally incompetent. The court specifies the scope and extent of the guardian's authority. Sometimes referred to as *partial guardianship.*

living (inter vivos) Trust   A Trust created during the lifetime of the person creating the Trust. A person may create a Trust by means of his or her Last Will and Testament. In that case, the Trust takes effect on the person's death.

living (inter vivos) v. testamentary Trusts   A *living Trust* is one that is created during the lifetime of the person creating the Trust (the creator, grantor, or maker). It can be either a revocable or an irrevocable Trust. Conversely, a *testamentary Trust* is created by the creator/grantor/maker's Last Will and Testament and takes effect at the grantor's death. Because of its nature, a testamentary Trust is irrevocable before the death of the creator/grantor/maker.

mental competence   The mental capability of people to make and communicate decisions.

natural guardian   The parent(s) of a child (i.e., by blood or adoption). In some states, under certain conditions, parents also are the natural guardians of their adult-age children with disabilities.

natural home   A residential option in which people continue to live with their natural families, most commonly with parent(s), but sometimes with other relatives.

net The gross value of property, minus expenses.

nursing home A residential option in which the main emphasis is on providing medical care to residents. Nursing homes are classified as either intermediate care facilities or skilled care facilities, depending on the extent of medical services provided.

permanent guardianship A situation in which the court subjects a ward to guardianship for an indefinite period. The guardianship remains in effect until somebody successfully petitions a court to remove it. There can be a temporary or interim guardianship—one for a limited period of time.

petitioner The person petitioning (asking) a court to adjudicate another person as having partial competence or complete mental incompetence. In most states, anybody may file such a petition.

plenary guardianship A situation in which a court gives the guardian full, complete, and unlimited authority to consent on the ward's behalf (for all matters personal and financial). Sometimes referred to as *complete guardianship*.

power of attorney A written document which gives one person (the agent) the authority to act on behalf of another (the principal). The power of attorney may be *general*, in which case the agent can act in all respects for the principal, or *special*, in which case the agent can only act in limited circumstances for the principal. Usually, a power of attorney must be signed by the person who gives (makes) it, notarized (acknowledged), and recorded in the public records of a clerk of court.

powers of a Trustee There are several different types of powers that a Trustee might have, such as:

express These are powers that are specifically stated in the Trust agreement, by court order, or by statute. Express powers generally include the power to sell the Trust property, to invest the proceeds thereof, and to pay income to beneficiaries.

implied Includes those unstated (unexpressed) powers that are essential to fulfilling the express purposes of the Trust.

mandatory The grantor instructs the Trustee to carry out certain acts. In doing so, the grantor creates a power in the Trustee and the duty of the Trustee to use the power.

discretionary The power of the grantor to allow the Trustee to use his or her judgment to decide whether a certain act should be performed. Even if the Trustee has discretionary powers, the use of these powers is still within the purview of the courts. However, the courts generally will not interfere with the Trustee's decisions, provided that the power is exercised in good faith and after consideration of the various factors involved. However, the courts may instruct the Trustee to change or reconsider the decision if the Trustee has acted in bad faith or arbitrarily.

Typical Trustee powers include the power to: sell property; make and carry out contracts; incur expenses; lease Trust property; mortgage or borrow money; compromise, arbitrate, or abandon claims against the Trust; exercise the powers of stockholders, including the power to vote; invest; distribute income; keep records; file tax returns; and give full information to the beneficiary.

presumption Previously determined rules of conduct or results that the law usually applies to all people in similar circumstances; e.g., adults are presumed to be mentally competent, and this presumption can be overcome (rebutted) de facto or de jure (in fact, or by a court).

prevocational activity centers Vocational options covering a wide range of settings and training programs. The main emphasis is on teaching vocational skills, with the goal of placing people with disabilities into other work settings. In centers, the training may include wages earned through work done on contracts that the center may have with businesses and industry.

probate 1. The judicial process which proves the validity of a person's Last Will and Testament and oversees its execution. 2. The court which oversees the administration of the estates of persons who are legally incompetent or deceased.

protective services Laws authorizing a court to allow state or local social service agencies (also called by other names) to consent to services on behalf of persons who, because of disability, are not able to provide for their own food, shelter, clothing, or medical care. Courts determine individual cases upon petition, usually by the agency. Protective services are usually for a limited period.

public guardian A public official (e.g., the superintendent of a state institution, or the director of a community social service agency) appointed by a court to serve as a guardian of another person.

qualifications of guardians To qualify to be a guardian, a person must be an adult, mentally capable, free of any convictions of serious crimes or crimes involving immoral behavior, willing and able to carry out the duties of a guardian, and willing and able to post a bond and take an oath to perform the duties of a guardian. The state may waive (excuse) the requirement that the person post a surety bond. Some states do not allow people from out of state to serve as guardians.

real property Land and improvements (buildings), and rights to the use of land (e.g., mining).

remainderman The person or other legal entity (e.g., a charity) entitled to the remainder of the Trust, that is, any property that remains in the Trust after the other beneficiaries of a Trust die or their interests expire. For instance, if A creates a Trust with income to B for life and a remainder to C, then B is an income beneficiary (life estate beneficiary) and C is the remainderman.

representative payee   A payee of government benefits. Usually appointed without a court adjudication that the beneficiary is mentally incompetent, the person is designated by a federal agency to receive the benefit payments from that agency on behalf of the person with a disability program (such as Social Security, Supplemental Security Income [SSI], and the Veteran's Administration) and to receive and manage the funds from that agency for another person who is deemed by the agency as unable to manage his own funds. The representative payee is appointed by the government agency. The appointment does not involve a court's determination of disability. The representative payee has no authority beyond the management of income from a particular agency.

reversibility   Along with risk, a component of the complexity of consent (decision-making). It describes the degree to which consequences or results can be changed or undone. For example, an operation to remove an appendix is not at all reversible once completed. However, a haircut represents a result that, with time, will be reversed completely.

revocable Trust   A Trust in which the grantor transfers assets to the Trustee, but retains the power to revoke, alter, or amend the Trust. The grantor also may retain the right to the Trust income during his or her lifetime.

revocable Trusts v. irrevocable Trusts   The distinction between revocable and irrevocable Trusts depends mainly on the intent of the person creating the Trust (grantor, maker, creator).
   In the case of a revocable Trust, the grantor retains the right to alter, amend, or terminate the Trust at any time before his or her death. The grantor can add or withdraw Trust property, change the Trustee, change beneficiaries, or do all three. A revocable Trust provides flexibility to the grantor or alters the terms of the Trust as the beneficiary's needs change, enables the grantor to monitor the Trustee while living, may entitle the grantor to receive Trust income, and keeps the Trust property as part of the grantor's taxable income. The grantor needs to include a provision for amendment or revocation when the Trust is created for it to be revocable. By contrast, an irrevocable Trust does not allow the grantor to terminate or amend its provisions.

risk   A component of the complexity of consent (decision-making). Refers to the danger or hazard that may result from a decision. Decisions with the potential for highly dangerous or hazardous consequences are said to be high-risk situations. Decisions with little or no potential danger associated with them are called low-risk.

sheltered workshops   Vocational options that include a wide range of settings. The common characteristic is that people with disabilities usually work in environments separate from the general community. Supervision and training is provided by paid staff who do not have disabilities. In most cases, work in these facilities is derived from contracts obtained from business and industry.

spendthrift Trusts   A Trust which prevents the beneficiary from transferring his rights to future payments and prevents his creditors from subjecting the beneficiary's interest in the Trust to their claims. Spendthrift Trusts are created to provide for the support of someone, but also to protect the income from that person's lack of thriftiness. Such a Trust is *not* created for the purpose of preventing the beneficiary from spending the money *after* the Trustee has given it to him or for the purpose of preventing his creditors from taking it thereafter. In short, a spendthrift Trust gives a beneficiary a right to future income, but he or she cannot assign (give or contract away) this right or apply it toward payment of debts before receiving the Trust funds.

substitute consent   A decision made by one person on behalf of another. The person giving substitute consent must have legal authority to do so, and must be the natural guardians of a person adjudicated to be mentally incompetent. Also called *third-party consent*.

supported employment   Vocational option in which people with disabilities work in community settings with different degrees of assistance provided by adult service agencies.

temporary guardianship   Guardianship created by a court to deal with specific situations of mental incompetence in which consent or refusal of consent is necessary (e.g., life-threatening emergencies, guardianship for a minor). The guardianship lasts only as long as necessary to deal with the specific situation.

testamentary   1) Pertaining to a Last Will and Testament; or, 2) an act that provides for the orderly passing of property at one's death or for any other function of a Will.

testamentary guardian   A person recommended as a guardian under another person's Last Will and Testament. The power to appoint rests with a court, but the guardian is suggested by the person's parents in their Last Will(s) and Testament(s). Although the final appointment is always made by a court, usually the court gives great weight to the parents' recommendation.

testator/testatrix   The decedent who leaves a Last Will and Testament. If male, the decedent is known as the testator, if female, as the testatrix.

Trust   A fiduciary relationship in which one party, the Trustee, holds the property for the benefit of another person, the beneficiary, and carries out the directions of the person who creates the Trust. The holding, management, protection, and disbursement of property by one person (Trustee) for the benefit of another (beneficiary) is the essence of a Trust. The person who creates the Trust is called the grantor, maker, trustor, or settlor. The elements of a Trust are:

grantor   The person who creates the Trust

trustee   The person who holds the Trust property for the beneficiary according the the provisions of the Trust

beneficiary   The person or other legal entity for whose benefit the Trust is created. There are two types of beneficiaries: life-estate and remainderman

principal, corpus, or res   The assets that are held by the Trustee for the beneficiary

Trust, or instrument   The document that sets forth the rights, duties, and interests of the parties

Trustee   Generally, any individual or corporation legally capable of taking title to the corpus of a Trust. Trust companies, banks, and individuals may be Trustees. The sole beneficiary of a Trust, however, cannot be the sole Trustee.

The grantor of a Trust normally selects the Trustee. To do so, the grantor need only show that a Trust is in existence and that someone is needed to administer it. A Trust, however, will not "fail" (be treated as nonexistent) merely because the grantor does not select a Trustee. The court will appoint a Trustee in such situations and also in those situations in which the named Trustee is unable to administer the Trust because of incompetence, disqualification, death, or refusal to accept the Trust. The grantor may provide for a substitute Trustee or give the power to others (in the Trust) to name a Trustee at the outset.

A *personal Trustee* is named by the grantor because he or she believes the Trustee to be the *only* person who can adequately administer the Trust. This situation occurs primarily in family circumstances in which the Trustee is a family member. A substitute Trustee normally will not be allowed if the personal Trustee is able to administer the Trust.

It is important to select a Trustee who understands the needs of the person with a disability (if the person is a beneficiary of the Trust), who will follow the grantor's directions, who can manage property, who probably will live as long as the beneficiary, and who has no conflict of interest with the beneficiary.

A grantor may name two or more Trustees who have equal and joint power to administer a Trust. This type of arrangement is called *co-Trusteeship*. The co-Trustees must agree on decisions concerning the administration of the Trust. If a co-Trustee acts without the agreement or knowledge of the other co-Trustee, the action is void. A grantor may want to consider allowing a majority of co-Trustees (three or more) to make decisions, or consider allocating certain duties among the Trustees.

A corporate Trustee is usually a bank or Trust company. There are three major advantages to having a corporation act as Trustee:

1. Corporate Trustees have the skills to manage and invest property.
2. They are generally impartial with respect to the beneficiaries.
3. There is no risk of an interrruption in the Trustee's service on account of disability because corporations have indefinite lives (exist for an indefinite period of time) and will continue to administer the Trust throughout the beneficiaries' lifetimes.

There are some disadvantages to having corporate Trustees. Most financial institutions require a minimum Trust of $50,000–$200,000. They also charge an annual fee for their services.

There also are advantages to having an individual Trustee. Often, an individual Trustee will be a close friend or relative who is concerned about the beneficiary's welfare and understands that person's special needs. In this case, there is no minimum Trust size. Also, the individual Trustee may not charge for services.

There are some disadvantages to having an individual Trustee. An individual Trustee may not have the skills to invest wisely. An individual Trustee may die within the beneficiary's lifetime. The beneficiary's interest may conflict with an individual Trustee's interest, for example, if a sibling is the Trustee.

vocational rehabilitation (VR)   Programs operating in each state that receives federal funds authorized under the Rehabilitation Act. The goals of the Act are to train and support people with disabilities in finding and keeping jobs, preferably in competitive employment. Services provided by VR include vocational counseling and evaluation, vocational training, job placement services, and other vocationally beneficial services. To quality him or her for the VR program, the person's disability must be a significant functional impairment to employment and there must be reasonable expectations that service will enhance the individual's employability. Determination of eligibility for VR is done case by case.

volunteer work   An employment alternative in which the worker is not paid.

whole-family approach   An approach to planning for the future that takes into consideration the needs and preferences of all family members who might be affected by decisions concerning a family member with a disability. The make-up of the *whole family* can vary greatly. Some people include extended family members, close friends, and others in their planning process. You will decide for yourself who has a stake in any decision made, that is, who is in your *whole family*.

Will (Last Will and Testament)   A Last Will and Testament is usually a written document, made by a mentally competent person, which directs how the testator/testatrix's property should be distributed when he or she dies. A Will allows a person to specify the people or institutions who should receive his or her property when he or she dies. A Will must be made in compliance with the laws of the state in which the person lives. To be valid, a Will usually must follow these guidelines:

1. The person making the Will must be 18 years of age.
2. The person must be legally mentally competent and act voluntarily.
3. The Will must be in writing and be dated.
4. The Will must be signed by the person making it and should be witnessed by other competent persons (the number is designated by state law) who usually must sign in the presence of each other and in the presence of the person making the Will. (You may write a Will without legal counsel, but this is not considered wise because you must comply with certain legal technicalities for the Will to be valid and effective.)

A Will cannot "expire" because it is a final document that becomes effective when the person who make the Will dies. Until death, the Will can be destroyed, canceled, and amended. The conditions of the Will can be changed at any time, as long as the person who made the will is legally competent at that time. An amendment can be made by writing a new Will or by writing a Codicil (amendment) to the Will. A person may want to change the conditions in a Will in case of changed economic or family circumstances, such as the death of a beneficiary, marriage, or the birth of additional children. Execution (signing) of a new Will cancels the old Will. If a person marries, separates, or divorces, that alone usually does not affect the validity of the Will.

If a person does not have a Will, he or she dies *intestate*. The state will intervene and essentially write a Will for the person. The state will distribute property according to its laws. This is called *intestacy distribution*. The intestate laws do not consider the conditions that a family may face if the family has a member with a disability, and intestacy laws therefore are intended for general purposes. If parents do not execute Wills, they lose control over the distribution of their property and become unable to assign a guardian for their minor child with disabilities (a testamentary guardian).

Other general characteristics of a Will usually include these: The testator may waive (i.e., excuse, require not to be paid) certain probate and administration costs (such as the bond posted by the executor, an inventory, and an appraisal of the estate). The testator may decide who will be the executor of the Will (the executor carries out the provisions of the Will). The testator also may select a trustee to manage property that the testator puts into a testamentary Trust. The testator usually may name a guardian for his or her minor children or (in some states) for adult children who are mentally incompetent. The testator also can avoid certain federal and state taxes if he or she prepares a Will properly.

As noted, the testator must be mentally competent at the time he or she executes a Will (signs, has witnessed, and acknowledges the Will). If there is doubt about the testator's mental capacity at the time of execution of the Will, the Will can be challenged in court. This means, among other things, that a person with mental retardation may be able to execute a Will but that the Will is more vulnerable to challenge.

The testator must act freely and voluntarily, that is, free of undue influence from another person, when executing the Will. This means, as well, that people who are mentally retarded may be able to execute a Will, but that such a Will is more vulnerable to challenge.

When a person dies and his or her Will is presented to the courts for probate, the executor must give notice to the creditors and beneficiaries of the testator, and they in turn have a certain period of time in which to file a claim against the estate or to challenge the provisions of the Will by filing a *caveat* (a challenge to the validity or terms of the Will) in court. If a creditor or beneficiary fails to file a claim or caveat within the time allowed by state law, the executor is not required to pay to claimant or beneficiary. After all claims have been filed and evaluated as to their validity, they must be paid from the assets in the decedent's estate. Some assets of the decedent are not counted as assets of an estate (e.g., *homestead* or *widow's allowances*). Following payment of valid claims and administrative expenses, including the fees of the executor and his or her attorneys, the estate is available for distribution, including distribution into a testamentary Trust.

work station/enclave Vocational option in which people with disabilities work in a group (with each other) in a business or industry setting (not in a sheltered workshop) under the supervision of adult service agency employees. The people with disabilities, while working in community settings, remain on the payroll of the adult service agency, and are not placed on the payroll of the business contracting for their services.

appendix two
PUBLIC, NATIONAL, AND PROFESSIONAL RESOURCES FOR FAMILIES ENGAGED IN FUTURE PLANNING

PUBLIC RESOURCES IN THE STATES AND OTHER U.S. JURISDICTIONS

The information in this appendix is provided through the kind assistance of the National Information Center for Handicapped Children and Youth, P.O. Box 1492, Washington, D.C. 20013. Listed by state are governmental units responsible for the following services:

> State department of education/special education services
> Office of the state coordinator of vocational education
> State mental retardation program
> Protection and advocacy agency

The names of agencies responsible for similar services vary among the states. The agency names listed under each state or other jurisdiction are those used in that particular governmental unit.

ALABAMA

Program for Exceptional Children and Youth
Department of Education
1020 Monticello Court
Montgomery, AL 36117

Special Needs Program
Division of Vocational Education Services
Department of Education
806 State Office Building
Montgomery, AL 36130

Department of Mental Health and Mental Retardation
200 Interstate Park Drive
Montgomery, AL 36193

Alabama Developmental Disabilities Advocacy Program
University of Alabama
P.O. Drawer 2847
Tuscaloosa, AL 35487

ALASKA

Department of Education
Pouch F
Juneau, AK 99811

Career and Vocational Education
Pouch F
Juneau, AK 99811

Division of Mental Health and Developmental Disabilities
Department of Health and Social Services
Pouch H-04
Juneau, AK 99811

P&A for the Developmentally Disabled, Inc.
325 E. 3rd Avenue, 2nd Place
Anchorage, AK 99501

ARIZONA

Division of Special Education
State Department of Education
1535 W. Jefferson
Phoenix, AZ 85007

Education Program Support
Department of Education
Division of Vocational Education
1535 W. Jefferson
Phoenix, AZ 85007

Department of Economic Security
Division of Developmental Disabilities
P.O. Box 6760
Phoenix, AZ 85005

Arizona Center for Law in the Public Interest
112 N. Central Avenue
Suite 400
Phoenix, AZ 85004

ARKANSAS

Special Education Division
Department of Education
Special Education Building
Room 105
Little Rock, AR 72201

Special Needs Programs
Department of Vocational Education
Executive Building, Suite 220
2020 W. 3rd Street
Little Rock, AR 72205

Developmental Disability Services
Department of Human Services
Waldon Building, Suite 400
7th & Main Streets
Little Rock, AR 72201

Advocacy Services, Inc.
Medical Arts Building
12th & Marshall Streets
Little Rock, AR 72202

CALIFORNIA

Special Education Division
Department of Education
P.O. Box 944272
Sacramento, CA 94244

Vocational Education Division
Department of Education
721 Capitol Mall, 4th Floor
Sacramento, CA 95814

Department of Developmental Services
Health and Welfare Agency
1600 9th Street NW, 2nd Floor
Sacramento, CA 95814

Protection and Advocacy, Inc.
2131 Capitol Avenue
Suite 100
Sacramento, CA 95816

COLORADO

Special Education
Department of Education
201 E. Colfax Avenue
Denver, CO 80203

Special Programs
Board of Community Colleges and Occupational
  Education
1313 Sherman Street, 2nd Floor
Denver, CO 80203

Division for Developmental Disabilities
Department of Institutions
3824 W. Princeton Circle
Denver, CO 80236

The Legal Center
455 Sherman Street, Suite 130
Denver, CO 80203

CONNECTICUT

**Bureau of Special Education and Pupil Personnel
  Services**
Department of Education
P.O. Box 2219
Hartford, CT 06145

**Vocational Programs for the Handicapped and
  Disadvantaged**
Department of Education
25 Industrial Park Road
Middletown, CT 06457

Department of Mental Retardation
90 Pitkin Street
East Hartford, CT 06108

**Office of Protection and Advocacy for Handicapped
  and Developmentally Disabled Persons**
90 Washington Street
East Hartford, CT 06106

DELAWARE

Exceptional Children/Special Programs Division
Department of Public Instruction
P.O. Box 1402
Dover, DE 19903

**Vocational Education/Exceptional Children
  Program**
Department of Public Instruction
P.O. Box 1402
Dover, DE 19903

Division of Mental Retardation
449 N. duPont Highway
Dover, DE 19901

**Developmental Disabilities Protection and
  Advocacy System**
913 Washington Street
Wilmington, DE 19801

FLORIDA

Bureau of Education for Exceptional Students
Department of Education
Knott Building
Tallahassee, FL 32301

Handicapped and Workstudy Program
Division of Vocational Education
Department of Education
Knott Building
Tallahassee, FL 32301

Developmental Services Program
Department of Health and Rehabilitation Services
1311 Winewood Boulevard, Building 5, Room 215
Tallahassee, FL 32301

**Governor's Commission on Advocacy for Persons
  with Disabilities**
Clifton Building, Room 209
2661 Executive Center Circle, W.
Tallahassee, FL 32301

GEORGIA

Program for Exceptional Children
State Department of Education
1970 Twin Towers East
205 Butler Street
Atlanta, GA 30334

Coordinator of Special Needs Program
Division of Secondary Vocational Instruction
1770 Twin Towers East
Atlanta, GA 30334

Division of Mental Health and Mental Retardation
Department of Human Resources
878 Peachtree Street, Room 306
Atlanta, GA 30309

Georgia Advocacy Office, Inc.
1447 Peachtree Street NE, Suite 811
Atlanta, GA 30309

HAWAII

Special Education Section
Department of Education
3430 Leahi Avenue
Honolulu, HI 96815

Occupational Development and Compensatory Education Section
Office of Instructional Services
Department of Education
941 Hind Iuka Drive
Honolulu, HI 96821

Division of Mental Health
Department of Health
P.O. Box 3378
Honolulu, HI 96801

Protection and Advocacy Agency
1580 Makaloa Street, Suite 860
Honolulu, HI 96814

IDAHO

Special Education Division
L. B. Jordan Building
650 W. State Street
Boise, ID 83720

Supervisor of Special Needs
Board of Vocational Education
650 W. State Street
Boise, ID 83720

Bureau of Developmental Disabilities
Division of Community Rehabilitation
Department of Health and Welfare
450 W. State Street, 10th Floor
Boise, ID 83720

Idaho's Coalition of Advocates for the Disabled, Inc.
1510 W. Washington Street
Boise, ID 83702

ILLINOIS

Department of Specialized Educational Services
100 N. First Street
Springfield, IL 62777

Department of Adult, Vocational, and Technical Education
Illinois State Board of Education
100 N. First Street
Springfield, IL 62777

Department of Mental Health and Developmental Disabilities
100 W. Randolph
Suite 6-400
Chicago, IL 60601

Protection and Advocacy, Inc.
175 W. Jackson Boulevard
Suite A-2103
Chicago, IL 60604

INDIANA

Department of Education
Division of Special Education
Room 229 State House
Indianapolis, IN 46204

Special Needs
401 Illinois Building
17 W. Market Street
Indianapolis, IN 46204

Division of Developmental Disabilities
Department of Mental Health
429 N. Pennsylvania Street
Indianapolis, IN 46204

Indiana Protection and Advocacy Service Commission for the Developmentally Disabled
850 N. Meridian Street
Suite 2-C
Indianapolis, IN 46204

IOWA

Division of Special Education
Department of Public Instruction
Grimes State Office Building
Des Moines, IA 50319

Special Programs
State Department of Public Instruction
Grimes State Office Building
Des Moines, IA 50319

Division of Mental Health, Mental Retardation, and Developmental Disabilities
Department of Human Services
Hoover State Office Building
Des Moines, IA 50319

Iowa Protection and Advocacy Services, Inc.
3015 Merle Hay Road
Suite 6
Des Moines, IA 50310

KANSAS

Division of Special Education
State Department of Education
120 E. 10th Street
Topeka, KS 66612

Vocational Education
State Department of Education
120 E. 10th Street
Topeka, KS 66612

Division of Mental Health and Retardation Services
State Office Building, 5th Floor
Topeka, KS 66612

Advocacy and Protective Services for the Developmentally Disabled, Inc.
513 Leavenworth Street, Suite 2
Manhattan, KS 66502

KENTUCKY

Office of Education for Exceptional Children
Capital Plaza Tower, 8th Floor
Frankfort, KY 40601

Unit Director
Special Vocational Programs Unit
2120 Capital Plaza Tower
Frankfort, KY 40601

Department for Mental Health/Mental Retardation
Cabinet for Human Resources
275 E. Main Street
Frankfort, KY 40621

Department of Public Advocacy
Division for Protection and Advocacy
151 Elkhorn Court
Frankfort, KY 40601

LOUISIANA

Special Education Services
State Department of Education
P.O. Box 94064
Baton Rogue, LA 70804

Vocational Education for the Handicapped
State Department of Education
P.O. Box 94064
Baton Rogue, LA 70804

Office of Mental Retardation
Department of Health and Human Resources
721 Government Street, Room 308
Baton Rogue, LA 70802

Advocacy Center for the Elderly and Disabled
1001 Howasrd Avenue, Suite 300A
New Orleans, LA 70113

MAINE

Division of Special Education
State Department of Educational and Cultural Services
State House, Station 23
Augusta, ME 04333

Handicapped Programs
Division of Program Services
Bureau of Vocational Education
State House, Station 23
Augusta, ME 04333

Bureau of Mental Retardation
Department of Mental Health and Mental Retardation
State Office Building, Room 411, Station 40
Augusta, ME 04333

Advocates for the Developmentally Disabled
P.O. Box 5341
Augusta, ME 04330

MARYLAND

Division of Special Education
State Department of Education
200 W. Baltimore Street
Baltimore, MD 21201

Special Programs Section
Division of Vocational-Technical Education
State Department of Education
200 W. Baltimore Street
Baltimore, MD 21201

Developmental Disabilities Division (Mental Retardation)
Department of Health and Mental Hygiene
201 W. Preston Street
Baltimore, MD 21201

Maryland Disability Law Center, Inc.
2510 St. Paul Street
Baltimore, MD 21218

MASSACHUSETTS

Division of Special Education
Quincy Center Plaza
1385 Hancock Street
Quincy, MA 02169

Bureau of Program Services
Division of Occupational Education
1385 Hancock Street
Quincy, MA 02169

Developmental Disabilities Law Center, Inc.
11 Beacon Street
Suite 925
Boston, MA 02108

Department of Mental Health
160 N. Washington Street
Boston, MA 02114

MICHIGAN

Special Education Services
Department of Education
P.O. Box 30008
Lansing, MI 48909

Special Populations, Programs, and Services
Vocational-Technical Education Service
P.O. Box 30009
Lansing, MI 48909

Program Development and Support Systems
Department of Mental Health
Lewis Cass Building, 6th Floor
Lansing, MI 48926

Michigan Protection and Advocacy Service
313 S. Washington Square
Suite 050
Lansing, MI 48933

MINNESOTA

Special Education Section
State Department of Education
Capitol Square Building
550 Cedar Street
St. Paul, MN 55101

Programs for the Handicapped
State Board of Vocational-Technical Education
Capitol Square Building
550 Cedar Street
St. Paul, MN 55101

Division of Retardation Services
Department of Human Services
Centennial Office Building, 4th Floor
St. Paul, MN 55155

Legal Aid Society of Minneapolis
222 Grain Exchange Building
323 Fourth Avenue, South
Minneapolis, MN 55415

MISSISSIPPI

Bureau of Special Education
Department of Education
P.O. Box 771
Jackson, MS 39205

Vocational Programs for the Handicapped
Department of Education
P.O. Box 771
Jackson, MS 39205

Bureau of Mental Retardation
Department of Mental Health
1100 Robert E. Lee Building
Jackson, MS 39201

Mississippi Protection and Advocacy System for the Developmentally Disabled
4793-B McWillie Drive
Jackson, MS 39206

MISSOURI

Division of Special Education
Department of Elementary and Secondary Education
P.O. Box 480
Jefferson City, MO 65102

Vocational Special Needs and Guidance Services
Department of Elementary and Secondary Education
P.O. Box 480
Jefferson City, MO 65102

Division of Mental Retardation/Developmental Disabilities

Department of Mental Health
P.O. Box 687
Jefferson City, MO 65102

Missouri Protection and Advocacy Services, Inc.
211-B Metro Drive
Jefferson City, MO 65101

MONTANA

Special Education Unit
Office of Public Instruction
State Capitol
Helena, MT 59620

Vocational Education Services
Office of Public Instruction
Helena, MT 59620

Developmental Disabilities Division/SRS
P.O. Box 4210
Helena, MT 59604

Montana Advocacy Program, Inc.
1219 E. 8th Avenue
Helena, MT 59601

NEBRASKA

Special Education Branch
State Department of Education
P.O. Box 94987
Lincoln, NE 68509

Vocational Special Needs Program
Division of Vocational Education
P.O. Box 94987
Lincoln, NE 68509

Office of Mental Retardation
Department of Public Institutions
P.O. Box 94728
Lincoln, NE 68509

Nebraska Advocacy Services for Developmentally Disabled Citizens, Inc.
522 Lincoln Center Building
215 Centennial Mall
Lincoln, NE 68508

NEVADA

Nevada Department of Education
Special Education Branch
Capitol Complex
400 W. King Street
Carson City, NV 89710

Vocational, Handicapped, and Disadvantaged
400 W. King Street
Capitol Complex
Carson City, NV 89710

Division of Mental Health/Mental Retardation
Department of Human Resources
1001 N. Mountain Street, Suite 2-A
Carson City, NV 89710

Developmental Disabilities Advocate's Office
2105 Capurro Way, Suite B
Sparks, NV 89431

NEW HAMPSHIRE

Special Education Section
State Department of Education
101 Pleasant Street
Concord, NH 03301

Vocational Special Services-Handicapped
Division of Vocational-Technical Education
101 Pleasant Street
Concord, NH 03301

Division for Community Developmental Services
Health and Welfare Building
Hazen Drive
Concord, NH 03301

Developmental Disabilities Advocacy Center, Inc.
6 White Street
P.O. Box 19
Concord, NH 03301

NEW JERSEY

Division of Special Education
Department of Education
225 W. State Street, CN 500
Trenton, NJ 08625

Division of Vocational Rehabilitation
Department of Labor and Industry
1005 Labor and Industry Building
John Fitch Plaza, CN 398
Trenton, NJ 08625

Division of Mental Retardation
Department of Human Services
222 S. Warren Street
Capitol Place One
Trenton, NJ 08625

Department of the Public Advocate
Division of Advocacy for the Developmentally
    Disabled, CN 850
Trenton, NJ 08625

NEW MEXICO

Division of Special Education
State Department of Education
300 Don Gaspar Avenue
Santa Fe, NM 87501

Handicapped Projects
State Department of Education Building
Santa Fe, NM 87503

Developmental Disabilities Bureau
HED-Behavioral Health Services Division
P.O. Box 968
Santa Fe, NM 87504

Protection and Advocacy System
2201 San Pedro NE
Building A, Suite 140
Albuquerque, NM 87110

NEW YORK

**Office for Education of Children with Handicap-
    ping Conditions**

State Department of Education
Education Building Annex, Room 1073
Albany, NY 12234

Office of Occupational and Continuing Education
Twin Towers Building
99 Washington Avenue, Room 1624
Albany, NY 12234

**Office of Mental Retardation/Developmental
    Disabilities**
44 Holland Avenue
Albany, NY 12229

Office of the Advocate for the Disabled
Agency Building 1, 10th Floor
Empire State Plaza
Albany, NY 12223

NORTH CAROLINA

Division of Exceptional Children
Department of Public Instruction
114 E. Edenton Street
Raleigh, NC 27611

Vocational Education for the Handicapped
Division of Vocational Education
Raleigh, NC 27611

**Division of Mental Health, Retardation, and
    Substance Abuse Services**
325 N. Salisbury Street
Raleigh, NC 27611

**Governor's Advocacy Council for Persons with
    Disabilities**
1318 Date Street, Suite 100
Raleigh, NC 27605

NORTH DAKOTA

Special Education Division
Department of Public Instruction
State Capitol
Bismarck, ND 58505

Supervisor of Special Needs
Board for Vocational Education
State Capitol
Bismarck, ND 58505

Developmental Disabilities Division
Department of Human Services
State Capitol
Bismarck, ND 58505

**Protection and Advocacy Project for the Develop-
    mentally Disabled**
State Capitol Annex, 1st Floor
Bismarck, ND 58505

OHIO

Division of Special Education
State Department of Education
933 High Street
Worthington, OH 43085

Ohio Rehabilitation Services Commission
4656 Heaton Road
Columbus, OH 43229

**Department of Mental Retardation/Develop-
mental Disabilities**
State Office Tower, Suite 1280
30 E. Broad Street
Columbus, OH 43215

Ohio Legal Rights Services
8 E. Long Street, 8th Floor
Columbus, OH 43215

OKLAHOMA

Section for Exceptional Children
State Department of Education
2500 N. Lincoln, Suite 263
Oklahoma City, OK 73105

Special Programs
Department of Vocational-Technical Education
1500 W. 7th Avenue
Stillwater, OK 74074

Developmental Disabilities Services
Department of Human Resources
P.O. Box 25352
Oklahoma City, OK 73125

**Protection and Advocacy Agency for Develop-
mental Disabilities**
9726 E. 42nd Street
Osage Building, Room 133
Tulsa, OK 74146

OREGON

Special Education and Student Services Division
Department of Education
700 Pringle Parkway SE
Salem, OR 97310

Vocational Rehabilitation Division
Department of Human Resources
2045 Silverton Road NE
Salem, OR 97310

**Program for Mental Retardation/Developmental
Disabilities**
Mental Health Division
Department of Human Resources
2575 Bittern Street NE
Salem, OR 97310

Oregon Developmental Disabilities Advocacy Center
400 Board of Trade Building
310 Southwest 4th Avenue
Portland, OR 97204

PENNSYLVANIA

Bureau of Special Education
333 Market Street
Harrisburg, PA 17126

Bureau of Vocational Education
333 Market Street
Harrisburg, PA 17126

Secretary for Mental Retardation
302 Health & Welfare Building
P.O. Box 2675
Harrisburg, PA 17105

Developmental Disabilities Advocacy Network, Inc.
3540 N. Progress Avenue
Harrisburg, PA 17110

RHODE ISLAND

Special Education Unit
Department of Education
Roger Williams Building, Room 200
22 Hayes Street
Providence, RI 02908

Vocational-Technical Education
22 Hayes Street
Providence, RI 02908

Division of Retardation
Department of Mental Health, Retardation, and
Hospitals
600 New London Avenue
Cranston, RI 02920

Rhode Island Protection and Advocacy System, Inc.
86 Weybosset Street, Suite 508
Providence, RI 02903

SOUTH CAROLINA

Office of Programs for the Handicapped
Koger Executive Center
100 Executive Center Drive
Santee Building, Suite A-24
Columbia, SC 29210

Vocational Rehabilitation Center
1410 Boston Avenue
P.O. Box 15
West Columbia, SC 29171

Department of Mental Retardation
2712 Middleburg Drive
P.O. Box 4706
Columbia, SC 29240

**South Carolina Protection and Advocacy System
for the Handicapped, Inc.**
2360-A Two Notch Road
Columbia, SC 29204

SOUTH DAKOTA

Section for Special Education
Division of Education
700 N. Illinois Street
Pierre, SD 57501

Special Needs
Division of Vocational Education
700 N. Illinois Street
Pierre, SD 57501

**Office of Developmental Disabilities and Mental
Health**
Department of Social Services

700 N. Illinois Street
Pierre, SD 57501

South Dakota Advocacy Project, Inc.
221 S. Central Avenue
Pierre, SD 57501

TENNESSEE

Division of Special Programs
132 Cordell Hull Building
Nashville, TN 37219

Special Vocational Programs
205 Cordell Hull Building
Nashville, TN 37219

Department of Mental Health and Mental Retardation
James K. Polk Building, 4th Floor
505 Deadrick Street
Nashville, TN 37219

Effective Advocacy for Citizens with Handicaps, Inc.
P.O. Box 121257
Nashville, TN 37212

TEXAS

Special Education Program
William B. Travis Building
1701 N. Congress Avenue
Austin, TX 78701

Occupational Education for Special Needs
William B. Travis Building
1701 N. Congress Avenue
Austin, TX 78701

Department of Mental Health and Mental Retardation
P.O. Box 12668
Austin, TX 78711

Advocacy, Inc.
7700 Chevy Chase Drive, Suite 300
Austin, TX 78752

UTAH

Special Education Section
State Office of Education
250 E. 5th South
Salt Lake City, UT 84111

Specialist for the Vocationally Handicapped
State Office of Education
250 E. 5th South
Salt Lake City, UT 84111

Division of Services to the Handicapped
Department of Social Services
P.O. Box 45500
Salt Lake City, UT 84145

Legal Center for the Handicapped
254 W. 400 South, Suite 300
Salt Lake City, UT 84101

VERMONT

Special Education Unit

Department of Education
120 State Street
Montpelier, VT 05602

Vocational Education for Disadvantaged and Handicapped Programs
120 State Street
Montpelier, VT 05602

Department of Mental Health
Community Mental Retardation Programs
103 S. Main Street
Waterbury, VT 05676

Vermont Developmental Disabilities Law Project
6 Pine Street
Burlington, VT 05401

VIRGINIA

Special Education and Professional Development
Department of Education
P.O. Box 6-Q
Richmond, VA 23216

Board of Vocational Rehabilitation Services
P.O. Box 11045
Richmond, VA 23230

Department of Mental Health and Mental Retardation
P.O. Box 1797
Richmond, VA 23214

Department for Rights of the Disabled
James Monroe Building
101 N. 14th Street, 17th Floor
Richmond, VA 23219

WASHINGTON

Division of Special Education
Superintendent of Public Instruction
Old Capital Building, F-G 11
Olympia, WA 98504

Division of Vocational Rehabilitation
State Office Building 2, (OB-21C)
Olympia, WA 98504

Division of Developmental Disabilities
Department of Social and Health Services
Mail Stop OB-42C
Olympia, WA 98504

The Troubleshooter's Office
1550 W. Armory Way, Suite 204
Seattle, WA 98119

WEST VIRGINIA

Office of Special Education
Capitol Complex
Building 6, Room B-309
Charleston, WV 25305

Disadvantaged, Handicapped, and Work-Study Programs
1900 Washington Street
Charleston, WV 25305

Developmental Disabilities Services
Division of Behavioral Health, Department of Health
1800 Washington Street
Charleston, WV 25305

West Virginia Advocates for the Developmentally Disabled, Inc.
1200 Quarrier Street, Suite 27
Charleston, WV 25301

WISCONSIN

Division for Handicapped Children and Pupil Services
125 S. Webster Street
P.O. Box 7841
Madison, WI 53707

Vocational Special Needs Programs
Bureau for Vocational Education
125 S. Webster Street
Madison, WI 53707

Developmental Disabilities Office
Division of Community Services
P.O. Box 7851
Madison WI 53707

Wisconsin Coalition for Advocacy, Inc.
16 N. Carroll, Suite 400
Madison, WI 53703

WYOMING

Special Programs Unit
State Department of Education
Hathaway Office Building
Cheyenne, WY 82002

Special Needs Programs
Hathaway Office Building
Cheyenne, WY 82002

Board of Charities and Reform
Herschlar Office Building
Cheyenne, WY 82002

Developmental Disabilties Protection and Advocacy Systems, Inc.
2424 Pioneer Avenue, Suite 101
Cheyenne, WY 82001

OTHER JURISDICTIONS

American Samoa

Special Education Division
Department of Education
Pago Pago, American Samoa 96799

Vocational Rehabilitation
P.O. Box 3492
Pago Pago, American Samoa 96799

No comparable mental retardation or protection and advocacy programs

District of Columbia

Division of Special Education and Pupil Personnel Services

District of Columbia Public Schools
10th & H Streets NW
Washington, DC 20001

Career Program for the Handicapped
Webster Building
10th & H Streets NW
Washington, DC 20001

Department of Human Services
Mental Retardation/Developmental Disabilities Administration
Randall Building, Room 200
1st & Eye Streets SW
Washington, DC 20024

Information Center for Handicapped Individuals
605 G Street NW
Washington, DC 20001

Guam

Special Education Section
Department of Education
P.O. Box DE
Agana, GU 96910

Vocational Rehabilitation
122 Harmon Plaza, Room B201
Harmon Industrial Park
Tamuning, GU 96911

Department of Mental Health and Substance Abuse
P.O. Box 8896
Tamuning, GU 96911

Advocacy Office for the Developmentally Disabled Citizen
P.O. Box 8830
Tamuning, GU 96911

Northern Mariana Islands

Special Education
Department of Education
Saipan, CM 96950
332-9812

Vocational Rehabilitation Services
Dr. Torres Hospital
Saipan, CM 96950
234-6538

NMI Catholic Services
P.O. Box 745
Saipan, CM 96950
234-6981

No comparable mental retardation agency

Puerto Rico

Special Education Program
Department of Education
P.O. Box 759
Hato Rey, PR 00919

Special Education Program
Vocational Area
P.O. Box 757
Hato Rey, PR 00919

Department of Social Services
P.O. Box 11398
Santurce, PR 00910

Protection and Advocacy
Department of Consumer Affairs
Minillas Governmental Center
P.O. Box 41059
Santurce, PR 00904

Virgin Islands

Division of Special Education
Department of Education
P.O. Box 6640
Charlotte Amalie
St. Thomas, VI 00801

Vocational-Technical Education
P.O. Box 6640
Charlotte Amalie
St. Thomas, VI 00801

Division of Special Education
P.O. Box 6640
Charlotte Amalie
St. Thomas, VI 00801

**Committee on Advocacy for the Developmentally
Disabled, Inc.**
31A New Street
Frederiksted, VI 00840

NATIONAL ORGANIZATIONS PROVIDING INFORMATION AND ADVOCACY

American Coalition of Citizens with Disabilities
1012 14th Street NW, Suite 901
Washington, DC 20005
(202) 628-3470

American Deafness Association
P.O. Box 55369
Little Rock, AR 72225
(501) 663-4617

American Foundation for the Blind
15 W. 16th Street
New York, NY 10011
(212) 620-2000

Association for Children with Down Syndrome
2612 Martin Avenue
Bellmore, NY 11710
(516) 221-4700

**Association for Retarded Citizens of the United
States**
2501 Avenue J
Arlington, TX 36011
(813) 640-0204
(800) 433-5255

Canadian Association for Community Living
Roehen Institute
Kingsmen Building, York University
4700 Kelle Street
Downsview, Ont., CANADA, M3JJ1P3
(416) 661-9611

Child Advocacy Center
1800 M Street NW, Suite 200
Washington, DC 20036
(202) 331-2200

Epilepsy Foundation of America
4351 Garden City Drive
Landover, MD 20785
(301) 459-3700

Fragile X Foundation
P.O. Box 300233
Denver, CO 80203
(800) 835-2246

Immune Deficiency Foundation
P.O. Box 586
Columbia, MD 21045
(301) 461-3127

National Autism Hotline
Autism Services Center
Douglas Educational Building
10th Avenue & Bruce
Huntington, WV 25701
(304) 525-8014

National Head Injury Foundation
P.O. Box 567
Framingham, MA 01701
(617) 879-7473

**National Information Center for Handicapped
Children and Youth**
P.O. Box 1492
Washington, DC 20013
(703) 522-3332

National Spinal Cord Injury Hotline
2201 Argonne Drive
Baltimore, MD 21218
(800) 526-3456

United Cerebral Palsy Association
66 E. 34th Street
New York, NY 10016
(212) 481-6300
(800) USA-1UCP

PROFESSIONAL ORGANIZATIONS

Alexander Graham Bell Association for the Deaf
3417 Volta Place NW
Washington, DC 20007
(202) 337-5220

American Academy for Cerebral Palsy
P.O. Box 11086
Richmond, VA 23230
(804) 355-0147

**American Association on Mental Retardation
(AAMR)**
1719 Kalorama Road NW
Washington, DC 20009
(202) 387-1968
(800) 424-3688

**American Association of University Affiliated
Programs**

8605 Cameron Street, Suite 406
Silver Spring, MD 20910
(301) 588-8252

American Bar Association
1800 M Street NW
Washington, DC 20036
(202) 331-2200

American Council for the Blind
1010 Vermont Avenue NW
Suite 1100
Washington, DC 20005
(202) 393-3666
(800) 424-8666

Association for Children and Adults with Learning Disabilities
4156 Library Road
Pittsburgh, PA 15234
(412) 341-1515, 341-8077

The Association for Persons with Severe Handicaps (TASH)
7010 Roosevelt Way NE
Seattle, WA 98115
(206) 523-8446

Autism Society of America
1234 Massachusetts Avenue NW
Suite 1017
Washington, DC 20005
(202) 783-0125

Council for Exceptional Children
1920 Association Drive
Reston, VA 22091
(703) 620-3660

Creative Management Associates
Robert J. Laux, President
P.O. Box 5488
Portsmouth, NH 03801
(603) 436-6308

Helen Keller National Center for Deaf-Blind Youth and Adults
111 Middleneck Road
Sands Point, NY 11050
(516) 944-8900 (TDD and Voice)

National Alliance of the Mentally Ill
1901 N. Fort Myer Drive
Suite 500
Arlington, VA 22209
(703) 524-7600

National Association of Developmental Disabilities Councils
1234 Massachusetts Avenue NW
Suite 103
Washington, DC 20005
(202) 347-1234

National Association of Private Residential Resources
(serving persons with mental retardation and developmental disabilities)
6400H Seven Corners Place
Falls Church, VA 22044
(703) 536-3311

National Association of Private Schools for Exceptional Children
1625 Eye Street NW, Suite 506
Washington, DC 20006
(202) 223-2192

National Association of Protection and Advocacy Systems
300 Eye Street NE
Suite 212
Washington, DC 20002
(202) 546-8202

National Down Syndrome Congress
1800 Dempster Street
Park Ridge, IL 60068
1-800-232-NDSC

National Easter Seal Society
1350 New York Avenue NW
Washington, DC 20005
(202) 347-3066

National Association of Social Workers
7981 Eastern Avenue
Silver Spring, MD 20910
(301) 565-0333

National Mental Health Association
1021 Prince Street
Alexandria, VA 22314
(703) 684-7722

Spina Bifida Association of America
1700 Rockville Pike
Suite 540
Rockville, MD 20854
(301) 770-SBAA

appendix three
PREFERENCE CHECKLIST

SECTION 1:   PREFERENCE AND CHOICE QUESTIONNAIRE

What are _____'s major means of communication?

_____ Speech   _____ Gestures (pointing, gazing, etc.)
_____ Signing   _____ Gestures and vocalization
_____ Communication device   _____ Vocalization
_____ Other (specify) _____

What are some ways that _____ expresses pleasure?

_____
_____
_____

What are some ways that _____ expresses displeasure?

_____
_____
_____

What are some of _____'s particular likes?

_____
_____
_____
_____

How do you know?

_____
_____
_____

What are some of _____'s particular dislikes?

_____
_____
_____
_____

How do you know?

_____
_____
_____

How does _____ generally indicate preference when given a choice between two or more activities, foods, objects, and so forth?

_____

_____

What kinds of choices does _____ characteristically have the opportunity to make?

_____

_____

On the average, how many times per day does _____ have the opportunity to make choices concerning where, when, and what to eat; where, when, and how to spend leisure time; when to get up and go to bed; what to wear; with whom to associate; how to spend money, etc.?

           Never   1–5 times   5–10 times   10–15 times   15+ times

When was the last time _____ had an opportunity to make a choice?

_____

_____

Who usually decides what clothes _____ wears each day?

___ The person	___ Mother and the person
___ Mother	___ Father and the person
___ Father	___ Both parents and the person
___ Both parents	___ Other (specify) _____

Who usually decides what _____ will do at any given time of day?

___ The person	___ Mother and the person
___ Mother	___ Father and the person
___ Father	___ Both parents and the person
___ Both parents	___ Other (specify) _____

Who usually decides how _____ will spend an allowance or other money?

___ The person	___ Mother and the person
___ Mother	___ Father and the person
___ Father	___ Both parents and the person
___ Both parents	___ Other (specify) _____

What was the last choice situation?

_____

_____

What home-management activities does _____ prefer to do or assist with?

___ Shopping	___ Shoveling	___ Mending
___ Setting the table	___ Cleaning	___ Gardening
___ Clearing the table	___ Dusting	___ Repairs
___ Washing dishes	___ Sweeping	___ Child care
___ Drying dishes	___ Mopping	___ Pet care
___ Emptying the trash	___ Cooking	___ Farm chores
___ Mowing the lawn	___ Ironing	___ Other _____

How does _____ prefer to spend leisure time at home?

_____

_____

How often does _____ participate in recreation and leisure activities in the community, such as movies, plays, shopping, dances, video arcades, bowling, concerts, eating out, sports events, and so forth?

           Frequently   Sometimes   Seldom   Never

What are some examples of the community-based recreation and leisure activities that _____ prefers?

Activities	How often does _____ participate in this activity?
_____	_____
_____	_____
_____	_____
_____	_____

What are _____'s special needs or preferences concerning

_____ Positioning? _____

_____

_____ Diet? _____

_____

_____ Health? _____

_____

At what time of day does _____ usually prefer to be active and productive?

_____

At what time of day does _____ usually prefer to rest and relax?

_____

Consider the following items. Which response might be most appropriate for your son, daughter, or other relative?

1. In most cases, when opportunities arise to make choices, _____ prefers to

| make choices independently | make choices with minimal help from others | make choices with moderate help from others | leave the choice completely to someone else |

2. In most cases, _____ prefers situations that offer

| unlimited choices | many choices | few choices | no choices |

3. In most cases, _____ prefers temperatures which are

| very warm | somewhat warm | somewhat cool | very cool |

4. In most cases, _____ prefers lighting which is

| very bright | somewhat bright | dim | virtually dark |

5. _____ prefers environments where there is

| lots of variety in activity from day to day | a moderate degree of change in daily activity | a low degree of change in daily activity | no change in activity from day to day |

Most of the time, _____ prefers to be

6.
| alone | with one other person | with a small group | with a large group |

7.
| very active | moderately active | relaxed | |

8.
| independent | supervised | dependent | |

9.
| with age peers | with older persons | with younger persons | |

Most of the time, _____ prefers to be

10.
| the center of attention | one of the crowd | seen but not heard | |

11. in the company of

| persons of the same sex | persons of the other sex | a mixed group | no preference |

12. involved in

| fast-paced activities | moderately-paced activities | slow-paced activities | |

13. engaged in

| highly repetitive activities | moderately repetitive activities | nonrepetitive activities | |

14. in environments where there is

lots of action	a moderate degree of action	limited action

Most of the time, _____ prefers to be

15.

in highly competitive situations	in moderately competitive situations	in noncompetitive situations

16.

in highly structured situations	in moderately structured situations	in loosely structured situations

17.

in unfamiliar new surroundings	in familiar surroundings	

18.

in highly visually stimulating environments	in moderately visually stimulating environments	in visually unstimulating environments

Most of the time, _____ prefers to be

19.

in noisy environments	in moderately noisy environments	in quiet environments

20. If you can think of any other particular preferences that _____ may have regarding everyday surroundings, environmental conditions, likes and dislikes, etc., please list them below.

_____

_____

_____

_____

Has _____ ever indicated a preference for a specific type of career? If yes, what?

_____

_____

_____

Has _____ ever indicated plans for the future? If yes, what are they?

_____

_____

_____

_____

SECTION 2:   THINGS THAT ARE IMPORTANT IN MY LIFE IN THE COMMUNITY

	Absolutely yes			Don't care			Absolutely no

A. About My Legal Rights and Programs

1. I may attend my own IEP, IPP, IHP, or other meetings.

	+3	+2	+1	0	−1	−2	−3

2. I may refuse to have certain goals or objectives included in my IEP, IPP, IHP or other programs if I feel that they are not right for me.

	+3	+2	+1	0	−1	−2	−3

3. My own programs and goals are fully explained to me.

	+3	+2	+1	0	−1	−2	−3

4. I have a say about the times I work on my programs and goals.

	+3	+2	+1	0	−1	−2	−3

		Absolutely yes			Don't care			Absolutely no
5.	I may see the records on my progress in my programs.	+3	+2	+1	0	−1	−2	−3
6.	I have a say over who can see my records.	+3	+2	+1	0	−1	−2	−3
7.	Only people who really need to know may see my records or files.	+3	+2	+1	0	−1	−2	−3
8.	Someone explains my rights to me about my own records or files.	+3	+2	+1	0	−1	−2	−3
9.	I may vote.	+3	+2	+1	0	−1	−2	−3
10.	I may work or campaign for a candidate of my choice.	+3	+2	+1	0	−1	−2	−3
11.	I may choose my own lawyer.	+3	+2	+1	0	−1	−2	−3
12.	I may join a self-advocacy group.	+3	+2	+1	0	−1	−2	−3
13.	I may join other support groups.	+3	+2	+1	0	−1	−2	−3
14.	I may go to classes or get advice about being my own advocate.	+3	+2	+1	0	−1	−2	−3
15.	I may go to classes or get advice about my voting rights and responsibilities.	+3	+2	+1	0	−1	−2	−3
16.	I may get advice about my duty to register for Selective Service.	+3	+2	+1	0	−1	−2	−3
17.	I may go to classes or get advice to help me understand laws about crimes, contracts, personal injuries, federal and state assistance, etc.	+3	+2	+1	0	−1	−2	−3
18.	I may go to classes or get advice about how to pay my income taxes.	+3	+2	+1	0	−1	−2	−3
19.	Someone acts as my advocate regarding my human rights.	+3	+2	+1	0	−1	−2	−3
20.	My family and friends may visit me at any time.	+3	+2	+1	0	−1	−2	−3
21.	My family and friends feel comfortable about making suggestions to the staff.	+3	+2	+1	0	−1	−2	−3
22.	My family and friends are told about my programs and goals.	+3	+2	+1	0	−1	−2	−3
23.	My family and friends have a say about the kinds of programs I may participate in.	+3	+2	+1	0	−1	−2	−3
24.	My family and friends are told about the good things I do as well as the problems I may have.	+3	+2	+1	0	−1	−2	−3
25.	The rights of my family to see my records are explained.	+3	+2	+1	0	−1	−2	−3
26.	There is a family support group available.	+3	+2	+1	0	−1	−2	−3
27.	The needs of my family are considered to be as important as my needs.	+3	+2	+1	0	−1	−2	−3
28.	The state or federal government pays for respite care for my family.	+3	+2	+1	0	−1	−2	−3
29.	_____	+3	+2	+1	0	−1	−2	−3
30.	_____	+3	+2	+1	0	−1	−2	−3
31.	_____	+3	+2	+1	0	−1	−2	−3

B. About My Health Needs and Rights

		Absolutely yes			Don't care			Absolutely no
1.	I may decide who will give me advice about my health needs.	+3	+2	+1	0	−1	−2	−3
2.	I may decide not to follow a diet that other people think I should.	+3	+2	+1	0	−1	−2	−3

	Absolutely yes			Don't care		Absolutely no	
3. I may decide not to do exercises that other people think I should.	+3	+2	+1	0	−1	−2	−3
4. I may decide who my doctor, dentist, and other specialist will be.	+3	+2	+1	0	−1	−2	−3
5. I may schedule my own appointments with a doctor or dentist.	+3	+2	+1	0	−1	−2	−3
6. I can decide not to see a doctor or dentist.	+3	+2	+1	0	−1	−2	−3
7. I have a say over who can see my medical records.	+3	+2	+1	0	−1	−2	−3
8. I am responsible for my own medications given by a doctor (e.g., pills for pain or seizures, pills to help me act calm).	+3	+2	+1	0	−1	−2	−3
9. I may decline to take any medications.	+3	+2	+1	0	−1	−2	−3
10. I may buy my own medicines at drug stores or supermarkets (e.g., aspirin; cough syrup; creams for insect bites, sunburn, rashes).	+3	+2	+1	0	−1	−2	−3
11. I may decide to have operations (like having my tonsils taken out, having tumors removed, or other operations if some part of my body has a problem) without advice from other people.	+3	+2	+1	0	−1	−2	−3
12. I may decide not to have an operation that a doctor or someone else, for example my parents, thinks I should have.	+3	+2	+1	0	−1	−2	−3
13. I may decide other things that a doctor may do for me (like fix a broken leg, or put a bandage on a bad cut).	+3	+2	+1	0	−1	−2	−3
14. I may decide not to let a doctor do anything to me.	+3	+2	+1	0	−1	−2	−3
15. I may decide to let a dentist pull a tooth.	+3	+2	+1	0	−1	−2	−3
16. I may decide not to let a dentist do anything to me.	+3	+2	+1	0	−1	−2	−3
17. _____	+3	+2	+1	0	−1	−2	−3
18. _____	+3	+2	+1	0	−1	−2	−3
19. _____	+3	+2	+1	0	−1	−2	−3

C. About How I Am Treated

	Absolutely yes			Don't care		Absolutely no	
1. I may talk and show both my good (positive) and bad (negative) feelings.	+3	+2	+1	0	−1	−2	−3
2. People respect my opinions.	+3	+2	+1	0	−1	−2	−3
3. I may make a deal about (negotiate) whether I will carry out what people tell me to do.	+3	+2	+1	0	−1	−2	−3
4. People take my feelings (such as loneliness, anger, sadness, happiness) seriously.	+3	+2	+1	0	−1	−2	−3
5. Somebody helps me to understand my emotions or feelings.	+3	+2	+1	0	−1	−2	−3
6. I may take moderate risks or chances.	+3	+2	+1	0	−1	−2	−3
7. I can have as much responsibility as I can handle.	+3	+2	+1	0	−1	−2	−3
8. I may decide how much I want to depend on other people.	+3	+2	+1	0	−1	−2	−3
9. I have control over my life.	+3	+2	+1	0	−1	−2	−3

		Absolutely yes			Don't care			Absolutely no
10.	Nobody checks on my incoming and outgoing mail or phone calls.	+3	+2	+1	0	−1	−2	−3
11.	No one may use the things I own without my permission.	+3	+2	+1	0	−1	−2	−3
12.	Nobody can take away my personal things as a punishment.	+3	+2	+1	0	−1	−2	−3
13.	I may choose what clothes I wear each day.	+3	+2	+1	0	−1	−2	−3
14.	I may buy clothing, food, and other things I want without someone else's okay.	+3	+2	+1	0	−1	−2	−3
15.	I may pick out the kinds of clothes I will buy.	+3	+2	+1	0	−1	−2	−3
16.	I may spend small amounts of money however I want to.	+3	+2	+1	0	−1	−2	−3
17.	I may handle my savings account or checking account by myself.	+3	+2	+1	0	−1	−2	−3
18.	Somebody else takes care of all my money.	+3	+2	+1	0	−1	−2	−3
19.	I may spend large amounts of money however I want to.	+3	+2	+1	0	−1	−2	−3
20.	_____	+3	+2	+1	0	−1	−2	−3
21.	_____	+3	+2	+1	0	−1	−2	−3
22.	_____	+3	+2	+1	0	−1	−2	−3

D. About My Free Time

		Absolutely yes			Don't care			Absolutely no
1.	I may practice my own religion, or no religion at all.	+3	+2	+1	0	−1	−2	−3
2.	I may do things that other people think are childlike.	+3	+2	+1	0	−1	−2	−3
3.	I may spend my free time doing quiet things like watching TV, playing cards, doing puzzles, reading, or listening to music.	+3	+2	+1	0	−1	−2	−3
4.	I may spend my free time doing nothing.	+3	+2	+1	0	−1	−2	−3
5.	I may go anyplace in my community that is open to the public.	+3	+2	+1	0	−1	−2	−3
6.	I may go anyplace in my community where I have been invited.	+3	+2	+1	0	−1	−2	−3
7.	The community where I live is easy to get around in. (Curb cuts, handicap parking, wheelchair ramps, etc., are present.)	+3	+2	+1	0	−1	−2	−3
8.	I may take part in any recreation in my community.	+3	+2	+1	0	−1	−2	−3
9.	I have chances to do fun things with people who do not have disabilities.	+3	+2	+1	0	−1	−2	−3
10.	I have chances to do fun things with people who have disabilities.	+3	+2	+1	0	−1	−2	−3
11.	I may schedule my own activities and fun things for weekends and evenings.	+3	+2	+1	0	−1	−2	−3
12.	I may smoke cigarettes, cigars, or pipes.	+3	+2	+1	0	−1	−2	−3
13.	I may drink alcoholic beverages if I am of legal age.	+3	+2	+1	0	−1	−2	−3
14.	I may go to taverns, bars, and night clubs.	+3	+2	+1	0	−1	−2	−3
15.	I may gamble if it is legal.	+3	+2	+1	0	−1	−2	−3

		Absolutely yes			Don't care			Absolutely no
16.	I may go shopping anywhere in my community.	+3	+2	+1	0	−1	−2	−3
17.	I may take part in or go watch sports events of any kind.	+3	+2	+1	0	−1	−2	−3
18.	I may go to any art event (like movies, arts and crafts, museums, concerts).	+3	+2	+1	0	−1	−2	−3
19.	I may go to classes to learn hobbies (like gardening, wood carving, collecting things).	+3	+2	+1	0	−1	−2	−3
20.	I may eat out anywhere in my community, if I can afford it.	+3	+2	+1	0	−1	−2	−3
21.	_____	+3	+2	+1	0	−1	−2	−3
22.	_____	+3	+2	+1	0	−1	−2	−3
23.	_____	+3	+2	+1	0	−1	−2	−3

SECTION 3: THINGS THAT ARE IMPORTANT IN MY RELATIONSHIPS WITH OTHER PEOPLE

		Absolutely yes			Don't care			Absolutely no
A.	**About My Family and Friends**							
1.	I may choose my friends.	+3	+2	+1	0	−1	−2	−3
2.	I may visit friends and family at any time it is okay with them.	+3	+2	+1	0	−1	−2	−3
3.	I have chances to meet and make friends with people who do not have disabilities.	+3	+2	+1	0	−1	−2	−3
4.	I have chances to meet and make friends with people who have disabilities.	+3	+2	+1	0	−1	−2	−3
5.	I have chances to meet and make friends with people outside my home and other homes like mine.	+3	+2	+1	0	−1	−2	−3
6.	My family and friends may, within reason, visit me at my house at any time.	+3	+2	+1	0	−1	−2	−3
7.	I may refuse to visit or be visited by friends and family at my home.	+3	+2	+1	0	−1	−2	−3
8.	My family and friends may take part in special events with me (like birthdays).	+3	+2	+1	0	−1	−2	−3
9.	I may decide how much I want to depend on other people.	+3	+2	+1	0	−1	−2	−3
10.	I may choose who will help me with my personal care.	+3	+2	+1	0	−1	−2	−3
11.	I may choose who will help me with my mail and telephone calls.	+3	+2	+1	0	−1	−2	−3
12.	People respect my opinions.	+3	+2	+1	0	−1	−2	−3
13.	I may make a deal about (negotiate) whether I will carry out what people tell me to do.	+3	+2	+1	0	−1	−2	−3
14.	People take my feelings (such as loneliness, anger, sadness, happiness) seriously.	+3	+2	+1	0	−1	−2	−3
15.	Somebody helps me understand my feelings.	+3	+2	+1	0	−1	−2	−3
16.	_____	+3	+2	+1	0	−1	−2	−3

	Absolutely yes			Don't care			Absolutely no

17. _____	+3	+2	+1	0	-1	-2	-3
18. _____	+3	+2	+1	0	-1	-2	-3

B. About My Sexual Needs

1. I may go to classes or get advice about sexuality.	+3	+2	+1	0	-1	-2	-3
2. I may go to classes or get advice about how to be a good parent.	+3	+2	+1	0	-1	-2	-3
3. I may go to classes or get advice about diseases I can get from having sex.	+3	+2	+1	0	-1	-2	-3
4. I may go to classes or get advice about homosexuality or lesbianism.	+3	+2	+1	0	-1	-2	-3
5. I may go to classes or get advice about masturbation.	+3	+2	+1	0	-1	-2	-3
6. I may go to classes or get advice about how to protect myself if somebody wants to be sexual with me and I don't want to.	+3	+2	+1	0	-1	-2	-3
7. I may go to classes or get advice about birth control.	+3	+2	+1	0	-1	-2	-3
8. I may make my own choice about birth control.	+3	+2	+1	0	-1	-2	-3
9. I may decide whether or not I want to get married.	+3	+2	+1	0	-1	-2	-3
10. I may decide whether or not to have my own children.	+3	+2	+1	0	-1	-2	-3
11. I have a private place where I may masturbate.	+3	+2	+1	0	-1	-2	-3
12. I may choose to look at "adult" books, magazines, and movies.	+3	+2	+1	0	-1	-2	-3
13. I may go on dates.	+3	+2	+1	0	-1	-2	-3
14. I may have sex with another person of the opposite sex if we both want to.	+3	+2	+1	0	-1	-2	-3
15. I may have sex with another person of my own sex if we both want to.	+3	+2	+1	0	-1	-2	-3
16. I may choose not to be sexual.	+3	+2	+1	0	-1	-2	-3
17. No one will pressure me to go on dates.	+3	+2	+1	0	-1	-2	-3
18. No one will pressure me to do sexual things with other people.	+3	+2	+1	0	-1	-2	-3
19. People respect my decisions about sexual things.	+3	+2	+1	0	-1	-2	-3
20. _____	+3	+2	+1	0	-1	-2	-3
21. _____	+3	+2	+1	0	-1	-2	-3
22. _____	+3	+2	+1	0	-1	-2	-3

C. About Other People and Things in My Life

1. I may ask for and get help (such as counseling) from persons other than my family or paid staff.	+3	+2	+1	0	-1	-2	-3
2. I may decline to take part in any special religious holidays or celebrations that the other people are doing together.	+3	+2	+1	0	-1	-2	-3
3. I may choose not to take part in group recreational and fun times.	+3	+2	+1	0	-1	-2	-3

	Absolutely yes			Don't care			Absolutely no
4. Lots of group activities are scheduled each month.	+3	+2	+1	0	−1	−2	−3
5. I have a say over who can see my records or files.	+3	+2	+1	0	−1	−2	−3
6. I have a say about the times I work on my programs and goals.	+3	+2	+1	0	−1	−2	−3
7. I may schedule my own activities and fun things for weekends and evenings.	+3	+2	+1	0	−1	−2	−3
8. I may do things that other people think are childish if I want to.	+3	+2	+1	0	−1	−2	−3
9. I may send and get mail (letters, cards, gifts) at any time.	+3	+2	+1	0	−1	−2	−3
10. I may take moderate risks or chances.	+3	+2	+1	0	−1	−2	−3
11. I may stay out as late as I want to.	+3	+2	+1	0	−1	−2	−3
12. I may go anywhere I want if I am of legal age.	+3	+2	+1	0	−1	−2	−3
13. _____	+3	+2	+1	0	−1	−2	−3
14. _____	+3	+2	+1	0	−1	−2	−3
15. _____	+3	+2	+1	0	−1	−2	−3

SECTION 4: THINGS THAT ARE IMPORTANT ABOUT THE PLACE WHERE I LIVE

	Absolutely yes			Don't care			Absolutely no
A. About the Things I May Do in My House							
1. I may have my own TV, stereo, and radio in my bedroom.	+3	+2	+1	0	−1	−2	−3
2. I may have my own furniture in my room.	+3	+2	+1	0	−1	−2	−3
3. I may put posters and pictures on my bedroom walls.	+3	+2	+1	0	−1	−2	−3
4. I may have my own bedroom.	+3	+2	+1	0	−1	−2	−3
5. I may have any other personal things that I want.	+3	+2	+1	0	−1	−2	−3
6. I have a say in how the rest of my house will be decorated.	+3	+2	+1	0	−1	−2	−3
7. I may have a larger pet (such as a cat or dog).	+3	+2	+1	0	−1	−2	−3
8. I may have smaller pets (such as birds, fish, or gerbils).	+3	+2	+1	0	−1	−2	−3
9. The staff that work in my house respect my opinions.	+3	+2	+1	0	−1	−2	−3
10. There is a place and time in my house where I can be by myself if I want to.	+3	+2	+1	0	−1	−2	−3
11. I may choose who takes care of my personal needs.	+3	+2	+1	0	−1	−2	−3
12. Someone of my sex takes care of my personal needs.	+3	+2	+1	0	−1	−2	−3
13. I may continue to use my family physician, dentist, and other specialists.	+3	+2	+1	0	−1	−2	−3
14. I have chances to meet and make friends with people outside my home and other homes like mine.	+3	+2	+1	0	−1	−2	−3

		Absolutely yes			Don't care			Absolutely no
15.	I may use the telephone whenever I want to.	+3	+2	+1	0	−1	−2	−3
16.	Nobody checks on my incoming and outgoing mail or phone calls.	+3	+2	+1	0	−1	−2	−3
17.	I may decline to take part in any special religious or holiday celebrations that other people in my house are doing together.	+3	+2	+1	0	−1	−2	−3
18.	I may pay my rent and utilities without someone else's okay.	+3	+2	+1	0	−1	−2	−3
19.	I may request special meals and diets.	+3	+2	+1	0	−1	−2	−3
20.	I may spend long periods of time away from the house with my family or friends (for vacations, trips, or special occasions).	+3	+2	+1	0	−1	−2	−3
21.	Punishments, if used, do not humiliate or embarrass me.	+3	+2	+1	0	−1	−2	−3
22.	The chores the staff ask me to do around the house are important or useful.	+3	+2	+1	0	−1	−2	−3
23.	I have a say about what chores or duties I do around the house.	+3	+2	+1	0	−1	−2	−3
24.	I may refuse to do any chores or duties around the house.	+3	+2	+1	0	−1	−2	−3
25.	My family and friends can become involved in boards and committees that supervise the running of the house.	+3	+2	+1	0	−1	−2	−3
26.	_____	+3	+2	+1	0	−1	−2	−3
27.	_____	+3	+2	+1	0	−1	−2	−3
28.	_____	+3	+2	+1	0	−1	−2	−3

B. About Where and With Whom I Will Live

		Absolutely yes			Don't care			Absolutely no
1.	I have a say in who my housemates will be.	+3	+2	+1	0	−1	−2	−3
2.	I have a say in who my roommates will be.	+3	+2	+1	0	−1	−2	−3
3.	Fewer than six people live in my house.	+3	+2	+1	0	−1	−2	−3
4.	The people who live with me are as capable as I am.	+3	+2	+1	0	−1	−2	−3
5.	Those living in the house are of different sexes.	+3	+2	+1	0	−1	−2	−3
6.	People in my house appear to care for one another.	+3	+2	+1	0	−1	−2	−3
7.	I may live in a house where nobody smokes.	+3	+2	+1	0	−1	−2	−3
8.	I do not have to follow the same schedule that everyone else has.	+3	+2	+1	0	−1	−2	−3
9.	I may stay in the house for several years without having to move.	+3	+2	+1	0	−1	−2	−3
10.	I may choose whether to move from one house to another.	+3	+2	+1	0	−1	−2	−3
11.	When I learn certain skills, I may move to another house where housemates are more independent.	+3	+2	+1	0	−1	−2	−3
12.	I may move back to my old house if the new place does not work out for me.	+3	+2	+1	0	−1	−2	−3
13.	If I get married, my spouse and I can still live in the house.	+3	+2	+1	0	−1	−2	−3

	Absolutely yes			Don't care			Absolutely no
14. If I have a nonmarital intimate relationship, my partner and I can still live in the same house.	+3	+2	+1	0	−1	−2	−3
15. I may live by myself.	+3	+2	+1	0	−1	−2	−3
16. The house is close to school and work.	+3	+2	+1	0	−1	−2	−3
17. The house is close to public transportation.	+3	+2	+1	0	−1	−2	−3
18. The house is close to shopping and recreational sites.	+3	+2	+1	0	−1	−2	−3
19. The house is in a neighborhood that is like my family's.	+3	+2	+1	0	−1	−2	−3
20. The house has a yard.	+3	+2	+1	0	−1	−2	−3
21. The house has space for a garden.	+3	+2	+1	0	−1	−2	−3
22. The house is in a safe neighborhood.	+3	+2	+1	0	−1	−2	−3
23. My house has a work program that is part of the overall program.	+3	+2	+1	0	−1	−2	−3
24. The staff at my house provides transportation to and from my job.	+3	+2	+1	0	−1	−2	−3
25. Most of my neighbors do not have a disability.	+3	+2	+1	0	−1	−2	−3
26. Most of my neighbors are friendly and helpful.	+3	+2	+1	0	−1	−2	−3
27. _____	+3	+2	+1	0	−1	−2	−3
28. _____	+3	+2	+1	0	−1	−2	−3
29. _____	+3	+2	+1	0	−1	−2	−3

C. About Staff and the Way My House is Run

	Absolutely yes			Don't care			Absolutely no
1. There is somebody in the house who knows how to give emergency first aid.	+3	+2	+1	0	−1	−2	−3
2. Someone in the house or the people who run the house act as an advocate of my human rights.	+3	+2	+1	0	−1	−2	−3
3. Someone in the house knows how to teach independent living skills.	+3	+2	+1	0	−1	−2	−3
4. Someone in the house knows how to handle behavior problems.	+3	+2	+1	0	−1	−2	−3
5. Staff are well-paid.	+3	+2	+1	0	−1	−2	−3
6. Staff take part in regular training to learn how to do their jobs better.	+3	+2	+1	0	−1	−2	−3
7. Staff members are employed over a long period of time; there is low staff turnover.	+3	+2	+1	0	−1	−2	−3
8. There are three or fewer staff changes within each week.	+3	+2	+1	0	−1	−2	−3
9. The house hires people of both sexes as staff.	+3	+2	+1	0	−1	−2	−3
10. Other (ancillary) services (such as physical and occupational therapy, respite care, personal care attendants) are reasonably available.	+3	+2	+1	0	−1	−2	−3
11. Staff meet all licensing requirements.	+3	+2	+1	0	−1	−2	−3
12. Staff or family members will not enter my bedroom or the bathroom when I close the door without knocking first and asking me if they can come in.	+3	+2	+1	0	−1	−2	−3

		Absolutely yes			Don't care		Absolutely no	
13.	If I am in the bedroom or bathroom and do not answer repeated knocks, someone will come in and check to see if I'm all right.	+3	+2	+1	0	−1	−2	−3
14.	The house is owned by a nonprofit organization.	+3	+2	+1	0	−1	−2	−3
15.	Smoking is not allowed in the house.	+3	+2	+1	0	−1	−2	−3
16.	The house is not closed during major holidays or during staff vacation times.	+3	+2	+1	0	−1	−2	−3
17.	The house has an active human rights committee with representatives from the community.	+3	+2	+1	0	−1	−2	−3
18.	My house is certified by an independent accreditation agency (such as ACMR-DD or CARF).	+3	+2	+1	0	−1	−2	−3
19.	The state or federal government pays for my living expenses.	+3	+2	+1	0	−1	−2	−3
20.	I have to pay less than $100 per month for my living expenses.	+3	+2	+1	0	−1	−2	−3
21.	The state or federal government pays for my personal care attendant.	+3	+2	+1	0	−1	−2	−3
22.	The total cost of living in the house is explained clearly and does not change from month to month.	+3	+2	+1	0	−1	−2	−3
23.	My family and friends can visit me any time.	+3	+2	+1	0	−1	−2	−3
24.	My family and friends feel comfortable about making suggestions to the staff who work in my house.	+3	+2	+1	0	−1	−2	−3
25.	My family and friends are told about my programs and goals.	+3	+2	+1	0	−1	−2	−3
26.	My family and friends have a say in the kinds of programs and goals I may have.	+3	+2	+1	0	−1	−2	−3
27.	My family and friends are told about the good things I do as well as about the problems I may have.	+3	+2	+1	0	−1	−2	−3
28.	My family and friends can become involved in boards and committees that supervise the running of the house.	+3	+2	+1	0	−1	−2	−3
29.	My family and friends may take part in special events with me (birthdays, celebrations, etc.).	+3	+2	+1	0	−1	−2	−3
30.	The rights of my family to see my records and files are explained.	+3	+2	+1	0	−1	−2	−3
31.	_____	+3	+2	+1	0	−1	−2	−3
32.	_____	+3	+2	+1	0	−1	−2	−3
33.	_____	+3	+2	+1	0	−1	−2	−3

SECTION 5: THINGS THAT ARE IMPORTANT ABOUT MY JOB

		Absolutely yes			Don't care		Absolutely no	
A.	**About the Kind of Job I Will Have**							
1.	I may choose the kind of work I want to do.	+3	+2	+1	0	−1	−2	−3

		Absolutely yes			Don't care			Absolutely no
2.	I may choose not to work.	+3	+2	+1	0	−1	−2	−3
3.	I may choose a nonwork activity program, like day recreation.	+3	+2	+1	0	−1	−2	−3
4.	I may work in a sheltered workshop.	+3	+2	+1	0	−1	−2	−3
5.	I may get the help of a job coach on my job.	+3	+2	+1	0	−1	−2	−3
6.	I may choose my own job coach.	+3	+2	+1	0	−1	−2	−3
7.	I may get a job in the community.	+3	+2	+1	0	−1	−2	−3
8.	I may go to a vocational training school instead of an actual job.	+3	+2	+1	0	−1	−2	−3
9.	I may work in a place where nobody smokes.	+3	+2	+1	0	−1	−2	−3
10.	I may quit my job.	+3	+2	+1	0	−1	−2	−3
11.	_____	+3	+2	+1	0	−1	−2	−3
12.	_____	+3	+2	+1	0	−1	−2	−3
13.	_____	+3	+2	+1	0	−1	−2	−3

B. About the Kind of Place Where I Will Work and the Things I Will Do

1.	I can get to work easily.	+3	+2	+1	0	−1	−2	−3
2.	I may use public transportation to get to my job.	+3	+2	+1	0	−1	−2	−3
3.	The place where I work is separate from the place where I live.	+3	+2	+1	0	−1	−2	−3
4.	My house has a work program that is part of the program.	+3	+2	+1	0	−1	−2	−3
5.	The staff at my house provide transportation to and from my job.	+3	+2	+1	0	−1	−2	−3
6.	I will work with the same people I live with.	+3	+2	+1	0	−1	−2	−3
7.	I will work with coworkers who do not have disabilities.	+3	+2	+1	0	−1	−2	−3
8.	I will work with coworkers who have disabilities.	+3	+2	+1	0	−1	−2	−3
9.	My coworkers respect my opinions.	+3	+2	+1	0	−1	−2	−3
10.	My coworkers are friendly and helpful.	+3	+2	+1	0	−1	−2	−3
11.	My coworkers are as capable as me.	+3	+2	+1	0	−1	−2	−3
12.	The place where I work is in a safe area.	+3	+2	+1	0	−1	−2	−3
13.	The place where I work follows all government rules (like health and safety, wage and hour, and affirmative action regulations).	+3	+2	+1	0	−1	−2	−3
14.	The place where I work hires people of both sexes.	+3	+2	+1	0	−1	−2	−3
15.	The jobs I do where I work are important.	+3	+2	+1	0	−1	−2	−3
16.	My job does not require hard physical work.	+3	+2	+1	0	−1	−2	−3
17.	I work in a quiet area.	+3	+2	+1	0	−1	−2	−3
18.	My workplace is clean and orderly.	+3	+2	+1	0	−1	−2	−3
19.	I may, within reason, decide what I wear on my job.	+3	+2	+1	0	−1	−2	−3
20.	There is a place just for me to keep my personal things safe while I work on my job.	+3	+2	+1	0	−1	−2	−3

	Absolutely yes			Don't care		Absolutely no	
21. My job has few changes in duties from day to day.	+3	+2	+1	0	−1	−2	−3
22. My job has the same scheduled hours every week.	+3	+2	+1	0	−1	−2	−3
23. I may, within reason, schedule my own work hours.	+3	+2	+1	0	−1	−2	−3
24. I may, within reason, schedule my own vacation times.	+3	+2	+1	0	−1	−2	−3
25. My work schedule will allow me to take part in social events and fun things at my house.	+3	+2	+1	0	−1	−2	−3
26. I will be protected from unkind remarks by other workers.	+3	+2	+1	0	−1	−2	−3
27. Somebody at the place where I work knows how to give emergency first aid.	+3	+2	+1	0	−1	−2	−3
28. Someone at the place where I work knows how to handle behavior problems.	+3	+2	+1	0	−1	−2	−3
29. My supervisor has had special training to work with people with disabilities.	+3	+2	+1	0	−1	−2	−3
30. My supervisor corrects my mistakes without humiliating or embarrassing me.	+3	+2	+1	0	−1	−2	−3
31. My supervisor respects my opinions.	+3	+2	+1	0	−1	−2	−3
32. My vocational teachers at the place where I work are employed over a long period of time; there is low staff turnover.	+3	+2	+1	0	−1	−2	−3
33. My vocational teachers are well paid.	+3	+2	+1	0	−1	−2	−3
34. The vocational teachers take part in regular inservice.	+3	+2	+1	0	−1	−2	−3
35. _____	+3	+2	+1	0	−1	−2	−3
36. _____	+3	+2	+1	0	−1	−2	−3
37. _____	+3	+2	+1	0	−1	−2	−3

C. About My Pay and Job Benefits

	Absolutely yes			Don't care		Absolutely no	
1. The amount I am paid will depend on how much work I do, even if it is less than minimum wage.	+3	+2	+1	0	−1	−2	−3
2. I will earn a salary that is the same that workers without disabilities get for doing the same job.	+3	+2	+1	0	−1	−2	−3
3. I will be paid weekly on my job.	+3	+2	+1	0	−1	−2	−3
4. I will be paid every other week on my job.	+3	+2	+1	0	−1	−2	−3
5. I will be paid monthly on my job.	+3	+2	+1	0	−1	−2	−3
6. I will have chances to work overtime and earn extra money on my job.	+3	+2	+1	0	−1	−2	−3
7. I can control how much I earn so I don't lose my Social Security Disability Insurance (SSDI) benefits.	+3	+2	+1	0	−1	−2	−3
8. I can control how much I earn so I don't lose my Supplemental Security Income (SSI) benefits.	+3	+2	+1	0	−1	−2	−3
9. I will get help in planning to use my SSI benefits for special job-related expenses.	+3	+2	+1	0	−1	−2	−3
10. I will have chances for advancement (promotions, raises in salary) in my job.	+3	+2	+1	0	−1	−2	−3

Disability and the Family

		Absolutely yes			Don't care			Absolutely no
11.	I get help if I am laid off from my job.	+3	+2	+1	0	−1	−2	−3
12.	A community agency will help me find another job if my competitive job doesn't work out.	+3	+2	+1	0	−1	−2	−3
13.	My job will provide me with special insurance (disability/worker's compensation) in case I get hurt.	+3	+2	+1	0	−1	−2	−3
14.	My job will provide me with health insurance.	+3	+2	+1	0	−1	−2	−3
15.	My job will provide me with dental insurance.	+3	+2	+1	0	−1	−2	−3
16.	I have the same rights to complain about things on my job that my coworkers without disabilities have.	+3	+2	+1	0	−1	−2	−3
17.	My job will provide me with retirement benefits.	+3	+2	+1	0	−1	−2	−3
18.	_____	+3	+2	+1	0	−1	−2	−3
19.	_____	+3	+2	+1	0	−1	−2	−3
20.	_____	+3	+2	+1	0	−1	−2	−3

appendix four
ASSESSING MENTAL COMPETENCE
FOR DECISION-MAKING (FIGURE 4.2.)

Appendix 4
Mental Competence for Decision-Making

		Concerning life in the community	Concerning relationships with other people	Concerning the place one lives	Concerning one's job	Concerning the acquisition of money	Concerning the spending of money
Defining the problem or need	Simple						
	Medium						
	Difficult						
Brainstorming	Simple						
	Medium						
	Difficult						
Evaluating and choosing alternatives	Simple						
	Medium						
	Difficult						
Communicating the decision to others	Simple						
	Medium						
	Difficult						
Taking action	Simple						
	Medium						
	Difficult						
Evaluating outcome of the action	Simple						
	Medium						
	Difficult						

Appendix 4
Mental Competence for Decision-Making

		Concerning life in the community	Concerning relationships with other people	Concerning the place one lives	Concerning one's job	Concerning the acquisition of money	Concerning the spending of money
Defining the problem or need	Simple						
	Medium						
	Difficult						
Brainstorming	Simple						
	Medium						
	Difficult						
Evaluating and choosing alternatives	Simple						
	Medium						
	Difficult						
Communicating the decision to others	Simple						
	Medium						
	Difficult						
Taking action	Simple						
	Medium						
	Difficult						
Evaluating outcome of the action	Simple						
	Medium						
	Difficult						

Appendix 4
Mental Competence for Decision-Making

		Concerning life in the community	Concerning relationships with other people	Concerning the place one lives	Concerning one's job	Concerning the acquisition of money	Concerning the spending of money
Defining the problem or need	Simple						
	Medium						
	Difficult						
Brainstorming	Simple						
	Medium						
	Difficult						
Evaluating and choosing alternatives	Simple						
	Medium						
	Difficult						
Communicating the decision to others	Simple						
	Medium						
	Difficult						
Taking action	Simple						
	Medium						
	Difficult						
Evaluating outcome of the action	Simple						
	Medium						
	Difficult						

Appendix 4
Mental Competence for Decision-Making

		Concerning life in the community	Concerning relationships with other people	Concerning the place one lives	Concerning one's job	Concerning the acquisition of money	Concerning the spending of money
Defining the problem or need	Simple						
	Medium						
	Difficult						
Brainstorming	Simple						
	Medium						
	Difficult						
Evaluating and choosing alternatives	Simple						
	Medium						
	Difficult						
Communicating the decision to others	Simple						
	Medium						
	Difficult						
Taking action	Simple						
	Medium						
	Difficult						
Evaluating outcome of the action	Simple						
	Medium						
	Difficult						

appendix five
RECOMMENDED READING

GENERAL RESOURCES

Braddock, D. (1987). *Federal policy toward mental retardation and developmental disabilities*. Baltimore: Paul H. Brookes Publishing Co. $29.95.

Federal policy equates to federal dollars. The lack of adequate funds continues to hamper the development of options for people transitioning from public school–based programs to the adult service system. Senator Bob Dole, in the foreword, summarizes this text: "This book is the single most useful document about federal government policy toward mental retardation and developmental disabilities produced in the 28 years that I have served in the United States Congress. Its preparation was a formidable task and the author has carried it out with great depth and objectivity" (p. xv).

Bruininks, R.H., & Lakin, K.C. (1985). *Living and learning in the least restrictive environment*. Baltimore: Paul H. Brookes Publishing Co. $26.00.

An excellent text, with contributions from leading professionals in the field of developmental disabilities. Fourteen chapters are divided into five sections that deal with the social changes in this country that led to greater participation in the community by people with disabilities. The broad areas investigated in detail are: historical and philosophical overview of service delivery, legal issues in the provision of habilitation services, community and family perspectives in integration, environmental issues, and a concluding chapter on the future. This book, while written primarily for professionals, would be of interest to many family members.

ERIC Clearinghouse on Handicapped and Gifted Children Information Bulletin. 1920 Association Drive, Reston, VA 22091.

Quarterly bulletin that can be received free of charge by anyone who asks to be placed on the house mailing list. The bulletin describes new books and publications that deal with a wide variety of disability issues. Among publications reviewed are some that may be ordered free of charge. Other news features include analyses of national policy trends and descriptions of model services nationwide. An excellent resource for families and professionals, ERIC will keep you informed of new developments in a timely manner.

Heal, L.W., Haney, J.I., & Novak Amado, A.R. (1988). *Integration of developmentally disabled individuals into the community* (2nd ed.). Baltimore: Paul H. Brookes Publishing Co. $24.95.

Covers all facets of community integration, from relevant legislation and litigation to research on the training of individuals for self-sufficient living.

Ludlow, B.L., Turnbull, A.P., & Luckasson, R. (1988). *Transitions to adult life for people with mental retardation: Principles and practices*. Baltimore: Paul H. Brookes Publishing Co. $30.00.

Addresses the challenge of guaranteeing an integrated life to persons with mental retardation in their adult years. In each of three areas—independent living, community participation, and employment—this book helps identify programming goals, shows how to implement a transition program, and provides an examination of legal and policy issues.

Summers, J.A. (Ed.). (1986). *The right to grow up: An introduction to adults with developmental disabilities*. Baltimore: Paul H. Brookes Publishing Co. $21.95.

A comprehensive text addressing the spectrum of needs of families and individuals with disabilities in the transition from school-based services to adult services. The 13 chapters of this book are written by leaders in the field of research and service delivery. Among the specific issues explained are: barriers to successful transitions; sexuality, marriage, and parenthood; residential services; vocational services; leisure and recreational needs; religious ministries; federal laws and policies; and aging. The book is written by professionals and targets a professional audience. For professionals in the field, this text is a compendium of necessary information.

The Exceptional Parent. Magazine published eight times a year. $16.00. Write to *Exceptional Parent*, 605
   Commonwealth Avenue, Boston, MA 02215.

A wonderfully informative magazine directed primarily at parents and other family members, but useful to
all professionals dealing with people with disabilities across the life cycle. Each issue of the magazine contains personal reports, descriptions of model programs and new teaching procedures, letters to the editor,
and many advertisements from firms providing various services and products. The magazine is liberally
illustrated and provides lively, informative news.

Transition Institute at Illinois. (1987). *Annotated bibliography on transition from school to work, Vol. II.*
   (1987). Champaign: University of Illinois. $6.50.

A comprehensive review of hundreds of publications dealing with all aspects of planning for transitions to
adult services by people with disabilities. The bibliography provides the information needed to secure reviewed publications. A title index, subject index, and author index provide easy access for readers. The
publications reviewed are useful to both lay and professional audiences.

Turnbull, A.P., & Turnbull, H.R. (1986). *Families, professionals, and exceptionality. A special partnership.*
   Columbus, OH: Charles E. Merrill. $17.95.

Family theory is reviewed, including resources, interaction styles, family functions, and life cycles. The role
of parents in special education and suggestions for building and maintaining positive parent-professional
interactions are described. While this book is written primarily for professionals working with families, it is a
good resource for parents and other family members.

FINANCIAL PLANNING AND GUARDIANSHIP

Abravamel, E.G. (1983). Discretionary support trusts. *Iowa Law Review, 66,* 273–304.

Useful for lawyers interested in a highly technical description of how to use Trusts to pass property from one
person to a second person in order to support that second person.

Apolloni, T., & Cooke, T.P. (Eds.). (1984). *A new look at guardianship: Protective services that support
   personalized living.* Baltimore: Paul H. Brookes Publishing Co.

Explains guardianship from a legal perspective, but focuses mainly on the collective guardianship model
developed throughout the United States. Contains a particularly helpful chapter on determining whether a
person is incompetent and should be subject to guardianship. Also useful for people who want to develop
their own protection, advocacy, and guardianship service systems.

Association for Retarded Citizens of the United States. (1984). *How to provide for their future.* Arlington,
   TX: Author. $2.00.

Discusses guardianship and basic factors that families should take into account in considering whether to
seek guardianship. Also discusses use of Wills, Trusts, and general estate planning, insurance, and government benefits. Useful as primer for families.

Brakel, S.J., Parry, J., & Weinen, B.W. (1985). *The mentally retarded and the law.* Chicago: American Bar
   Foundation. No price given.

A comprehensive review of legal issues, with references to applicable judicial decisions and federal and state
statutes involving persons with disabilities. Chapters on incompetency, guardianship, and restoration to
competency, decision-making rights, family laws, and entitlements to services are particularly helpful. Useful primarily to lawyers.

Burgdorf, R.L., Jr. (1980). *The legal rights of handicapped persons: Cases, materials, and text.* Baltimore:
   Paul H. Brookes Publishing Co.

Reproduces important judicial decisions and legal commentary concerning guardianship (among other issues involving law and people with developmental disabilities). Commentaries and editor's notes concerning
guardianship deal largely with question of whether guardianship is appropriate as a prosthetic device or
inappropriate as a means to strip away a person's rights. Material on incompetency, guardianship, and autonomy is provocative. Useful principally to lawyers.

Burgdorf, R.L., Jr., & Spicer, P.P. (1983). *The legal rights of handicapped persons: Cases, materials, and
   text, 1983 supplement.* Baltimore: Paul H. Brookes Publishing Co.

Brings Burgdorf's 1980 work up to date as of 1983.

Frolick, D. (1979). Estate planning. *University of Pittsburgh Law Review, 40,* 305–357.

Comprehensive article on estate planning. Earliest comprehensive article on the matter, and to date, the
best. Discusses the nature of private and public assets available to a family, including Social Security. Describes how to put together a package of private and public benefits by using carefully drawn Trusts. Discusses some of the legal perils that Trusts may face. Focuses primarily on Pennsylvania law. Useful to lawyers
and other estate planners in all states.

Fruge, D.L., & Green, K.O. (1982). *Estate planning for retarded persons and their families.* Oxford: Mississippi Law Research Institute, University of Mississippi Law Center. No price given.

Discusses guardianship and other legal procedures for providing for personal and financial care of person with mental retardation. Tied closely to Mississippi law, but the considerations concerning guardianship apply to families in all states. Complete discussion of federal benefit programs, techniques of estate planning, Wills and Trusts, life insurance, annuities, and Trusts to benefit future generations. Sets out sample Trust provisions. Contains good resource guide for further information. Useful for lay persons and professionals (lawyers and financial planners).

Holdren, D.P. (1985). *Financial planning for the handicapped.* Springfield, IL: Charles C Thomas.

Comprehensive description of the use of all possible financial planning tools and strategies, including finance, investments, health and disability insurance, life insurance, federal taxation, Social Security benefits, retirement income and expenses, fundamentals of estate planning, and Wills and Trusts. Useful for experienced financial planners.

Human Development Program and University Affiliated Facility. (1983). *A guide to federal benefits and programs for adults with developmental disabilities.* Lexington: University of Kentucky. No price given.

Describes major federal programs providing financial benefits, directly or indirectly, for people with disabilities. Contains descriptions of programs in community development, education and rehabilitation, employment, income assistance, housing support services, research, staff development, and rights in public education. Each program description contains statement of program objective, uses and restrictions on funds, eligibility, application procedures, federal agency jurisdiction, whom to contact, and statutory authorization. Useful in determining what federal programs might be available. Best used by person familiar with benefits packaging.

Massay, J. (1981). Protecting the mentally incompetent child's trust interest from state reimbursement claims. *Denver Law Journal, 58,* 557–566.

Primarily discusses Colorado law, but also that of other states on how to use a Trust to provide private funds to a person with a disability while preventing a state from requiring the Trust to be used to support a person with a disability who receives care from the state. Useful to lawyers.

Russell, L.M. (1983). *Alternatives: A family guide to legal and financial planning for the disabled.* Evanston, IL: First Publications. No price given.

Discusses guardianship and multiple considerations families must face in deciding whether to seek guardianship. Uses hypothetical families to illustrate considerations. Contains sample court forms for use in guardianship in Cook County, Illinois. Contains good advice on how to work with lawyers on guardianship proceedings. Presents useful information on Wills, Trusts, government benefits, taxes, insurance, and financial planning (investments). Useful for lay persons and professionals (lawyers, financial planners).

Sales, B.S., Powell, D.H., & Van Duizend, R. (1982). *Disabled persons and the law: State legislative issues.* New York: Plenum.

Contains model statutes for states in areas of guardianship, among others. Explains legal issues involved in guardianship, cites relevant judicial decisions, proposes model state law on guardianship, and gives rationale for proposed model law. Useful primarily to lawyers.

Townsend, M.G. (1980). Avoiding an unwanted invasion of trust. *Albany Law Review, 45,* 237–259.

Primarily discusses New York law, but also that of other states, on how to use a Trust to provide funds to a person with a disability while preventing a state from requiring the Trust to be used to support a person with a disability who receives care from the state. Useful to lawyers.

SOCIAL-INTERPERSONAL

Cornelius, D.A., Chipouras, S., Makas, E., & Daniels, S.M. (1982). *Who cares?: A handbook on sex education and counseling services for disabled people* (2nd ed.). Baltimore: University Park Press. $18.50.

An excellent resource for professionals and family members interested in the socio-sexual needs of people with disabilities. Procedures for identifying the educational needs of people with disabilities concerning sexuality are thoroughly explained. Options for delivering counseling and education are discussed, along with methods for evaluating results. Issues surrounding the establishment of service agency policies in the area of sexuality are also discussed. The resource sections at the back of the book list organizations and other reference materials addressing socio-sexuality and people with a disability.

Foxx, R., & McMorrow, M. (1983). *Stacking the deck: A social skills game for retarded adults.* Champaign, IL: Research Press. $19.95.

The teaching model presented relies on a game format that can enhance attention to relevant social skills issues for people with disabilities. It targets professionals, paraprofessionals, and family members as teachers of people with disabilities. New skills can be taught and existing skills can be refined using the innovative game approach. Targeted skills are broken into three broad categories: general social skills, social/vocational skills, and social/sexual skills.

Haavik, S.F., & Menninger, K.A. (1981). *Sexuality, law, and the developmentally disabled person: Legal and clinical aspects of marriage, parenthood, and sterilization.* Baltimore: Paul H. Brookes Publishing Co.

A comprehensive text that deals with the spectrum of issues relating to sexual needs and the expression of those needs by people with disabilities. The issues, many of which are highly complicated, are explained from clinical and legal perspectives. Options in the areas of marriage, procreation, and sterilization are described. Policy issues and personal rights are investigated in detail. This is a must reference for professionals dealing with the adult needs of people with disabilities.

Schleien, S.J., & Ray, M.T. (1988). *Community recreation and persons with disabilities: Strategies for integration.* Baltimore: Paul H. Brookes Publishing Company. $25.95.

This publication specifically addresses the recreation and leisure needs of people with disabilities. Following a brief historical overview of the progress of community-based recreation programs, the authors quickly proceed to the nitty-gritty of evaluating individual needs, establishing integrated programs, and monitoring effectiveness. Numerous survey and evaluation instruments that can help identify such things as ecological and personal barriers to successful programs, skill deficits, and personal preferences are offered. This is an excellent text that would be useful to a wide range of professionals as well as family members.

Valletutti, P., & Bender, M. (1982). *Teaching interpersonal and community living skills.* Austin, TX: PRO-ED. $21.00.

Describes a model for teaching interpersonal and community living skills to adolescents and adults with developmental disabilities. The model presented can be easily tailored to individual needs. The skills are addressed to the individual's role as a worker, consumer, resident, citizen, learner, and participant in community life. A useful resource for both professional and nonprofessional audiences.

Wehman, P., & Schleien, S. (1981). *Leisure programs for handicapped persons.* Austin, TX: PRO-ED. $21.00.

Explores the recreational and leisure needs of children, adolescents, and adults with a disability. Many practical models for developing individualized recreational programs are described. A reference that can be used easily by both professional and nonprofessional audiences.

RESIDENTIAL

Bruininks, R.H., Hill, B.K., Lakin, K.C., & White, C. (1985). *Residential services for adults with developmental disabilities.* Logan: Utah State University, Developmental Center for Handicapped Persons. $10.00.

This technical report represents the cooperative efforts of several nationally renowned researchers and practitioners in the provision of residential services to people with disabilities. The report addresses the historical evolution of service delivery and provides an introduction to the philosophical principles underpinning residential services for people with disabilities. The different models of residential options currently available are described along with data indicating the prevalence of the models. A number of exemplary programs across the nation are featured. Unique aspects of these state-of-the-art programs are identified. One chapter is devoted to describing barriers to residential services, and the following chapter offers recommendations to service professionals and policymakers to overcome barriers and establish programs that meet individual and family needs. Although primarily for a professional audience, this book is very readable, and of value to parents and other family members.

Fifield, M., & Smith, B. (1985). *Personnel training for serving adults with developmental disabilities.* Logan: Utah State University, Developmental Center for Handicapped Persons. $12.50.

An excellent review of the personnel training needs of the adult services system. The book offers the central premise that expanding existing options depends on the availability of properly trained staff. It then describes training strategies that are appropriate for residential staff as well as for personnel who will work in other areas in the adult service field. One chapter is devoted to the training needs of parents and others in advocacy roles.

Halpern, A.S., Close, D.W., & Nelson, D.J. (1986). *On my own: The impact of semi-independent living programs for adults with mental retardation.* Baltimore: Paul H. Brookes Publishing Co. $16.95.

This book provides a detailed study of more than 300 adults with mental retardation who live in semi-independent residential programs in four states. The book reports individual cases, providing an insight into the needs, successes, and failures of real people. The issues surrounding residential services are honestly and sensitively reviewed. Must reading for adult service providers and suggested reading for families and advocates. The language at times tends to be technical, but the warmth generated by the people it studies makes this book highly readable for most audiences.

Janicki, M.P., Krauss, M.W., & Seltzer, M.M. (Eds.). (1987). *Community residences for persons with developmental disabilities: Here to stay.* Baltimore: Paul H. Brookes Publishing Co. $39.95.

Provides practical answers to questions about the successful management of community residences. Provides an in-depth look at administrative duties, staff training, liability and safety, and other issues that affect residential management decisions.

Summers, J.A., & Reese, R.M. (1986). Residential services. In J.A. Summers (Ed.), *The right to grow up: An introduction to adults with developmental disabilities* (pp. 119–148). Baltimore: Paul H. Brookes Publishing Co. $21.95.

Provides a comprehensive overview of residential services for people with disabilities. Begins with a review of the historical foundations of the move from large institutional settings to small community facilities that meet residential needs. The chapter proceeds to describe the range of individual needs that residential programs must address. Finally, different residential models are described. The framework used in this chapter to organize residential models is the basis for the organizational framework used in this book, which makes this chapter particularly consistent with the information offered in this book.

EMPLOYMENT

Barnett, S.S., & Smith, A.M. (Eds.). (1986). *Employment options for young adults with deaf-blindness.* New York: Helen Keller National Center, Technical Assistance Center. $15.00.

This publication contains contributions from leading professionals in the field of transition. The emphasis is on people who have deaf-blindness disabilities. People providing services to this population will find a wealth of information and practical suggestions that can be used in adult service programs. Among the issues addressed are the coordination of strategies, behavior problems and proposed interventions, vocational training strategies, and policy analysis. This is possibly the best single resource specifically about people with deaf-blindness.

Bellamy, G.T., Rhodes, L.E., Mank, D.M., & Albin, J.M. (1988). *Supported employment: A community implementation guide.* Baltimore: Paul H. Brookes Publishing Co. $19.95.

Provides practical advice on how to implement supported work programs, and describes the perspectives and needs of each party involved in the development and maintenance of these programs: local service providers, parents, professional staff, public agencies, teachers, and employers.

Chadsey-Rusch, J., Hanley-Maxwell, C., Phelps, L.A., & Rusch, F.R. (1986). *School-to-work transition issues and models.* Champaign: University of Illinois, Transition Institute at Illinois. $6.50.

Investigates the barriers encountered by people with disabilities in their transition to work settings from an innovative angle—the premise presented is that systems and not individuals cause problems. The four sections of this book present strong recommendations on how to deal with system problems. Section II, which investigates job termination causes, is insightful and exciting reading. In less than 100 pages, the authors capture the essence of the changes needed for successful transitions to employment by people with disabilities.

Harnish, D.L., Chaplin, C.C., Fisher, A.T., & Tu, J. (1987). *Transition literature review on educational, employment, and independent living options.* Champaign: University of Illinois, Transition Institute at Illinois.

Thoroughly reviews current literature on transition issues affecting adolescents and adults with disabilities. Organized in an easy-to-follow conceptual framework. The annotated bibliographies will be of value to adult service providers and interested researchers. This is a tremendously important work by a group of researchers at the vanguard of the field.

Mcloughlin, C.S., Garner, J.B., & Callahan, M.T. (1987). *Getting employed, staying employed: Job development and training for persons with severe handicaps.* Baltimore: Paul H. Brookes Publishing Company. $22.95.

This is a step-by-step "how to" manual for those interested in developing and maintaining community-based employment opportunities for people with disabilities. In Section I, the authors make a convincing argument against traditional sheltered and segregated work programs for people and document the appropriateness of pursuing supported and competitive employment models. Section II describes the process of developing new jobs from initial planning, to obtaining an appointment with prospective employers, to negotiating for placements. Section III offers advice on the training of prospective employees, ongoing assessment, and long-term monitoring. Professionals, potential employers, and interested family members will find this a valuable resource.

Moon, S., Goodall, P., Barcus, M., & Brooke, V. (Eds.). (1985). *The supported work model of competitive employment for citizens with severe handicaps: A guide for job trainers.* Richmond: Virginia Commonwealth University, Rehabilitation Research and Training Center. $9.00.

This book is written for direct service staff working with people with disabilities in vocational programs. It addresses job development, placement strategies, on-site job training techniques, and follow-up services. The target for job placements are existing industries and businesses furthering integration in community settings. Useful forms for documentation purposes are provided along with a detailed resource section. The straightforward language and innovative suggestions make this an excellent resource for a general audience.

Rusch, F.R. (Ed.). (1986). *Competitive employment issues and strategies.* Baltimore: Paul H. Brookes Publishing Co. $36.00.

Offers 24 chapters by leading experts in the field of vocational options for people with disabilities. The first chapter reviews the obstacles to competitive employment and offers procedures for overcoming them. Descriptions of successful competitive programs in five settings are presented in the subsequent chapters in Section I. Section II thoroughly explores state-of-the-art methodology for establishing successful vocational programs. Section III looks at issues that affect successful job placements, such as support networks, consumer satisfaction, personnel training, and parent and family involvement. This is the definitive text on competitive employment issues.

Wehman, P. (1981). *Competitive employment: New horizons for severely disabled individuals.* Baltimore: Paul H. Brookes Publishing Co. $18.50.

Explores the issue of employment for people with severe disabilities in community settings, rather than traditional sheltered programs. Procedures for successful training, placement, and support are described. Public perceptions are discussed in detail and recommendations for influencing the community at large are offered. Several model programs are described that provide information that is useful to both family members and professionals.

Wehman, P., Moon, M.S., Everson, J.M., Wood, W., & Barcus, J.M. (1988). *Transition from school to work: New challenges for youth with severe disabilites.* Baltimore: Paul H. Brookes Publishing Co. $23.95.

Paul Wehman has been a forceful leader in research efforts and program development in the area of vocational opportunities for people with disabilities. In this book, Wehman and his colleagues offer an in-depth look at the world of work and people with disabilities. Model vocational programs from across the country are described and conceptual models for delivering services are offered. One chapter is devoted to parent-professional roles and responsibilities, and strategies for building strong partnerships are presented. The book is geared toward a professional audience. A truly important resource for those working with people with disabilities who are transitioning from the education system to the adult world.

ADVOCACY

Bronicki, G.J., & Turnbull, A.P. (1987). Family-professional interactions. In M. Snell (Ed.), *Systematic instruction of persons with severe handicaps* (pp. 7–35). Columbus, OH: Charles E. Merrill. $33.95.

Provides an overview of family systems theory and parental rights under the Education for All Handicapped Children Act. The information provided in this chapter can help parents and other family members deal with school system professionals in the individualized education program process for students in special education. Understanding individual rights and acting on them is a key element of advocating within established systems. Education professionals are provided with a view of the students within the context of the family. Armed with common knowledge, families and professionals can form true partnerships to address common goals.

Gardner, N.E.S. (1980). *The self-advocacy workbook.* Lawrence: The University of Kansas, Kansas University Affiliated Facility. $13.00.

Intended to be used by people with disabilities who are interested in developing skills needed to be self-advocates. Introduces the "road" concepts behind the self-advocacy movement and in subsequent chapters provides suggestions aimed at helping people form their own self-advocacy groups. The issues covered include: forming a group, running meetings, choosing advisors, developing group goals, getting community support, and formal incorporation procedures. The book is presented in a large-print format but the language level may make it inappropriate for some people. In these cases, others with higher reading skills could be called on to help.

Goldfarb, L., Brotherson, M.J., Summers, J.A., & Turnbull, A.P. (1986). *Meeting the challenge of disability or chronic illness: A family guide.* Baltimore: Paul H. Brookes Publishing Co. $14.95.

This book addresses family coping mechanisms. It reviews the wide array of daily family needs, and provides a detailed description of a practical problem-solving process. The six-step process described can be used by families in a myriad of situations. Advocacy entails identifying problems that may exist in current programs or services, and taking action to affect change. This book can be a valuable aid to family members in their advocacy efforts within existing systems and when engaged in activities aimed at establishing alternative options.

Turnbull, H.R. (Ed.). (1978). *The consent handbook.* Washington: American Association on Mental Deficiency. $9.00.

An exhaustive review of the legal and ethical issues surrounding consent and people with disabilities. The components needed for legal consent are presented and everyday examples are offered for further clarification. The text is useful for legal professionals as well as family member in planning for the adult futures of people who may not be competent to provide consent in all life areas. The book represents a valuable resource for people considering guardianship for a relative or friend with a disability.

Turnbull, H.R. (Ed.). (1981). *The least restrictive alternative: Principles and practices.* Washington, DC: American Association on Mental Deficiency. $3.75.

A comprehensive review of an important and often misunderstood principle is presented in a manner that renders this book useful to a wide array of professionals and family members. The editor and other contributors trace the historical development of the least restrictive alternative (LRA) principle and provide the reader with references for further study. The impact of the LRA principle on the lives of people with disabilities in various settings is discussed. Recommendations for policy changes are also offered.

Turnbull, H.R. (1986). *Free appropriate public education.* Denver: Love Publishing. $34.95.

A comprehensive review of the issues surrounding the education of students with disabilities is presented. The text is divided into four sections. Section I offers an introduction to the American judicial system and a historic overview of the education of students with disabilities. Section II outlines the major principles of federal legislation dealing with the education of students with disabilities. Section III deals with enforcement efforts, and Section IV views education within the context of the American value system. The text provides references to pertinent case law and statutes.

Turnbull, H.R., & Turnbull, A.P. (Eds.) (1985). *Parents speak out: Then and now.* Columbus, OH: Charles E. Merrill. $12.95.

This book is a follow-up to the first edition, which consisted of personal essays by parents and other family members describing real life events dealing with their sons, daughters, and relatives with disabilities. This edition presents the original stories first published in 1978, along with essays describing the successes and failures experienced years later. Three new personal stories are also added. This is a book written by parents, but the target audience is not limited to parents. Professionals and nonfamily members working in the field of disabilities will find this real life acount worthwhile also.

Tymchuk, A.J. (1985). Effective decision making for the developmentally disabled. Portland, OR: EDNICK. $15.95.

The book describes a detailed curriculum for teaching decision-making skills to people with mental disabilities. May be used by family members, teachers, or adult service providers. It details teaching strategies that have proven successful with a wide range of people in a variety of situations. The book provides detailed worksheets that enable teachers to track the progress of their students. Teaching decision-making to people with disabilities enables them to assume greater control of their lives and enhance life's quality. While some may find the book's language too technical, it represents one of the few such texts addressing an important life skill.

Williams, P., & Shoultz, B. (1982). *We can speak for ourselves.* London: Souvenir Press. $10.95

The first part of this book offers a thorough review of the history of the self-advocacy movement in this country. The general principles of self-advocacy are described and its goals are discussed. Considerable attention and space is given to suggestions for organizing and sustaining local self-advocacy groups. The self-advocacy movement in Great Britain is surveyed in later chapters. It becomes clearly evident that people with disabilities share common aspirations for their lives in the community. The appendices provide valuable how-to, step-by-step hints that can be used in all aspects of self-advocacy. This book is must reading for people interested in empowerment for people with disabilities.

appendix six
SAMPLE ENABLING DOCUMENTS FOR FAMILY-DIRECTED AGENCIES

ARTICLES OF INCORPORATION
OF
FULL CITIZENSHIP, INC.

We, the undersigned, being natural persons of the age of 21 years or more, for the purpose of forming a nonprofit corporation under the General Corporation Code of Kansas, do hereby adopt the following Articles of Incorporation.

Article I

The name of the corporation is FULL CITIZENSHIP, INC.

Article II

The address of the corporation's registered office in Kansas is 1560 Alvamar Drive, Lawrence, Kansas 66046, in Douglas County, Kansas. The telephone number is (913) 841-1989.

Article III

The name of the corporation's registered agent at the address of its registered office is H. Rutherford Turnbull, III.

Article IV

This corporation is organized as a nonprofit corporation and exclusively for charitable, educational, and scientific purposes, including, among others, to develop and operate state-of-the-art, community-based, and maximally integrated vocational, residential, and social programs and services for people with mental retardation or other developmental disabilities (hereinafter, "people with disabilities") by such methods consistent with the corporation's nonprofit, charitable, educational, and scientific purposes as the directors may deem advisable from time to time, all for the purpose of securing for people with disabilities the same basic rights held by all other Americans and full citizenship in America.

No part of the net earnings, income, or assets of the corporation shall be distributed or distributable to or inure to the benefit of any individual, member, director, officer, or other private person, except that the corporation shall be authorized and empowered to pay reasonable compensation for services rendered and to make payments and distributions in furtherance of the purposes set forth in Article V hereof.

No substantial part of the corporation's activities shall consist of the carrying on of propaganda, or otherwise attempting to influence legislation; nor shall the corporation participate in, or intervene in (including the publication or distribution of statements) any political campaign on behalf of any candidate for public office.

Article V

The corporation shall have the following powers, which shall be exercised only to advance its nonprofit, charitable, educational, and scientific purposes:

1. To provide people with disabilities, regardless of their age, sex, race, color, or creed, with opportunities for the same basic rights that are held by people without disabilities. These opportunities include the rights of consent and choice consistent with those persons' inherent or augmented abilities, and opportunities for vocational, residential, and social-interpersonal services, programs, and facilities specially designed to meet their physical, educational, habilitation, medical, mental, emotional, psychological, and

behavioral needs. These services, programs, and facilities shall be based on principles of nonaversive active treatment; shall be data-based and research-validated; shall develop or replicate models and state-of-the-art services, programs, and facilities; shall develop or employ the latest technological advances relevant to such persons; shall encourage and enable research by students, staff, and faculty at the University of Kansas and at other universities or colleges in the United States or elsewhere; shall contribute to the development, use, dissemination, and evaluation of similar services, programs, or facilities throughout Kansas, other states, and other countries by other universities, colleges, service providers, associations, corporations, partnerships, other business entities, or individuals; and at all times and in all ways will be centered on and advance the quality of life of people with disabilities.

2. To apply for, receive, administer, evaluate, and do all other relevant activities associated with federal, state, or local governmental, or with privately organized corporate, foundation, association, or partnership grants, contracts, awards, fellowships, practica, stipends, or other financial benefits.

3. To enter into all necessary or desirable contracts, obligations, agreements, or other undertakings with, for, or in association with any agencies of federal, state, or local governments or with privately organized corporate, foundation, association, or partnership entities, including without limitation universities, colleges, vocational, community, or junior colleges, and public or private residential, vocational, or social-interpersonal programs for people with disabilities.

4. To do and perform all acts reasonably necessary or desirable to accomplish the purposes of the corporation, including the execution of a Regulatory Agreement or other agreements with the Secretary of the United States Department of Housing and Urban Development and the execution and delivery of such other instruments and undertakings as may be necessary to enable the corporation to secure the benefits of financing under Sections 8 or 202 of the Housing Act of 1959 as amended. Such Regulatory Agreements and other instruments and undertakings shall remain binding upon the corporation, its successors, and assigns so long as mortgage on the corporation's property is held by the Secretary of Housing and Urban Development.

5. To enter into regulatory or any other agreements with the Secretaries or any other officials of any department or agency of the United States or of any agency of any state or local government, including without limitation the United States Department of Housing, the United States Department of Health and Human Services, the United States Department of Education, the United States Department of Labor, the Kansas Department of Social and Rehabilitation Services, the Kansas Department of Education, and the Kansas Department of Human Resources, with any of the National Institutes, such as the National Institute of Health, National Institute of Disability and Rehabilitation Research, National Institute on Stroke and Communicative Disorders, and with any other governmental or quasigovernmental departments, agencies, bureaus, or entities, and with the successors, assigns, or designees of any of the aforesaid entities.

6. To encourage and enable students at the University of Kansas to engage in practica, clinical or field experiences, and in any other academic experience and training with people with disabilities.

7. To encourage and enable research to be conducted in connection with activities of the corporation, subject to the prior approval of the directors or their designees.

8. To help develop, organize, operate, fund, enable, and advance the activities of self-advocacy by individuals or groups of individuals with disabilities.

9. To create, operate, and engage in all activities necessary or desirable for the creation of a system of personal or financial limited or plenary guardianship, including congregate guardianship or conservatorship, pooled financial trusteeship, or other advocacy, on behalf of people with disabilities.

10. To work closely with parents, siblings, other relatives, and friends of people with disabilities in carrying out activities of the corporation and, by such activities as the directors from time to time may deem appropriate, to develop, organize, operate, fund, enable, and advance parental, sibling, and other relational activities that carry out the purposes of the corporation, including, among others, activities that sponsor parent, sibling, peer, and teacher awards.

11. To work with public and private preschools, and elementary, junior high, and high schools in carrying out the purpose of the corporation.

12. To solicit, receive, or manage general or special donations, bequests, gifts, devises, or legacies, for the purposes of carrying out the corporation's activities.

13. To charge fees for services rendered or to be rendered.

14. To enter into fee-for-services contracts with federal, state, or local governmental authorities.

15. To enter into any desirable or necessary contracts, obligations, agreements, or other undertakings with any corporations, associations, partnerships, or other business entities, whether profit or non-profit, and with any individuals, that relate in any way to the employment of people with disabilities.

16. To borrow money and issue evidence of indebtedness in furtherance of any or all of the objects of its business and to secure the same by mortgage, pledge, or other lien on the corporation's property.

17. To buy, own, sell, assign, mortgage, or lease any interest in real or personal property, and to construct, maintain, and operate improvements thereon necessary or incident to the accomplishment of the purposes as set forth in the Articles of Incorporation and all amendments thereto.

18. To purchase, receive, take by gift, devise, or bequest, or otherwise acquire, and to own, hold, retain, use, improve, lease as lessor or lessee, manage, operate, control, sell, exchange, convey, assign, and

otherwise dispose of, encumber, affect, or deal in and with any real or personal property, or any interest therein, situated within or without the State of Kansas, as may be necessary and proper for carrying on its legitimate affairs.

19. To borrow money in furtherance of any or all of the objects of its business, to make and issue notes, bonds and other evidences of such indebtedness, and to secure the same by mortgage, deed of trust, pledge, or other lien or encumberance upon any part or all of its real or personal property.

20. To issue, execute, draw, accept, discount, pledge, sell, exchange, or otherwise deal in or dispose of promissory notes, drafts, bills of exchange, warrants, bonds, debentures, and other negotiable or non-negotiable instruments and evidences of indebtedness, whether secured or unsecured.

21. To acquire and take over as a going concern and thereafter to carry on the business of any person, firm, association, corporation, or other entity whose business this corporation is authorized to conduct.

22. To acquire, by subscription, purchase, contract, or otherwise, and to sell, exchange, mortgage, pledge, and otherwise dispose of or turn to account the stocks, bonds, debentures, obligations, and other securities of every character and description, issued or created by any corporation or other entity, whether or not engaged in any business which this corporation is authorized to conduct, or by any federal, state, or local government, whether domestic or foreign, and to exercise any and all rights, powers, and privileges of individual ownership or interest in respect of any and all such securities, including the right to vote thereon and to consent and otherwise act with respect thereto.

23. To lend and advance money or give credit to any person, firm, or corporation, with or without security.

24. To make donations in furtherance of any of its purposes.

25. To belong to, join, or otherwise participate in and with, as a member or sponsor or in any other capacity, in any category of membership or sponsorship or otherwise, any voluntary professional, parent/family, or self-advocacy association, corporation, partnership, or other business entity, whether organized for profit or not, in the field of disabilities, in the United States or any other country.

26. To assess regular or special dues, subscriptions, assessments, levies, or charges against its members in such amounts and at such times as its directors may deem appropriate and to create, amend, or terminate any classifications of membership as its directors may deem appropriate, all without limitation.

27. To engage in any lawful act or activity for which nonprofit corporations may be organized under the Kansas General Corporation Code to effect any or all of the purposes for which the corporation is organized.

PROVIDED, however, that:

1) The corporation shall not have or exercise any power or authority either expressly, by interpretation, or by operation of law, nor shall it engage directly or indirectly in any activity, that would prevent the corporation from qualifying and continuing to qualify as an organization described in Section 501(c)(3) of the Internal Revenue Code, as amended.

2) The corporation shall never be operated for the primary purpose of carrying on a business or trade for profit.

3) No compensation, reimbursement, or payment shall ever be paid to any member, officer, director, trustee, creditor, or organizer of this corporation, or to any substantial contributor to it, except as an allowance for actual expenditures or services actually made or rendered to or for the corporation; and neither the whole nor any portion of the net earnings or assets of the corporation shall ever be distributed to or divided among such persons.

4) In the event of the dissolution of the corporation, the resolution of its affairs, or other liquidation of its assets, the corporation's property shall not be conveyed to any organization created or operated for profit or to any individual for less than the fair market value of such property, and all assets remaining after the payment of the corporation's debts shall be conveyed or distributed only to an organization or organizations created and operated for nonprofit purposes similar to those of the corporation; PROVIDED, however, that the corporation shall at all times have the power to convey any and all of its property to the Secretary of Housing and Urban Development or other valid lienholder, mortgage, trustee, or pledgee.

Article VI

The category into which this corporation's activities are to fall, so far as its activities are concerned, is that which is defined by Section 501(c)(3) of the Internal Revenue Code, as amended.

Article VII

This corporation shall not have authority to issue capital stock, but in lieu of stockholders the corporation shall have members, according to the terms and conditions therefor set forth in bylaws.

Article VIII

All members of the corporation shall have equal voting rights and there are no limitations on the voting rights of any of the members.

Article IX

The names and addresses of the incorporators are:

Susan A. Fowler
2708 Stone Barn Terrace
Lawrence, Kansas 66046

Jean Ann Summers
441 Michigan Street
Lawrence, Kansas 66044

Jerry T. Hannah
3200 Riverview Drive
Lawrence, Kansas 66044

Ann P. Turnbull
1560 Alvamar Drive
Lawrence, Kansas 66046

Jan Sheldon
1701 Tennessee Street
Lawrence, Kansas 66044

H. Rutherford Turnbull, III
1560 Alvamar Drive
Lawrence, Kansas 66046

Article X

The first board of directors shall consist of the following persons, who shall be vested with the power and authority to adopt the initial bylaws of the corporation and who shall hold office until their successors are duly elected and qualified, all as provided in the bylaws. Thereafter, the number of directors shall be as specified in the bylaws and the directors shall be elected or appointed in the manner and for the terms stipulated in the bylaws.

The names and addresses of the persons constituting the first board of directors are:

Benjamin Behr
2804 Tomahawk Drive
Lawrence, Kansas 66046

Jean Ann Summers
441 Michigan Street
Lawrence, Kansas 66044

Susan A. Fowler
2708 Stone Barn Terrace
Lawrence, Kansas 66046

Ann P. Turnbull
1560 Alvamar Drive
Lawrence, Kansas 66046

Jerry T. Hannah
3200 Riverview Drive
Lawrence, Kansas 66044

H. Rutherford Turnbull, III
1560 Alvamar Drive
Lawrence, Kansas 66046

Jan Sheldon
1701 Tennessee Street
Lawrence, Kansas 66044

The directors and board of directors shall have all powers granted by Kansas law and statutes.

Article XI

Each director and officer of the corporation shall be indemnified by the corporation against all reasonable costs and expenses, including counsel fees, actually and necessarily incurred by or imposed upon him or her or her estate in connection with the defense of any action, suit, or proceeding to which he or she shall be made a party by reason of his or her being or having been a director or officer of the corporation (whether or not he or she continues to be a director or officer at the time when such costs or expenses are incurred), except in relation to any matter as to which he or she shall be adjudged in any such action, suit, or proceeding, without such judgment being reversed, to have been liable for negligence or misconduct in the performance of his or her duties as such director or officer. In the event of the settlement of any such action, suit, or proceeding prior to the final judgment, the corporation shall also make reimbursement for payment of the costs, expenses, and amounts paid or to be paid in settling any such action, suit, or proceeding which such settlement appears to be in the interests of the corporation in the opinion of the majority of the directors who are not involved, or, if all are involved, in the opinion of independent legal counsel selected by the board of directors. No director or officer of the corporation shall be liable to any other director or officer or other person for any action taken or refused to be taken by him or her as director or officer with respect to any matter within the scope of his or her official duty except such action or neglect or failure to act as shall constitute negligence or misconduct in the performance of his or her duties as director or officer.

To the maximum extent allowed by law, members of the corporation shall have no personal liability for corporate debts or for other actions of the corporation that cause or may cause liability to the corporation.

Article XII

The term for which this corporation is to exist is perpetual.

IN WITNESS WHEREOF, we have hereunto subscribed our names this ____ day of January, 1987.

Susan A. Fowler
Susan A. Fowler

Jean Ann Summers
Jean Ann Summers

Jerry T. Hannah
Jerry T. Hannah

Ann P. Turnbull
Ann P. Turnbull

Jan Sheldon
Jan Sheldon

H. Rutherford Turnbull III
H. Rutherford Turnbull, III

STATE OF KANSAS))
) SS:
COUNTY OF DOUGLAS))

On this, the 13th day of January, 1987, there personally appeared before me, the undersigned, a Notary Public, in and for the State of Kansas, Douglas County, the above named, Susan A. Fowler, Jerry T. Hannah, Jan Sheldon, Jean Ann Summers, Ann P. Turnbull, and H. Rutherford Turnbull, III, who are personally known to me to be the same persons who executed the foregoing written Articles of Incorporation of Full Citizenship, Inc., and they duly acknowledged the execution of the same.

IN TESTIMONY WHEREOF, I have hereunto subscribed my name and affixed my official seal this the 13th day of January, 1987.

Mary Beth Johnston
Notary Public

[SEAL]

My appointment expires: 3/30, 19 90.

BYLAWS FOR
FULL CITIZENSHIP, INC.

Article 1

Offices

Section 1. *Principal Office.* The principal office for the transaction of the business of the corporation is hereby located at 1560 Alvamar Drive, Lawrence, Kansas 66046.

Section 2. *Registered Office.* The corporation, by resolution of its board of directors, may change the location of its registered office as designated in the Articles of Incorporation to any other place in Kansas. By like resolution, the resident agent at such registered office may be changed to any other person or corporation, including itself. Upon adoption of such a resolution, a certificate certifying the change shall be executed, acknowledged, and filed with the Secretary of State, and a certified copy thereof shall be recorded in the office of the Register of Deeds for the county in which the new registered office is located (and in the old county, if such registered office is moved from one county to another).

Section 3. *Other Offices.* Branch or subordinate offices may at any time be established by the board of directors at any place or places where the corporation is qualified to do business.

Article II

Membership

Section 1. *Membership.* Members shall be selected from the general public by a majority vote of a quorum at an annual or special meeting of the directors. Initial members shall be selected by a majority vote of the directors.

Members shall be individuals who are committed to and actively engaged in activities that advance the purposes of the corporation as set out in the Articles of Incorporation.

All members are voting members unless otherwise specified in the Articles of Incorporation.

Section 2. *Application for Membership.* Applications for membership shall be made in the manner prescribed by the board of directors. Honorary memberships shall be determined under terms and conditions as specified by resolution of the board of directors.

Section 3. *Resignation From Membership.* A resignation from membership shall be presented to the board of directors, but shall not relieve any member from any liability for any dues, assessments, or other obligations to the corporation which are unpaid at the time such resignation is filed or which may arise prior to the acceptance of the resignation.

Section 4. *Termination or Suspension.* If any member of the corporation shall commit any act prejudicial to the conduct of the affairs of the corporation or the purposes for which it is formed, or shall have changed his or her status so as to be ineligible for membership, such person shall be notified in writing to appear personally before the board of directors at a designated time not less than thirty (30) days after such notification and, at such time, be given a hearing. By a majority vote of all the directors present at the meeting, the membership of such person in the corporation may be terminated or suspended. Suspension is not appropriate where the person has ceased to be a person in the category of persons eligible for membership. If either suspension or termination is decided upon, the terms and conditions of same shall be specified in writing and delivered to the suspended or terminated member.

Written notices hereunder shall be delivered by registered mail to the member's last known address.

Section 5. *Transfer of Memberships.* Memberships in the corporation shall be nontransferrable. There shall be no transfer or alienation by inter vivos or testamentary device otherwise.

Section 6. *Fines and Penalties.* Fines or penalties are not permitted. The penalty for misconduct is suspension or termination as provided above.

Section 7. *Place of Meetings.* All annual meetings of members and all other meetings of members shall be held at the principal office of the corporation unless another place within or without the State of Kansas is designated either by the board of directors pursuant to authority hereinafter granted to said board, or by the written consent of all members entitled to vote thereat, given either before or after the meeting and filed with the secretary of the corporation.

Section 8. *Meetings of Voting Members and Other Membership Matters.* The annual meetings of the voting members shall be held on the 20th day of December, in each year at 10 a.m. of said day; provided, however, that should said day fall upon a Saturday or Sunday, then such annual meeting of voting members shall be held at the same time and place on the Friday preceding such designated meeting date. At such meeting, directors shall be elected, reports of the affairs of the corporation shall be considered, and any other business may be transacted which is within the power of the members.

Written notice of each annual meeting shall be given to each member entitled to vote, either personally or by mail or other means of written communication, charges prepaid, addressed to such member at his address appearing on the books of the corporation or given by him to the corporation for the purpose of notice. If a member gives no address, notice shall be deemed to have been given if sent by mail or other means or written communication addressed to the place where the principal office of the corporation is situated, or if published at least once in some newspaper of general circulation in the county in which said office is located. All such notices shall be sent to each member entitled thereto not less than ten (10) days nor more than fifty (50) days before each annual meeting, and shall specify the place, the day and the hour of such meeting, and shall state such other matters, if any, as may be expressly required by statute. If this bylaw as to the time and place of election of directors is changed, such notice shall be given to members at least twenty (20) days prior to such meeting.

Section 9. *Special Meetings.* Special meetings of the members, for any purpose or purposes whatsoever, may be called at any time by the president or by the board of directors, or by one or more members holding not less than one-fifth of the voting power of the corporation. Except in special cases where other express provision is made by statute, notice of such special meetings shall be given in the same manner as for annual meetings of members. Notices of any special meeting shall specify the place, day, and hour of such meeting, and the general nature of the business to be transacted.

Section 10. *Voting.* Unless the board of directors has fixed in advance by resolution a record date for purposes of determining entitlement to vote at the meeting, the record date for such determination shall be as of the close of business on the day next preceding the date on which the meeting shall be held. Such vote may be *viva voce* or by ballot; provided, however, that all elections for directors must be by ballot upon demand made by a member at any election and before the voting begins. Each voting member shall have one (1) vote for directors and all other matters which may properly come before the members at any annual or special meeting.

Section 11. *Quorum.* The presence in person or by proxy of a majority of voting members shall constitute a quorum for the transaction of business. The voting members present at a duly called or held meeting at which a quorum is present may continue to do business until adjournment, notwithstanding the withdrawal of enough voting members to leave less than a quorum.

Section 12. *Consent of Absentees.* The transactions of any meeting of members, either annual or special, however called and noticed, shall be as valid as though had at a meeting duly held after regular call and notice, if a quorum be present either in person or by proxy, and if, either before or after the meeting, each of the members entitled to vote, not present in person or by proxy, signs a written waiver of notice, or a consent to the holding of such meeting, or an approval of the minutes thereof. All such waivers, consents, or approvals shall be filed with the corporate records or made a part of the minutes of the meeting.

Section 13. *Proxies.* Every person entitled to vote or execute consents shall have the right to do so either in person or by one or more agents authorized by a written proxy executed by such person and filed with the secretary of the corporation; provided that no such proxy shall be valid after the expiration of six (6) months from the date of its execution, unless the person executing it specifies therein the length of time for which such proxy is to continue in force.

Section 14. *Inspection of Corporate Records.* The membership ledger, the books of account, and minutes of proceedings of the members, the board of directors, and of executive committees of directors shall be open to inspection upon the written demand of any member within five (5) days of such demand during ordinary business hours if for a purpose reasonably related to his interests as a member. A list of members entitled to vote shall be exhibited at any reasonable time and at meetings of the members when required by the demand of any member at least twenty (20) days prior to the meeting. Such inspection may be made in person or by an agent or attorney authorized in writing by a member, and shall include the right to make abstracts. Demand of inspection other than a members' meeting shall be made in writing to the president or secretary of the corporation.

Section 15. *Inspection of Bylaws.* The corporation shall keep in its principal office for the transaction of business the original or a copy of these bylaws as amended or otherwise altered to date, certified by the secretary, which shall be open to inspection by the members at all reasonable times during ordinary business hours.

Article III

Directors

Section 1. *Powers.* Subject to limitations of the Articles of Incorporation, and of the Kansas Corporation Code as to action which shall be authorized or approved by the members, and subject to the duties of directors as prescribed by the bylaws, all corporate powers shall be exercised by or under the authority of, and the conduct and affairs of the corporation shall be controlled by, the board of directors. Without prejudice to such general powers, but subject to the same limitations, it is hereby expressly declared that the directors shall have the following powers, to wit:

First—To alter, amend, or repeal the bylaws of the corporation.

Second—To select and remove all the other officers, agents, and employees of the corporation, prescribe such powers and duties for them as may not be inconsistent with law or with the Articles of Incorporation or the bylaws, fix their compensation, and require from them security for faithful service.

Third—To conduct, manage, and control the affairs and conduct of the corporation, and to make such rules and regulations therefor not inconsistent with the law, or with the Articles of Incorporation or the bylaws, as they may deem best.

Fourth—To change the principal office and registered office for the transaction of the conduct of the corporation from one location to another as provided in Article I hereof; to fix and locate from time to time one or more subsidiary offices of the corporation within or without the State of Kansas, as provided in Article I, Section 2 hereof; to designate any place within or without the State of Kansas for the holding of any members' meeting or meetings except annual meetings; to adopt, make, and use a corporate seal, to prescribe the forms of certificates of membership, and to alter the forms of such seal and of such certificates from time to time as in their judgment they may deem best, provided such seal and such certificate shall at all times comply with the provisions of law.

Fifth—To borrow money and incur indebtedness for purposes of the corporation, and to cause to be executed and delivered therefor, in the corporate name, promissory notes, bonds, debentures, deeds of trust, mortgages, pledges, hypothecations or other evidences of debt and securities therefor.

Sixth—To appoint an executive committee and other committees, and to delegate to such committees any of the powers and authority of the board in the management of the conduct and affairs of the corporation, except the power to adopt, amend, or repeal bylaws. Any such committee shall be composed of one or more directors.

Section 2. *Number and Qualification of Directors.* The authorized number of directors of the corporation shall be not more than twenty-five (25) and not less than three (3) until changed by amendment to this bylaw. Directors must be members.

Section 3. *Election and Term of Office.* The directors shall be elected at each annual meeting of voting members, but if any such annual meeting is not held, or the directors are not elected thereat, the directors may be elected at a special meeting of voting members held for that purpose as soon thereafter as convenient. All directors shall hold office for a period of three years, and they may be re-elected to an unlimited number of successive terms, until their respective successors are elected. Directors shall serve staggered terms, the terms to be determined by lot at the September, 1987, meeting of the Board, with the then-existing directors to be elected for one-, two-, and three-year terms and their respective successors to serve for three-year terms. A director may be removed from office at any time for good cause, however, by a majority vote of the voting members, and he may be removed without cause by a two-thirds vote of the voting members.

Section 4. *Vacancies.* Vacancies of the board of directors may be filled by a majority of the remaining directors. If at any time, by reason of death, resignation, or other cause, the corporation should have no directors in office, then any officer or any member may apply to the District Court for a decree summarily ordering election as provided for by the Kansas Corporation Code. Each director so elected shall hold office until his successor is elected at an annual or special meeting of the members.

A vacancy or vacancies on the board of directors shall be deemed to exist in case of the death, resignation, or removal of any director, or if the authorized number of directors be increased, or if the members fail at any annual or special meeting of voting members at which any director or directors are elected, to elect the full authorized number of directors to be voted for at the meeting, or if any director or directors elected shall refuse to serve.

The members holding at least twenty percent (20%) of the outstanding membership certificates may call a meeting at any time to fill any vacancy or vacancies not filled by the directors, or if the board of directors filling a vacancy constitutes less than a majority of the whole board as constituted immediately prior to any increase in the number of directors. If the board of directors accepts the resignation of a director rendered to take effect at a future time, the board or the members shall have power to elect a successor to take office when the resignation is to become effective.

No reduction of the authorized number of directors shall have the effect of removing any director prior to the expiration of his term of office.

Section 5. *Place of Meeting.* Regular and special meetings of the board of directors shall be held at any place within or without the State of Kansas which has been designated from time to time by resolution of the board or by written consent of all members of the board. In the absence of such designation, all meetings shall be held at the principal office of the corporation.

Section 6. *Regular Meetings.* Immediately following each annual meeting of members, the board of directors shall hold a regular meeting for the purpose of organization, election of officers, and the transaction of other business. Notice of such meeting is hereby dispensed with.

Section 7. *Other Regular Meetings.* Other regular meetings of the board of directors shall be held without call at such time as the board of directors may from time to time designate in advance of such meeting. Notice of all such regular meetings of the board of directors is hereby dispensed with.

Section 8. *Special Meetings.* Special meetings of the board of directors for any purpose or purposes shall be called at any time by the president, or if that person is absent or unable or refuses to act, by the secretary or by any other director. Notice of such special meetings, unless waived by attendance therat or by written consent to the holding of the meeting, shall be given by written notice mailed at least twelve (12) days before the date of such meeting or be hand-delivered or notified by telegram at least ten (10) days before the date such meeting is to be held. If mailed, such notice shall be deemed to be delivered when deposited in the United States mail with postage thereon addressed to the director at his residence or usual place of business. If notice be given by telegraph, such notice shall be deemed to be delivered when the same is delivered to the telegraph company.

Section 9. *Notice of Adjournment.* Notice of the time and place of an adjourned meeting need not be given to absent directors if the time and place be fixed at the meeting adjourned.

Section 10. *Waiver of Notice.* The transactions of any meeting of the board of directors, however called and noticed or wherever held, shall be as valid as though had at a meeting duly held after regular call and notice, if a quorum be present, and if, either before or after the meeting, each of the directors not present signs a written waiver of notice, or a consent to holding such meeting, or an approval of the minutes thereof. All such waivers, consents, or approvals shall be filed with the corporate records or made a part of the minutes of the meeting.

Section 11. *Quorum.* A majority of the total number of directors shall be necessary to constitute a quorum for the transaction of business, except to adjourn as hereinafter provided. Every act or decision done or made by a majority of the directors present at a meeting duly held at which a quorum is present shall be regarded as the act of the board of directors, unless a greater number be required by law or by the Articles of Incorporation. The directors present at a duly called or held meeting at which a quorum is present may continue to do business until adjournment, notwithstanding the withdrawal of enough directors to leave less than a quorum.

Section 12. *Meetings by Telephone.* Members of the board of directors of the corporation, or any committee designated by such board, may participate in a meeting of the board of directors by means of conference telephone or similar communications equipment, by means of which all persons participating in the meeting can hear one another, and such participation in a meeting shall constitute presence in person at the meeting.

Section 13. *Adjournment.* A majority of the directors present may adjourn any directors' meeting to meet again at a stated day and hour or until the time fixed for the next regular meeting of the board.

Section 14. *Fees and Compensation.* Directors shall not receive any stated salary for their services as directors, but, by resolution of the board, adopted in advance of, or after the meeting for which payment is to be made, a fixed fee, with or without expenses of attendance, may be allowed one or more of the directors for attendance at each meeting. Nothing herein contained shall be construed to preclude any director from serving the corporation in any other capacity as an officer, agent, employee, or otherwise, and receiving compensation therefor.

Article IV

Officers

Section 1. *Officers.* The officers of the corporation shall be a president, vice president, a secretary, and a treasurer. The corporation may also have, at the discretion of the board of directors, a chairman of the board, more than one vice president, and such other officers as may be appointed in accordance with the provisions of Section 3 of this Article IV. Any number of offices may be held by the same person.

Section 2. *Election.* The officers of the corporation, except such officers as may be appointed in accordance with the provisions of Section 3 or Section 5 of this Article IV, shall be chosen annually by the board of directors, and each shall hold his office until he shall resign or shall be removed or otherwise disqualified to serve, or his successor shall be elected and qualified.

Section 3. *Subordinate Officers, Etc.* The board of directors may appoint such other officers as the conduct of the corporation may require, each of whom shall have authority and perform such duties as are provided in these bylaws or as the board of directors may from time to time specify, and shall hold office until he shall resign or shall be removed or otherwise disqualified to serve.

Section 4. *Compensation of Officers.* Officers and other employees of the corporation shall receive such salaries or other compensation as shall be determined by resolution of the board of directors, adopted in advance or after the rendering of the services, or by employment contracts entered into by the board of directors. The power to establish salaries of officers, other than the president or chairman of the board, may be delegated to the president, chairman of the board, or a committee.

Section 5. *Vacancies.* A vacancy in any office because of death, resignation, removal, disqualification, or any other cause shall be filled in the manner prescribed in these bylaws for regular appointments to such office.

Section 6. *Removal and Resignation.* Any officer may be removed, either with or without cause, by a majority of the directors at the same time in office, at any regular or special meeting of the board, or, except in case of an officer chosen by the board of directors, by any officer upon whom such power of removal may be conferred by the board of directors.

Section 7. *Chairman of the Board.* The chairman of the board, if there be such an officer, shall, if present, preside at all meetings of the board of directors, and exercise and perform such other powers and duties as may be from time to time assigned to him by the board of directors or prescribed by these bylaws.

Section 8. *President.* Subject to such supervisory powers, if any, as may be given by the board of directors to the chairman of the board, if there be such an officer, the president shall be the chief executive officer of the corporation and shall, subject to the control of the board of directors, have general supervision, direction, and control of the conduct and officers of the corporation. He shall preside at all meetings of the members and, in the absence of the chairman of the board, at all meetings of the board of directors. He shall be a nonvoting *ex officio* member of all the standing committees, including the executive committee (on which the president shall be a voting ex officio member), if any, and shall have the general powers and duties of management usually vested in the office of president of a corporation, and shall have such other powers and duties as may be prescribed by the board of directors or these bylaws.

Section 9. *Vice President.* In the absence or incapacity of the president to perform the duties of that office, the vice president or vice presidents, if there be such an officer or officers, in order of their rank as fixed by the board of directors, or if not ranked, the vice president designated by the board of directors, shall perform all the duties of the president, and when so acting shall have all the powers of, and be subject to all the restrictions upon, the president. The vice presidents shall have such other powers and perform such other duties as from time to time may be prescribed for them respectively by the board of directors or these bylaws.

Section 10. *Secretary.* The secretary shall keep, or cause to be kept, a book of minutes at the principal office or such other place as the board of directors may order, of all meetings of directors and members, with the time and place of holding, whether regular or special, and if special, how authorized, the notice thereof given, the names of those present at directors' meetings, the members present or represented at members' meetings and the proceedings thereof.

The secretary shall keep or cause to be kept at the principal office a membership list showing the names of the members and their addresses, and the number and date of membership certificates issued, and the date of suspension, termination or resignation of every membership certificate surrendered for cancellation.

The secretary shall give notice, or cause notice to be given, of all meetings of the members and of the board of directors required by these bylaws or by law to be given, and shall keep the seal of the corporation in safe custody, and shall have such other powers and perform such other duties as may be prescribed by the board of directors or these bylaws.

Section 11. *Treasurer.* The treasurer shall keep and maintain, or cause to be kept and maintained, adequate and correct accounts of the properties and business transactions of the corporation, including accounts of its assets, liabilities, receipts, disbursements, gains, losses, capital, and surplus. The books of account shall at all reasonable times be open to inspection by any director.

The treasurer shall deposit all monies and other valuables in the name and to the credit of the corporation with such depositories as may be designated by the board of directors. He shall disburse the funds of the corporation as may be ordered by the board of directors, shall render to the president and directors, whenever they request it, an account of all of his transactions as treasurer and of the financial condition of the corporation, and shall have such other powers and perform such other duties as may be prescribed by the board of directors or these bylaws. He shall be bonded, if required, by the board of directors.

Article V

Miscellaneous

Section 1. *Dues.* The dues required for initial membership and annually or otherwise shall be as specified by written resolution of the board of directors. Such dues may be changed from time to time except that once a member has paid his original membership fee, if any, and becomes a member, no subsequent increase or decrease in the membership fee shall warrant an assessment or require a refund as to such fee with respect to such member. Nonpayment of dues shall be a proper cause for suspension or revocation of membership hereunder. All dues shall be payable as specified by the board of directors. Annual dues shall be in the same amount for all members of the same membership class. The annual dues may vary for each membership class where there is more than one such class.

Section 2. *Use of Roberts Rules of Order.* The most current revision of Roberts Rules of Order shall be used for the conduct of all members' and directors' meetings, except as otherwise provided hereunder or in the Articles of Incorporation.

Section 3. *Indemnification of Directors and Officers.* When a person is sued, either alone or with others, because he or she is or was a director or officer of the corporation, in any proceeding arising out of his or her alleged duties or out of any alleged wrongful act against the corporation or by the corporation, he or she shall be indemnified for his or her reasonable expenses, including attorney's fees incurred in the defense of the proceeding, if both of the following conditions exist:

    (a) The person sued is successful in whole or in part, or the proceeding against him or her is settled with the approval of the court.

    (b) The court finds that his conduct fairly and equitably merits such indemnity.

The amount of such indemnity which may be assessed against the corporation, its receiver, or its trustee, by the court in the same or in a separate proceeding, shall be so much of the expenses, including attorney's fees incurred in the defense of the proceeding, as the court determines and finds to be reasonable. Application for such indemnity may be made either by the person sued or by the attorney or other person rendering services to him or her in connection with defense, and the court may order the fees and expenses to be paid directly to the attorney or other person, although he or she is not a party to the proceeding. Notice of the application for such indemnity shall be served upon the corporation, its receiver, or its trustee, and upon the plaintiff and other parties to the proceeding. The court may order notice to be given also to the members in the manner provided in Article II, Section 2, for giving notice of members' meetings, in such form as the court directs.

Section 4. *Checks, Drafts, Etc.* All checks, drafts or other orders for payment of money, notes or other evidences of indebtedness, issued in the name of or payable to the corporation shall be signed or endorsed by such person or persons and in such manner as, from time to time, shall be determined by resolution of the board of directors.

Section 5. *Annual Report.* No annual report to members shall be required, but the board of directors may cause to be sent to the members reports in such form and at such times as may be deemed appropriate by the board of directors.

Section 6. *Contracts, Deeds, Etc., How Executed.* The board of directors, except as in these by-laws otherwise provided, may authorize any officer or officers, agent or agents, to enter into any contract or execute any instrument in the name of and on behalf of the corporation, and such authority may be general or confined to specific instances; and unless so authorized by the board of directors, no officer, agent, or employee shall have any power or authority to bind the corporation by any contract or engagement or to pledge its credit or to render it liable for any purpose in any amount, provided, however, that any deeds or other instruments conveying lands or any interest therein shall be executed on behalf of the corporation by the president or vice president if there be one.

Section 7. *Membership Certificates.* A certificate of membership shall be issued to each member when any such member so requests, and no such certificate shall be issued when initial membership fees are required until such fees are paid in full, unless the board of directors specifically authorizes installment payments. All such certificates shall be signed by the president or vice president, and the secretary, or an assistant secretary.

Where different classes of membership are provided hereunder, the membership certificates shall be clearly captioned with the type of membership which they represent.

Section 8. *Fiscal Year.* The board of directors shall have the power to fix and from time to time change the fiscal year of the corporation. In the absence of action by the board of directors, however, the fiscal year of the corporation shall end each year on the date which the corporation treated as the close of its first fiscal year, until such time, if any, as the fiscal year shall be changed by the board of directors.

Article VI

Amendments

Section 1. *Power of Directors.* New bylaws may be adopted or these bylaws may be amended or repealed by a majority vote of the board of directors at any regular or special meeting thereof, provided, however, that the time and place fixed by the bylaws for the annual election of directors shall not be changed within sixty (60) days preceding the date on which such elections are to be held. Notice of any amendment of the bylaws by the board of directors shall be given to each member having voting rights within ten (10) days after the date of such amendments by the board.

CERTIFICATE OF SECRETARY

I, the undersigned, do hereby certify:

1. That I am duly elected acting secretary of FULL CITIZENSHIP, INC., a Kansas nonprofit corporation; and
2. That the foregoing bylaws, comprising eleven (11) pages, constitute the original bylaws of said corporation, as duly adopted at the meeting of the board of directors thereof duly held on the 18th day of May, 1987.

IN TESTIMONY WHEREOF, I have hereunto subscribed my name and affixed the seal of the said corporation this 18th day of May, 1987.

_____
Secretary

(SEAL)

INDEX